Handbook of
Chinese Medicine
and **Ayurveda**

Handbook of
Chinese Medicine
and **Ayurveda**

An Integrated Practice of
Ancient Healing Traditions

Bridgette Shea, L.Ac., MAcOM

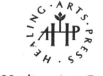

Healing Arts Press
Rochester, Vermont

Healing Arts Press
One Park Street
Rochester, Vermont 05767
www.HealingArtsPress.com

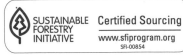

Text stock is SFI certified

Healing Arts Press is a division of Inner Traditions International

Note to the reader: This book is intended as an informational guide. The
remedies, approaches, and techniques described herein are meant to supplement,
and not to be a substitute for, professional medical care or treatment. They should
not be used to treat a serious ailment without prior consultation with a qualified
health care professional.

Library of Congress Cataloging-in-Publication Data
Names: Shea, Bridgette, 1973– author.
Title: Handbook of Chinese medicine and ayurveda : an integrated practice of
    ancient healing traditions / Bridgette Shea, MAcOM.
Description: Rochester, Vermont : Healing Arts Press, [2018] | Includes
    bibliographical references and index.
Identifiers: LCCN 2017052352 (print) | LCCN 2017046695 (ebook) |
    ISBN 9781620556160 (hardback) | ISBN 9781620556177 (ebook)
Subjects: LCSH: Integrative medicine—Handbooks, manuals, etc. | Medicine,
    Chinese—Handbooks, manuals, etc. | Medicine, Ayurvedic—Handbooks,
    manuals, etc. | BISAC: HEALTH & FITNESS / Alternative Therapies. |
    MEDICAL / Alternative Medicine.
Classification: LCC R733 (print) | LCC R733 .S5325 2018 (ebook) |
    DDC 615.5/38—dc23
LC record available at https://lccn.loc.gov/2017046695

Printed and bound in the United States by Lake Book Manufacturing, Inc.
The text stock is SFI certified. The Sustainable Forestry Initiative® program promotes
sustainable forest management.

10 9 8 7 6 5 4 3 2 1

Text design and layout by Priscilla Baker
This book was typeset in Garamond Premier Pro with Nutmeg, Avant Garde, Gill
    Sans, and Legacy Sans used as display typefaces
Artwork by William Crane

To send correspondence to the author of this book, mail a first-class letter to the
author c/o Inner Traditions • Bear & Company, One Park Street, Rochester, VT
05767, and we will forward the communication, or contact the author directly via
her website at **www.agelessinsaratoga.com**.

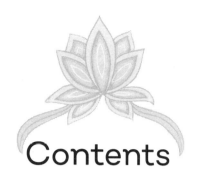

Contents

PART I

Foundations

PART II

Heal Thyself and Others

PART III

In the Clinic

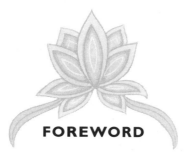

Finding the Calm Within

John Douillard, D.C., CAP

In the *Handbook of Chinese Medicine and Ayurveda,* these ancient medicinal systems come from roots steeped in a time-tested study of nature—something to which we, as a culture, have lost our connection.

These traditional systems of medicine evolved over thousands of years of studying the most subtle aspects of nature—Mother Nature and human nature. These studies concluded that the most profound aspects of the human body and the most powerful aspects of nature were not the most obvious, they were the most subtle. It was in the most subtle aspects of nature that researchers found the true operating system behind the human body and life itself.

For example, modern science tells us that the genes of the human microbiome, which we cannot see with the naked eye, outnumber the genes in the human genome by about one hundred to one, and 90 percent of the cells of the human body, while silently governing all of the body's physiological functions, are actually microbial. These ancient sciences understood that gentle manipulation or therapeutic corrections at the most refined and subtle aspects of the body would deliver the most powerful healing and, ultimately, transformational change.

While healing and optimal health was always a major theme in both systems of medicine, it was never the goal. The goal was to first restore balance to the body, so that the mind could gain the awareness needed to make deep mental, emotional, and spiritual transformational change. Healing was a means to a greater end. They were seeking truth; the same, nonchanging, reliable truth they witnessed in nature, season after season, year after year, and generation after generation.

While nature provided a safe and reliable canvas for life, life itself took advantage of nature's predictable cycles by evolving on every level from the most subtle to the most blatant. The human body was also evolving, and the potential was unlimited. Much of human evolution was linked to a growing level of awareness that allowed humans to potentially shed what Ayurveda termed "the cause of disease" and the obstacles to full human potential. In Ayurveda, the cause of disease was referred to as *pragya parad,* which translates as "the mistake of the intellect." This is where the mind starts thinking of itself as separate, better than, and disconnected from the field of intelligence or consciousness from which we came.

This same field of intelligence that the ancients experienced in nature, they also experienced in the human body, coming to the conclusion that, at the most subtle level, they were experiencing the same field everywhere. Connecting to and becoming aware of this field of intelligence or consciousness was the key to nature's sustainability, the healing of the human body, and the evolution of human potential.

Removing the mistake of the intellect would first require a heightening in the state of awareness and then the ability to employ transformational actions or therapies such as dietary modifications, lifestyle changes and herbal and energetic support at the most effective level. More specifically, becoming conscious would elicit awareness of the subtle circadian cycles that underwrite both the human body and nature itself. Science suggests that we must live in harmony with these circadian rhythms for optimal health, and many experts believe that the field called "circadian medicine" will revolutionize medicine as we know it. Both Chinese medicine and Ayurveda are based on a lifestyle that is in balance with daily, monthly, and seasonal light/dark circadian cycles. These are prerequisites for spiritual evolution.

In ancient times, as in modern times, people were distracted by their senses, looking outside themselves for ways to be more content, less hungry, and safe from the illusion of wealth and material gain. Chinese medicine and Ayurveda were developed to reconnect their respective cultures to something more real. It was clear that the fascination with sensory stimulation was the source of pragya parad and the onset of disease (mental, physical, and emotional). Vedic science, Chinese medicine, kung fu, tai chi, and many other eastern martial art forms were based on living in truth. The word *Veda* means "truth," and *ayus* means "life," so the most accurate definition of Ayurveda is a system of medicine designed to reveal the "truth of your life."

From the perspective of healing, both Chinese medicine and Ayurveda believe in supporting the body's ability to heal itself rather than doing the healing for the body, as we see done in Western medicine and many forms of natural medicine today. Restoring and heightening the body's self-awareness enables the body to clearly recognize health problems as problems and, in a spontaneous and effortless manner, heal itself.

Humans maximize their potential by adhering to a law of nature called the "coexistence of opposites," in which a deep awareness of silence is coexistent with dynamic activity of the body and mind. In nature the coexistence of opposites demonstrates some of its most powerful forms—think atoms and solar systems with silent centers and things spinning around them. In a hurricane, the bigger the eye of the hurricane, the more powerful the winds, suggesting that the source of the hurricane's power comes from the calm, silent center. The winds of the storm and the calm must coexist in order for the hurricane to reach its full strength. Likewise, humans must establish an awareness of peace and calm in the midst of their busy, stressful lives in order to reach their full human potential.

Ayurveda and Chinese medicine employ martial art techniques that center around the mastery of the bow and arrow. The bow is a metaphor for the coexistence of opposites. When you pull back the bow, you must pull it all the way back and establish the bowstring in a deep experience of calm and silence for an accurate and transformational flight of the arrow. Any small movement or deviation of the bowstring once pulled back will have an exponentially distorted effect on the flight of the arrow. The more fully you can pull the bow back and establish it in a space of physical and mental peace and calm, the more accurate your shot will be. And the more often you take action in your life from this calm place, the more transformational your experience of life will be.

Fundamentally, these ancient systems of medicine so eloquently described by Bridgette Shea in the *Handbook of Chinese Medicine and Ayurveda* not only help us heal our injuries and physical imbalances, but they also provide the transformational opportunities to completely free ourselves from the ignorance of a mind that easily attaches itself to the material world, which unknowingly separates us from the truth and our full potential. Close your eyes, pull back the bow, be still, breathe, connect with nature, and then from this place, open your eyes and take action!

DR. JOHN DOUILLARD, D.C., CAP, is the best-selling author of *Eat Wheat* and *The 3-Season Diet,* a former NBA nutritionist, and the creator of LifeSpa .com—proving ancient wisdom with modern science—and has over 6 million YouTube views.

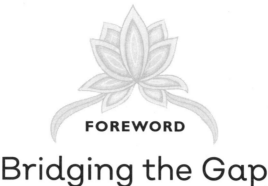

Bridging the Gap

Kim Beekman

have had the great privilege to learn from Bridgette Shea for more than ten years as a client and a student. I have gained wisdom ranging from the life-changing connection to my breath to the depth of theory and practice of Ayurveda and Reiki. Bridgette's ability to convey the higher wisdom of Ayurveda into a practical day-to-day application of wellness has always been impressive and invaluable. Not everyone is blessed to have her living in their hometown, so it is a true gift to have her practical wisdom documented here for all to experience.

Bridgette has developed a unique work with this practical comparison of traditional Chinese medicine and Ayurveda. No other author has bridged the fundamental aspects of Chinese medicine and Ayurveda with a detailed focus on the similarities of these ancient traditions. She has created an accessible and digestible guide to help practitioners, students, and clients of either modality to understand the overlapping benefits of each tradition.

Personally, the connection between Ayurveda and Chinese medicine has always eluded me. Although I am a longtime student of Yoga philosophy and an Ayurveda wellness counselor, yoga teacher/trainer, Reiki master, meditation teacher, and spiritual author, I have never been able to answer my students' question, "How does Ayurveda compare to

Chinese medicine?" Because of the difference in the way the two systems view the elements, prana/qi, and consciousness, it was never clear to me how to map the fundamentals and share the common and unique aspects of the two traditions. All other sources seemed to show the differences between the two as opposed to the similarities in theory and treatment.

Doing a thorough review of Chinese medicine was too much for me because I wasn't interested in learning a new system, so I would shrug without much to say to those who would ask. However, Bridgette's comparison provides such a straightforward side-by-side comparison, focusing on the similarities of the two sciences, it has allowed me to bridge my Ayurvedic understanding to Chinese medicine. This has deepened my understanding of Ayurveda and opened me up to what Chinese medicine has to offer.

This book is a must-read for any practitioner or student of Chinese medicine or Ayurveda, Yoga, Reiki, or any other healing art. Healing is the understanding of how to bring the body and its energies back into balance. An understanding of the two most profound healing sciences provides the basis for any healer on the path of bringing people back into alignment with their higher consciousness, whether it's in the body, energetics, mind, or spirit. The way in which Bridgette presents the ancient wisdom will open your consciousness to a deeper understanding of your body, energy, and the phenomenal intelligence of the natural world. Her perspective will bring new insight into nature's ability to heal and restore balance.

KIM BEEKMAN is an Ayurveda wellness counselor, yoga teacher/trainer, Reiki master, meditation teacher, and author of *Awaken Your Potency: A Practical Guide to the Law of Attraction, Ayurveda, and Meditation.*

Introduction

What do we find more interesting, wondrous, and magical than the inner workings of ourselves? What we are, who we are, why we are here, and what our purpose is in this life. How incredible nature is! If we have a cut, it heals, if we have an emotionally turbulent time, we go deeper into the why of our being and higher into the truth of a grander whole, and we emerge stronger, more pieced together. Chinese medicine and Ayurveda, two of the oldest healing systems of the world, offer us tangible, and oftentimes transcendent, "bigger-picture" insights into who we are as individuals, as living beings, in relationship to ourselves, to others, to the environment, the world, and existence in general. And both continue to make an ever-increasing contribution to the health and well-being of people around the world.

Chinese medicine has become increasingly popular because of the widespread positive results arising from its bodywork modality, acupuncture. These include alleviating pain, providing emotional comfort, increasing fertility, reducing stress, and addressing a long list of other issues for millions of people worldwide. Acupuncture is now recognized in the United States by many insurance companies, and many people have access to it, whether it's at a methadone treatment facility, a fertility clinic, on a military base, on-site at a disaster, on a cruise ship, in a doctor's office, or with an acupuncturist in private practice. The interest in how it works is growing, even in those who have yet to receive its benefits. It's fascinating and quickly becoming a part of our daily lives.

Ayurveda, too, is increasing in popularity by leaps and bounds as it follows yoga into mainstream consciousness. Ayurveda segments on Dr. Oz and numerous references to it by such respected experts in the field of mind/body medicine as Deepak Chopra and Andrew Weil have certainly aided in its spread. Ayurveda fills in the gaps in Chinese medicine, particularly in relationship to diet and cleansing. Many people are absolutely obsessed with food and dieting, and Ayurveda offers the most complete, time-honored system available for understanding food at the level of consciousness as well as the level of the physical body. It is the natural go-to method for anyone seriously interested in using simple lifestyle modification, diet, and detoxification as tools for wellness and weight loss.

My own treatment practice involves a blend of Chinese and Ayurvedic medicine, maximizing the ways in which they supplement and enhance each other. However, most of the books on the market only cover one or the other, and the very few that discuss both do so in a way that does not necessarily emphasize their similarities or how they can be used together in a clinical practice. Also, it is often the case that introductory books in Chinese medicine offer a lot of good information but are either far too simplistic, or, like many books in Ayurveda, too complex and esoteric for a beginner. I've been frustrated throughout my career by the lack of a good single resource I can suggest to my clients. Instead I've recommended books I know won't really meet their needs and given away tons of handouts. I know many other practitioners who end up doing the same.

There is a need for a clear, simple explanation of the deep knowledge of human health preserved in these systems, combined with accessible, immediately usable recommendations for a healthy diet and lifestyle. This book provides just such a resource for practitioners, patients, or anyone interested in either Chinese medicine or Ayurveda. I present the material in such a way as to clearly illustrate the ideas in both traditions without being too simplistic or overly complex.

Whatever your starting point, this book will help you to understand the theory behind the actions outlined in both practices. Uniquely, it offers a blend of the two systems, while staying true to the roots of each discipline. It also includes dietary guidance, food lists, and a constitutional self-analysis questionnaire, which will guide you in utilizing the key concepts in the medicines to enhance mental, emotional, and physical balance. It is also a seamless introduction for the practitioner wishing to cross over into using a complementary field for understanding life and medicine in a different yet familiar and useful way.

Why is it important to blend Chinese medicine and Ayurveda, and why have I chosen these two fields to highlight? The story of how I came to combine them in my own practice offers some significant insights with wide applicability.

I became formally interested in ancient healing modalities in 1992 while visiting the original Aesclepion (a healing temple sacred to Aesclepius, the god of medicine) in Old Epidaurus, Greece. Having been a vivid dreamer my whole life, I had a natural fascination with the ancients' development of transformational dream healing clinics. While there, I was introduced to stelae (stone slabs) that depicted priestesses hovering their hands over patients, and a few years later I found myself practicing and teaching Reiki, qigong, yoga, and other energetic healing arts modalities. While I was receiving zero balancing energy work,* I was given the "audible vision" of the word *astanga,* which means "eight-limbed" and is used to identify certain schools of yoga instruction. It is also used more specifically to refer to the foundational Yoga philosophy compiled by the ancient sage Patanjali. This led me to study Patanjali's Yoga and later to go to India to pursue a deep study of *asana* (posture) and *pranayama* (breath control), *mudra* (ritual gesture), Sanatana Dharma (eternal truth),† Sanskrit, and a little Ayurveda. While I was in India, through the same energy work modality of zero balancing, I received similar guidance to become an acupuncturist.

I ended up in Seattle a year and a half later studying Chinese

---

*Zero balancing is a body-mind therapy that uses skilled touch to balance the relationship between body energy and structure to amplify wellness.

†*Sanatana Dharma* is the actual term for what is generally referred to as the Hindu religion; the word *Hindu* was originally a slang term for the peoples of the Indus Valley region.

medicine at Seattle Institute of Oriental Medicine (SIOM), one of the more rigorous Chinese medical schools in the country. Becoming a practitioner of Chinese medicine—which includes herbal medicine and acupuncture—is an involved and demanding process. After three to four years of undergraduate study and prerequisites similar to that of someone applying to medical school, you can apply to Chinese medicine school. Programs include a minimum of three years of full-time year-round study and result in a master's degree.

The program I was in is the only one in the United States requiring extensive training in the Chinese language. At SIOM students are taught to translate both simplified and classical characters. This means that the participants not only study the foundational texts that define the medicine but also translate them so that they are not solely relying on someone else's interpretation. This is very rare in the Western acupuncture world, and it grants participants a view of the medicine that not everyone has direct access to.

Through this in-depth exposure I found that the theory underlying the medicine is very vague and often confusing. I felt a lack of continuity and explanation in the material with regard to foundational principles. Because of this, I had difficulty connecting to the soul of the medicine and acquiring an experiential awareness of its underpinnings. I was left with more questions than answers and felt that my understanding lacked grounding. Because of this feeling of disconnect, I returned to my earlier interest in Ayurveda.

There is an enormous body of knowledge on Ayurvedic medicine that is also thousands of years old yet lacks the gaps I experienced in the Chinese tradition. This is not to say the same wisdom is lacking in Chinese medicine. It's just that the information on Ayurveda's core principles is much more accessible and it feels more complete to me. I started reading and contemplating the ancient Ayurveda texts, including the foundational works of the Indian physicians Charaka and Sushruta. There is a flow to them and to modern authors' renderings of their teachings that caused me to think about what I was studying in Chinese medical school and go, "Oh, so *that's* what this is saying."

As I continued my course at SIOM, I also attended workshops

with Dr. Vasant Lad. Dr. Lad is probably the most well-known and well-loved Indian Ayurveda vaidya living in the West. His Ayurvedic Institute produces many of the textbooks used by students in not only the United States but elsewhere in the Western world. When he isn't instructing from his home base in New Mexico or taking students to India to observe clinical practice, Dr. Lad travels the world teaching Ayurveda. In addition to attending various workshops, whenever I could, I intensively studied the ancient texts and teachings of Ayurveda and began an apprentice-like training with a Seattle-based Ayurveda practitioner, Kumudini Shoba.

In addition to what I was learning through external resources, I engaged daily in thought experiments. I would internalize the concepts of Ayurveda as much as possible and use them to decipher the code of Chinese medicine. Every now and again I would feel a tremendous sense of accomplishment when a respected teacher would verify the conclusions I had come to on my own. This helped keep me going in the process. I utilized my knowledge of Ayurveda to help me understand Chinese medicine at a deeper level and eventually integrated both systems into a comprehensive traditional medicine practice.

Without the influence of Ayurveda, I'd be practicing Chinese medicine with less depth of understanding in its foundational principles. The way the truth of the medicine from India is presented resonated more with me—it made more initial "aha" sense. Being able to apply this knowledge, once I had ingested and assimilated it, helped me to see where the Chinese were coming from in a new light. Instead of feeling like I was on the fringes of Chinese medicine, I could more readily integrate its concepts and truths into my perception in the clinic, and in life overall. Honestly, I'd have felt somewhat like an automaton in my learning and in my practice had it not been for my early applied understanding of Ayurveda. I'm sure this isn't true for everyone, and for some it may be the other way around. They may feel that Chinese theory helps them understand Ayurveda. I've met many Chinese medicine practitioners who naturally have a deep connection to and integrated experience of their art.

Having said that, some of the most remarkable, spirited, contented folks I've come across are Ayurvedic practitioners who apply its teachings to their daily lives. This has made me step back and really think about how Chinese medicine is being passed down, at least in the Western world, and the effect this may have on the everyday application of its teachings for its practitioners. Although many enjoy their work, it seems as though there is less support for utilizing what it has to offer as a way of life. This may be especially so in small towns and more remote areas where there are fewer practitioners who can meet up and discuss case studies or support one another in other ways, for example, through exchanging treatments or attending internal cultivation sessions. This may have something to do with why job retention for acupuncturists is remarkably low five years post-graduation. There are a number of reasons for this and I see it happen. In fact, the way the whole acupuncture clinic scene is set up isn't for everyone. But practitioners may not know it until they've already run the gamut of schooling, loans, and becoming small business owners. However, among people who have studied Ayurveda—at least in the West—I recognize a deep experiential understanding and appreciation for Ayurveda and an awareness that the practice of it isn't a job so much as it is a way of life. In fact, the word *Ayurveda* can be translated as "the wisdom of life."

The meaning of the word *Taoism*—Chinese medicine's foundational cosmological philosophy—isn't that far removed. It roughly means "not interfering with the natural course of events." We need to know the natural course of events so as not to interfere with their process. At their roots, both of these modalities emphasize the knowledge of nature or life. Whatever the system, the practitioner's capacity to have an internal experiential awareness of the concepts inherent in the medicine and therefore in life creates not only a better practitioner but a natural resonance of trust between the practitioner and the person they are treating. Conversely, the lack of this awareness may present as an obstacle to practice.

This book offers a clear view of the backbone of each of these systems, so as not to be overwhelming to the beginner. It is an excellent manual to offer patients because it contains all the information that they will need to understand what they're being treated for and why and can provide more detail than we typically have time for in sessions. This can be indispensable for helping people keep themselves balanced between treatments.

At the same time the book offers a profound resource for the experienced practitioner of either system who gets bound up in the complexity that can arise when contemplating the medicine or a specific case. And it is a useful aid for accessing information from a related discipline that may be the key to unlocking unanswered questions or may offer another tool with which to treat oneself or others. It can also aid practitioners who integrate both systems into their practice by offering a firm foundation in all the necessary concepts in both traditions.

Part I of this book places Chinese medicine and Ayurveda in the context of other ancient medicines, providing the reader with a better understanding of the complexity and scientific nature of medical systems developed thousands of years before our own. From this starting point, we merge into a parallel explanation of Chinese medicine and Ayurveda. I know of no other book that lays out the principal tenets of these two systems side by side. This approach reveals the similarities between the foundational theories of both and makes the concepts easier to follow.

For example, in a single chapter on the five elements, central to both medicines, the discussion proceeds idea by idea rather than presenting two separate elemental theories. This speaks to the interconnectedness of these approaches to well-being, while also making it easy for the reader to learn more about a particular topic in one place rather than having to flip through the book for answers.

Part I also includes chapters that focus on constitution, anatomy, and consciousness, again, as they are understood in both systems. Chapter 4 contains a simple self-quiz to assess your constitution or current body-mind makeup. Using this and the health recommendations for each type presented in Part II, you can more clearly decide for yourself or for your clients what course of action is recommended for a specific presentation.

Part II provides information on how to balance yourself. It contains a discussion on taste and which foods are optimal for which body-mind type along with basic dietary guidance that is practical and easy to implement but that the average person has probably never considered. Indeed some of the information contained here may even be news to practitioners. This is one of the beauties of combining these disciplines for the benefit of our patients. Also in this section is a chapter on a simple, safe, effective home cleanse.

Part III is geared toward the practitioner. That is not to say the layperson will not derive benefit from it, but it is written in a slightly different voice and with a little more assumption that the reader has a solid grasp of at least one of the two disciplines. It offers treatment suggestions useful for practitioners from many disciplines that incorporate some Chinese medicine or Ayurveda into their practice, as well as generalized herb recommendations, acupressure guidance, and cross-discipline treatment protocols.

Finally, the book includes a glossary of commonly used terms from both traditions.

In this text I have done my best to incorporate the very best of both traditions and to emphasize what I judged at the time of writing to be the most useful points from both. In some places I have taken the liberty of oversimplifying some concepts or focusing on a general theme instead of delving more deeply into the material. Many details have been left out in an effort to offer a general introduction to both systems that isn't too complicated. In some places I have drawn from my own perspective and experience, rather than adhering to traditional or textual ways of explaining concepts. Some of the terminology could be presented differently or more completely, as could all of the theory and concepts. To do this would be an undertaking involving many more years of practice, contemplation, study, and writing. I invite others to jump off from here and carry this work forward.

All of that being said, it is my intention that this book can help you change your life for the better, and I have constructed it in such a way as to help you enjoy the process. The common questions of practitioners, patients, and students that I have encountered are largely addressed here in an easily accessible format. This book can be a lifelong resource of basic information on both Chinese medicine and Ayurveda. It contains a vast wealth of knowledge that a person can use to help maintain his or her well-being and to help bring the body and mind into greater balance.

One of India's foundational medical texts, the Charaka Samhita, states: "Good health stands at the very root of virtuous acts, acquirement of wealth, gratification of desire, and final emancipation."[1] May this book contribute to the improved health and well-being of you, your loved ones, and those who trust you to support them on the healing journey.

PART I

Foundations

1

The Magic of Ancient Medicine

The history of medicine is a fascinating topic because it is our history. Mystery, horror, and magic abound when contemplating how ancient humans developed the complex systems of medicine that we have at our disposal today. Imagine being one of those ancient people, living in the Stone Age or earlier and having a tooth abscess or delivering a baby without any antibiotics or pain relief. Imagine breaking a bone or getting a laceration or a fever and being exposed to the elements the way primitive humans were. Or think of living in a village, struggling with unreliable crop yields, harsh weather conditions, and poor sanitation while loved ones were fighting off a mysterious, perhaps fatal, illness. How did ancient humans know what to do in these situations? Through trial and error, observation, experimentation, and intuition they figured it out. Just as we are, to a large extent, still figuring it out.

Long before medical doctrines were put into written language, people were learning how to care for one another when something went wrong. Medicine evolved from the insight of intuitive, wise men and women, shamans, and barefoot doctors and was passed down from practitioner to apprentice over the course of millennia. Ancient peoples believed that exogenous pathogenic factors, spirits, ancestors, ghosts, and internal factors, such as mental and emotional issues, as well as causes from past lives or past actions in this life contributed to the development of a myriad of symptoms and disease processes.

The ancients were able to deduce a large amount of information about how the body operated and how it related to its environment. These findings included details about the gross physical body as well as the mental, emotional, spiritual, and energetic dimensions of a living being. The ancient medical traditions viewed a human being as a whole in and of itself and inseparable from the rest of existence. Ancient humans recognized the cause and effect between where and how people lived and their good health, or lack of it. They evolved this knowledge to include a complete vision of how the universe operates, and how we operate within it. Cosmology not only included the dawn of time but also the moment of conception. At least one culture completely understood embryology, in some ways even better than we understand it today.

Practitioners' areas of expertise often overlapped with that of artists, calligraphers, astrologers, palm readers, augurers, and exorcists. Many were great thinkers and scientists, able to blend their beliefs with rationality. The ancient practitioners established elaborate models of pathogenesis, diagnosis, prognosis, and treatment strategies. They systematized medical education and specialized in certain areas. They dissected corpses, developed bodywork modalities, performed surgeries, and prescribed medications.

Some of the ancient traditions are widely in use to this day, while others have left a lasting legacy of tools or approaches. Two of the more refined and widely accessible traditions come from India and China. Before examining these elaborate living traditions, let's explore some of the other forms of prehistoric medicine that evolved simultaneously in different parts of the ancient world, such as Mesopotamia, Egypt, and Greece. It is probable that none of these systems of traditional medicine developed in isolation. It is difficult to know which came first when looking at Greek, Indian, and Chinese medicine. The oldest written medical texts that contain information on the humors and elements come from Greece and are dated to around 400 BCE, while the medical canons of India and China date to around 250–100 BCE. However, the systems from India and China are much more complex and well-documented.

ANCIENT MEDICAL TRADITIONS OF MESOPOTAMIA AND EGYPT

The Sumerians of Mesopotamia are widely recognized as being the first civilization to have developed a written language, called cuneiform. Many cuneiform tablets exist to this day, several hundred of them having to do with medicine. The ancient Sumerian system of medicine included diagnosis, prognosis, and treatment. Many of the treatments outlined in the tablets discuss courses of action that would still be taken to this day. Some of the ailments addressed include skin diseases, bleeding, worms and flukes, neurological disorders, and fever.

Several medical papyri from ancient Egypt have been found, such as the Kahun Gynaecological Papyrus, dated to between 2100 and 1900 BCE, which focuses on gynecology and obstetrics. The Edwin Smith Papyrus dates to 1600 BCE, but there is some evidence it is only a copy of an original text that dates to 2500 BCE, when the Giza pyramids are believed to have been built. It contains a description of the brain, pulse diagnosis, and forty-eight surgical cases. It also outlines which ailments can be treated and which cannot.[1] Diagnosis and prognosis are just two of the skills Egyptian physicians had in common with their Chinese and Indian counterparts.

The Ebers Papyrus dates to 1555 BCE. It describes 876 remedies and 500 medicinal substances and talks about cutting into the body and cauterization. It also discusses ailments involving the stomach, liver, heart, veins, ears, tongue, and teeth and includes information on treating coughs, colds, bites, accidents, diseases of the head, burns, itching, musculoskeletal ailments, and tumors. It also provides a section on women's health and beauty preparations.[2]

The ancient Egyptians thought that humors were the primary cause of disease in the body. They called them air, blood, urine, mucus, semen, and feces and believed they all flowed in channels from the heart and through the body and terminated at the anus.[3] These ideas are aligned with the medical theory of the ancient Greeks, as well as that of Ayurveda and Chinese medicine, which all describe a humoral system and channels that distribute energy, nutrition, food, fluids, and information.

The Egyptian toolkit contained linen (adhesive/sutures), copper needles, metal shears, surgical knives, saws, probes, spatulas, hooks, forceps, cauteries, and scalpels.[4] As one can surmise from this information, Egyptian medicine has greatly influenced our own medicine today.

ANCIENT GREEK MEDICINE

The roots of modern allopathic medicine are said to have originated in ancient Greek medicine, most notably with Hippocrates and Galen. Hippocrates, who lived from about 460–377 BCE, is credited with teaching that the focus in medicine should be on the person. Most people have heard of the Hippocratic oath, a variation of which is taken by modern medical doctors. It was originally a religious oath ensuring that the doctor was operating for the greater good of the community. Its values—particularly, respecting one's teachers and honoring patient confidentiality—persist today.*

Greek medicine started largely as superstition. Good health was seen as a gift from the gods and ill health as a form of divine punishment. Around 400 BCE there was a paradigm shift toward reason, inquiry, and cause and effect. It was observed that lifestyle, heat, cold, and trauma all contributed to health and disease. People became concerned with diet and the treatment of disease. Hippocrates stressed the importance of nutrition and air quality. He believed we should not interfere too strongly when bringing the body back to health. He had

---

*A translation of the complete oath can be found in the appendix.

a "less is more" approach. He preached removing any excess humor and allowing the body to do the rest. Hippocrates's *On Ancient Medicine* reads very much like a lecture on Ayurveda or Chinese medicine theory and emphasizes the role of diet in health and disease.

Other interesting parallels between Greek and Eastern medicine are the concepts of depletion and repletion and the environmental factors of hot, cold, moist, and dry as being present in the body and potentially injurious to it. Bitter, salty, sweet, acidic, sour, and bland are the six tastes in Greek medicine. Ayurveda also has six; Chinese medicine has five. The Greeks believed the tastes needed to be mixed because straight tastes could cause damage. Methods of diagnosis in Greek medicine included inquiry into diet, bowel, and sleep habits, as well as pulse and facial diagnoses. Popular treatments included herbs, amulet adornment, sneezing therapy, enemas, and bloodletting.[5] Bloodletting was used more moderately in Ancient Greece than in later years (starting in the Middle Ages and extending to as recently as the 1800s), when it was overused and harmful.

Galen of Pergamum is perhaps the next most popular Greek medical practitioner and philosopher who had an influence on the roots of Western medicine. He lived from about 129 to 216 CE. Unlike previous thinkers, he recognized that humoral imbalance can also exist more specifically in the internal organs. His main interest was anatomy. Animal dissection had come into vogue, and through it he was able to identify the seven cranial nerves and heart valves. He found that arteries indeed carried blood, not air, and he tied off the laryngeal nerve in an effort to prove that the brain, not the heart, controlled the body.[6]

Galen described three systems in the body: the brain and nerves were believed to control sensation and thought, the heart and arteries were responsible for life-giving energy, and the liver and veins were in charge of nutrition and growth. These assessments are not far off. Blood and air were thought to be at their most refined when they produced *pneuma*, the subtle "material that is the vehicle of sensation."[7] Pneuma was synonymous with the concepts of breath, spirit, or soul and was recognized as air in motion, or an internal wind.

This idea of pneuma is a very real phenomenon in Chinese medicine and Ayurveda—it is called *qi* (pronounced "chi") and *prana vayu*,* respectively—and is associated with the breath, air, and sensation. In fact, it is the primary substance/force associated with vitality and wellness, as well as disease origin and formation. In addition to sharing strong parallels with Ayurveda and Chinese medicine, Greek medicine had an influence on Tibetan medicine and is also the basis of Unani, which is discussed in the next section.

UNANI

Unani, also known as Islamic or Arabian medicine, was largely adapted from Greek medicine in the seventh century and based heavily on the teachings of Galen, including his humoral theory. Practitioners aimed to restore the humors to the balance that existed before the imbalanced disease state. There are several branches of Unani medicine. Some doctors are experts in anatomy and physiology, some in surgery, and others in ophthalmology and internal medicine. Unani practitioners believed, and many probably still do, that astrology was/is directly related to the health and well-being of an individual.

Hunain ibn Ishaq was a famous Unani practitioner from the late ninth century. He was the first to document that images entered the lens of the eye. It was previously believed that the eyes radiated light, and this light went out from the eyes and was reflected back to them from the object of vision.[8] Cataract surgery, using suction through a needle, was practiced in the ninth and tenth centuries and was not utilized in Europe for another thousand years. Unani medicine continues to exist, particularly on the Indian subcontinent, but now includes modern methods of diagnosis, such as X-rays and ultrasound. Unani is recognized for its successful treatment of leukoderma, rheumatism, arthritis, sinusitis, jaundice, and elephantiasis.[9] Like Chinese medicine and Ayurveda, Unani is a living tradition.[10]

Vayu is Sanskrit for "wind."

CHINESE MEDICINE

We believe Chinese medicine has its roots in prehistory, but its origin and its influence on other emerging medical systems in antiquity are unknown. Many ideas exist concerning the development of Chinese medical theory. The 1991 discovery of a 5300-year-old frozen corpse in the Alps revealed that some knowledge of acupuncture existed before it was written down, and it occurred outside of China. Known as Otzi, the iceman, he is believed to have been a farmer who died in his forties, having suffered from many ailments. His body displayed more than fifty tattoos that correspond to acupoints that would be used today to treat his health conditions.[11] This ancient Chinese information found on an Alpine man who lived thousands of years before its written documentation is just one example of the knowledge shared between cultures and the extent to which acupuncture's origins remain a mystery.

Many practitioners speculate on just how such detailed awareness of the body and its subtle pathways and inner workings came about. Some believe it was the result of cause and effect. For example, if someone had a headache, ancient man may have realized that pressing certain points would help to alleviate it. However, it doesn't seem possible that this random discovery provides the whole picture of how the medicine emerged. Another theory may seem fantastical to many modern readers but is completely plausible to those involved in the esoteric sciences, internal martial arts, or meditation. That theory is that people in some kind of altered state, be it meditative or otherwise, were able to visualize the invisible pathways of energy or qi, which brings vitality to all bodily tissues. In fact, there are many ancient medical diagrams depicting these pathways.

Some ancient Chinese may have told a different story: one of divine intervention. There are three primary divine beings said to be responsible for the origin of the Chinese medical system, among other things. Their date of being is unknown, as their mythical existence is part of a cultural memory from beyond the first written accounts. Fu Xi, the originator of the *bagua* (or *pakua*),* is responsible for elemental and yin/yang theory, Shen Nong is credited with the development of herbalism, and Huang Di is thought to have established acupuncture and diagnostic techniques.

In Chinese medicine, acupuncture and herbs are two separate disciplines. The first written treatise on acupuncture dates to before the earliest written works on herbal medicine. This may suggest that acupuncture theory developed first, or it may just mean we don't have access to an earlier text on herbal medicine yet. The Nei Jing, or the Yellow Emperor's Classic of Internal Medicine, is dated to around 250 BCE. It contains the earliest explanation we have on acupuncture, meridian theory, the five elements, and yin and yang. It is written in the format of a conversation between the divine emperor, Huang Di (the Yellow Emperor), and his court physician, Qi Bo. There are numerous translations of the two primary books in this text. Some of the information it contains is pretty straightforward if you know Chinese medical theory, but most of it is either vague or completely veiled, requiring either a full understanding of the Chinese language at the time the text was written combined with complete knowledge of Taoist thought, or the guidance of a seasoned practitioner over the course of many years.

In addition to the work of these mythical figures, there are preserved writings from various doctors. Zhang Zhong Jing is one such person. He is famous for his text, the Shang Han Lun, or the Treatise on Cold Damage, which outlines the differentiation of syndromes through six stages. This poor man struggled to treat an epidemic that caused a large portion of his village, including many of his close family members, to suffer and die. He developed the theory of cold pathogens: how they enter the body, where they can manifest in the body, and how to treat them with herbs and some acupuncture. To this day Chinese medicine practitioners successfully use Zhang Zhong Jing's formulas for diseases as insignificant as the common cold to

---

*A bagua is a circular arrangement of eight trigrams used in Taoist cosmology to represent the eight fundamental principles of reality, which are also known as the eight forces of nature.

those as serious as the flu, as well as dysentery-like ailments and other life-threatening disorders.

Another important contribution to the history and practice of Chinese medicine is that of the Wen Bing Xue (Warm Disease theory). The primary doctors responsible for its development and codification are Wu You Ke, Ye Tian Shi, Xue Sheng Bai, Wu Ju Tong, and Wang Meng Ying. Warm disease has a different diagnostic parameter—known as the four levels—than cold damage. This school of thought teaches that communicable diseases are primarily of a warm nature, or turn warm once they enter the body. What we now call pathogens were called *pestilential qi* by original Wen Bing practitioners, as well as by Chinese medicine practitioners today. Originators of the theory proposed that pestilential qi enters the body through the mouth and nose and wreaks a fairly predictable havoc on the system, depending upon where it lands. The four levels explain disease manifestation in terms of superficial qi levels and entry to bodily fluids and organ systems. It is a highly developed theory and still in use today.

Herbal medicine is a highly sophisticated branch of the Chinese system that probably accounts for the majority of treatment protocols worldwide. Traditional Chinese medicine is a huge industry in China. Its annual revenue, just for herbal preparations, was estimated at 17 billion dollars, and that amount is expected to almost triple by 2025.[12] In 2012, Bin Li of Morgan Stanley explained that in China, even physicians trained in the West are using Chinese medicine as a first line of treatment 30 percent of the time. And 46 percent of Western doctors either use Chinese medicine instead of Western medicine, or treat using both systems. He explains that there is a growing population in China using Chinese medicine to treat chronic diseases.[13] In addition, the government of Taiwan has committed to spending millions to boost its Chinese medicine industry, including incorporating testing standards and making sure herbs are pure.

In China, some hospitals have a traditional medicine wing. I remember one of my professors in Chinese medicine school talking about how one of her favorite, and more profound, experiences with the medicine while studying in China was watching the delivery of herbs to the hospital. She said huge shipments would come in vehicles like dump trucks and empty their contents of thousands of pounds of herbs at the hospital on a weekly basis. She recalled marveling at this, something we may never experience living in the West, and at seeing the medicine's profound effects on oncology patients at the hospital.

Chinese medicine is also growing in popularity by leaps and bounds in the Western world. Bayer HealthCare Pharmaceuticals purchased the Chinese medicine company Dihon Pharmaceutical Group in 2014 for over half a billion dollars.[14] Herbal remedies from China may have a bad rap due to pesticides, tampering, and toxicity, but many reputable Western Chinese herb manufacturers from the United States are producing safe, clean, effective remedies for clients in the West. Chinese herbal medicine was recently a hot news item when Tu Youyou was awarded the 2015 Nobel Prize for using the Chinese herbal remedy artemisia in the development of an antimalarial pharmaceutical.[15]

Chinese medicine is considered a different discipline than acupuncture in China. Chinese medicine practitioners are pretty much considered doctors of herbology and almost like Western internal medicine practitioners. Acupuncturists practice a different craft, focusing on meridian theory as opposed to organ theory. Today in the West acupuncturists are not necessarily trained in herbal medicine, but most Chinese medicine practitioners are trained in acupuncture.

AYURVEDA

Ayurvedic medicine is the leading traditional medical practice in India. Unlike Chinese medicine, Ayurveda has survived severe censorship for millennia. There is a complete system of pathogenesis, diagnosis, and treatment, as there is in Chinese medicine. Although individual doctors may take issue with an interpretation of the original texts here and there, there doesn't seem to be quite the same controversy over key concepts in the medicine as there is in Chinese medicine. I'd say the primary concern among well-trained Ayurvedic doctors is the Westernization, misunderstanding, and dumbing down of key concepts in the medicine. We will explore these ideas in more detail below.

The oldest mention of any form of medicine in Indian texts exists in the *Atharva Veda* (the knowledge of everyday procedures), which dates to anywhere from 1500 to 900 BCE. It contains potions, spells, and incantations used to treat various illnesses and to charge objects used to treat disease.[16] After this, the next major writing on Ayurveda occurs with the appearance of the Charaka and Sushruta Samhitas, dating from around 200 BCE.

Common to most ancient medical treatises are the vague dates associated with their origins. In order to date manuscripts, scholars look at particular word, character, or phrase choices. Just like today, the ancients had their versions of sayings like, "cut off your nose to spite your face" or "my bad" that came in and out of style. Often scholars find such time-sensitive phrases that are much older—sometimes hundreds of years older—than the attributed date of authorship of a text. This makes it very difficult to know for sure when a medicine or a book about it originated. Also, the knowledge was often shared for generations through an oral tradition in which entire texts' worth of information was transmitted to students who then memorized it. This is why verses were constructed in a certain way. Much like a rhyme helps us remember certain things, the Sanskrit teachings had a specific cadence that made them easier to memorize.

So, Charaka may not have been the only author of the Charaka Samhita, nor Sushruta of his namesake. Either way, Charaka was believed to be an enlightened doctor, and Sushruta a master surgeon. Their two texts form the clinical foundation of Ayurvedic medicine and include every explanation you can conceive of about health and life. These include but are not limited to an appropriate daily regimen; our bodies' attunement to the natural world; prevention; disease causation and treatment; various diseases; surgical procedures; fetal development, childbirth, and postpartum care; rejuvenative and cleansing practices;

pathogenesis; prognosis and treatment; and using food to harmonize the body, mind, and spirit.

Sushruta, a skilled surgeon, went as far as to outline which *marmani* (vital points) should not be cut through, as injury to them could cause serious complications and make healing much more difficult. He described over a thousand illnesses, herbs, and prescriptions. The Sushruta Samhita explains cataract surgery, cesarean section, prostate removal, and intestinal blockage management to name a few. The Astanga Hridayam, a later text, is also used in Ayurvedic education.

Today in India, the training to become an Ayurvedic doctor with the degree of Bachelor of Ayurvedic Medicine and Surgery (BAMS) is a state-regulated program that takes five-and-a-half years to complete and includes a year of clinical rotation. Prior to being accepted into a BAMS program, candidates take biology, chemistry, and physics and must score well on a premed exam. Ayurvedic physicians in India are usually in private practice or work in clinics or Ayurvedic hospitals. Others may teach or work in India's billion-dollar-a-year Ayurveda pharmaceutical industry.

Other Ayurvedic physicians may work in panchakarma facilities. Panchakarma—a worldwide growing industry—is part of a unique specialty in Ayurvedic medicine and is perhaps what sets Ayurveda most apart from any other medicine in the world. *Panchakarma* means "five actions." These refer to five cleansing categories, which one may need to experience in order to detoxify, heal, and rejuvenate. The panchakarma practices involve many oiling techniques, including specialized two-person massage, pouring of oil over the forehead, vamana (vomiting therapy), sudation (sweat therapy), and purgation. A milder form of panchakarma that only involves the more pleasant of the above practices is popular in Western spas around the world.

According to *Frontline World*, two-thirds of India's rural population uses Ayurveda as their primary medical care. And it is growing in popularity in the West. In the United States for example, as of 2004, more than 750,000 people had experienced some kind of Ayurvedic treatment.[17] Most of us are fascinated with one of the primary tenets of Ayurveda: having a constitutional type. When we know our type, we are better equipped, theoretically, to take care of ourselves in a way that helps us look and feel better and, we hope, last longer. In Ayurveda, the term used to address constitutional types is *dosha*. The word *dosha* indicates something that is flawed or has the potential to go awry.

There are three doshas: *vata, pitta,* and *kapha.* Some equate vata to kinetic energy, pitta to thermal energy, and kapha to potential energy. The easiest way to understand this concept is by looking at how the ancient seers viewed existence. In Sanatana Dharma, or eternal wisdom, there are three fundamental forces involved with the cyclical ongoings of the universe that manifest not only cosmically, but locally and internally, and they are personified in Indian religious belief as Brahma, Vishnu, and Shiva. Brahma is the kinetic energy of creation; Shiva is the force that breaks down the old in the process of transformation to make way for the new; and Vishnu is the potential energy of the sustainer. In Ayurveda, they translate to vata, pitta, and kapha, respectively. Vata is associated with the universal principle of movement, pitta with the universal principle of transformation, and kapha with the universal principle of stability and sustainability. These three forces aren't just principles or vague concepts in Ayurveda; they are natural laws.

POLITICAL INFLUENCE ON THE DEVELOPMENT OF CHINESE AND AYURVEDIC MEDICINES

One of the reasons I believe that there can be a great synergy between Chinese medicine and Ayurveda is because of the influence politics has had over the development of what we now know as Chinese medicine. Prior to the early 1900s, Chinese medicine was the official medicine of the Chinese people. With the Nationalist movement, people began to believe that the old ways of the isolated Chinese people were holding back their progress in science. Because of this, the practice of Chinese medicine was made illegal.[18]

Later, the Communists started to allow it again because of the shape the people were in after Mao's Great Leap Forward. But by the 1960s, Mao decided to blame the old ways of the Chinese for the country's problems. As a result, the Cultural Revolution emerged. During this time, traditional medicine was again outlawed and many master practitioners were imprisoned or killed. This led to a dramatic loss in the number of people trained traditionally in the medicine.[19]

Once the government decided to reinstate some form of China's traditional medicine, they did it with an emphasis on combining it with Western medical theory. This shifted even acupuncture theory, as Western anatomical teaching was adopted and esoteric subtle anatomy was discarded. According to the Association for Traditional Studies (ATS), the Communists allowed only the anatomy that was in agreement with Western anatomy, specifically the neurological system, to be included in the curriculum. In fact, any information that was not in line with Communist-approved teaching was eliminated from Chinese medicine textbooks.[20]

This led to a massive shift toward combining conflicting medical paradigms, which emphasized the power of Western medicine and greatly watered down the traditional teachings. After some time the government recognized the effectiveness of traditionally trained practitioners and solicited them to teach the up-and-coming generation of students. ATS states that countrywide, only 500 traditionally trained teachers existed who were willing or able to take on students. For many logistical reasons this program failed, and the hybridization of Chinese medicine and Western medicine continues to this day.[21] It is what we know in the West as "traditional Chinese medicine."

Traditional Chinese medicine (TCM) is a standardized form of Chinese medicine that follows specific guidelines across the board for diagnosis and treatment. In this way, it differs from what many practitioners simply refer to as, "Chinese medicine." Standardized TCM is more scripted and doesn't always totally account for the intricacies inherently present in an individual and his or her presentation. An example of this would be giving an acupuncture treatment based on the disease as opposed to the person. Unlike TCM, Chinese medicine incorporates more out-of-the-box diagnosis and treatment, empirical knowledge, and lineage wisdom. Although it is still medicine, it is more of an intuitive art.

Luckily, there are many Western people who are passionate enough about the original teachings of the medicine and have the means to go to China, Taiwan, Korea, or Japan to seek out one of these truly traditionally trained elders or their direct disciples/students. These Westerners, along with some Chinese students of these practitioners who have left China for the West, are slowly helping with the reemergence of the original teachings of the medicine.

One positive development from this hybridization is that it probably contributed to Chinese medicine being more accepted by and accessible to Westerners, as a treatment modality to both receive and practice. The incorporation of Western medical concepts into the training has helped practitioners better understand lab results, diseases, and how to communicate with a Western medical team. It also has influenced the face of Chinese medicine in that the educational model and therefore practice is clinical in nature, which is something we in the West are generally comfortable with and have come to expect in medical establishments. This has given Chinese medicine credibility in the American psyche above and beyond many other holistic or energy-based practices.

Ayurveda did not undergo quite the same gutting that Chinese medicine did, but it did face suppression that was worse in some areas than others. During the Middle Ages, Muslim invaders burned Indian institutions, including Ayurveda universities. Unani was largely practiced at this time, but the Indians never stopped using Ayurveda, and the traditional knowledge of it was never lost. Fortunately, the Muslim invaders did not completely take over in the mountainous regions of the northwest, Assam, or the deep south. In Goa, the Portuguese, and later the British, suppressed traditional medicine for some time. Today, however, Westerners are supporting the popularity of Ayurveda in India and abroad. Because Ayurveda has been passed down more intact than Chinese medicine, there is an essence and a completion to it that can enhance the practice of Chinese medicine. There are conceptual gaps in Chinese medicine that we can fill in with Ayurveda. Likewise, because Chinese medicine practitioners in the West undergo a clinical training not present in Western Ayurveda practitioner programs, the practice of Chinese medicine has much to offer to the approach of modern Ayurveda practitioners outside of India. It also offers training in formula construction that is unparalleled in Ayurveda training outside of BAMS programs.

2

In the Beginning

The Roots of Ayurveda and Chinese Medicine

Chinese medicine and Ayurveda are both built upon several thousand years of cultural belief systems and philosophies. Although these theories of life may differ in tone and focus, there are universal themes that run through both traditions' roots. Both have in common a cosmology, a constitutional theory, a concept of the elements, a science of taste and diet, and observational diagnostic tools like tongue and pulse diagnosis. What differs is the lens through which the originators perceived the world, both its seen and unseen aspects. That lens has influenced how each system unfolded. In this chapter we will look at these underlying beliefs and cosmologies.

Interestingly, both systems have emerged from a primary cosmology that applies to all life and beyond life to everything that exists. Each system's cosmology applies to the birth and function of our universe, our minds, and our cells. The origin theory that underpins Chinese medicine is Taoism. Taoism is the philosophy underlying the study and practice of energy cultivation systems such as tai chi, qigong, and Chinese martial arts and is inherent in the arts of calligraphy, feng shui, music, and meditative practice.

Ayurveda is based largely on Sankhya philosophy, one of the main underlying systems of thought in India. It is the foundation for much of the yoga philosophy and practice so popular throughout India and the West today, and it is the root theory for understanding matter in many Indian disciplines including *vastu* (a traditional Indian science of architecture, similar to feng shui), Vedic astrology, meditation, and yoga.

PHILOSOPHY

The origins of any medicine are a product of many years of trial and error, observation, learning, thinking, sharing, experience, and practice. How we perceive, as is true of those who came before us, is heavily steeped in what we believe. These beliefs are rooted in the dominant philosophical paradigm of the day. Below is a brief discussion of the predominant philosophies that had an influence on the development of both Chinese medicine and Ayurveda as we know them today.

Taoism

Taoism is recognized as one of the six main religions in China and is believed to have evolved out of a pre-Taoist shamanistic tradition or conglomeration of traditions. Its source text is Lao-tzu's Tao Te Ching, thought to have been written in either the fifth or sixth century BCE. Adherents would probably categorize Taoism as a philosophy and a way of life rather than a religion. Its fundamental premise is that each individual should live according to their own true nature, according to the Tao. The Tao (or Dao) means "way" or "path," but it is actually not definable beyond that. As it says in the first verse of the Tao Te Ching, the way that can be named is not the way. It is nameless, formless, and eternal. It is the origin of all that is, and it is all that is. It is nothing and it is everything. It is doing and not doing. The following is a direct translation of the verse.

體 道	*Embodying the Way*
道可道	*The way that can be the way*
非常道	*Is not the upheld way*
名可名	*The name that can be named*

非常名	*Is not the upheld name*
無名天地之始	*Without name the beginning of heaven and earth*
有名萬物之母	*Having name the mother of the myriad things*
故常無欲	*Thus upholding without desire*
以觀其妙	*To observe the subtlety*
常有欲	*Upholding having desire*
以觀其微	*To observe the boundary*
此兩者	*These two*
同出而異名	*Together emerging but differently named*
同謂之玄	*Together called the mysterious*
玄之又玄	*The mysterious of the mysterious*
衆妙之門	*The gate of crowding subtlety*

VERSE 1 OF TAO TE CHING
(TRANSLATED BY TIM BAGLIO, MAcOM, L.Ac.)

The supreme ultimate Tao manifests as two polar energies, yin and yang, whose fluctuations are considered to be the cause of the universe. Their concrete manifestations are Earth and Heaven. From the inter-mingling of yin and yang arise five elements, which in turn are the basis of all phenomena (also known as the "ten thousand things").

When one is not living in harmony with the Tao, the mind and body are askew. This is when disease can arise. Bringing one back into resonance with the Tao, by way of the Tao, allows internal forces to self-regulate and create homeostasis. Taoism honors nature and speaks of the relationship between Earth and Heaven. In Chinese medicine, Earth and Heaven are also present in the living being and should have good interaction and connection to one another in order for all aspects of the person to be harmonious.

Confucianism

Confucius was a Chinese philosopher who was thought to have lived between 551 and 479 BCE. Some say his passion was for tradition, as he was responsible for reanimating Chinese cultural beliefs, attitudes, and practices from antiquity. These include an emphasis on the family and social harmony and a reverence for ancestors. The teachings of Confucius contain a code of ethics, but they are more like a cultural value system than an organized religion. Most people are familiar with Confucius's *Analects*, a compilation of his quotes and teachings that reflect his overall message.[1] The New Culture Movement in China attempted to obliterate Confucianism,[2] but Confucius's reverence for tradition as a cultural value crossed millennia and can be witnessed in the reemergence of Chinese medicine.

Sankhya

Sankhya is one of the six orthodox philosophical systems in India. It is variously believed to have emerged sometime between 1500 and 300 BCE. Sankhya cosmology explains the journey of consciousness into matter, the qualities of matter, the senses, and the mind. Many other traditions in India, such as yoga, have their roots in Sankhya philosophy. Sankhya is a rational philosophy that contends that there are three ways of acquiring knowledge: perception, inference, and the testimony of others. These three proofs are used in Ayurveda during examination and diagnosis. Sankhya is also pertinent to the study of Ayurveda because it is the first system to describe the fundamental principles of material nature.

Sankhya philosophy is one of cosmic dualism. When two completely separate principles create friction with one another, the whole of existence emerges. This is similar to the yin/yang principle of Taoist cosmology. According to Sankhya, two primordial entities—*purusha* (consciousness) and *prakriti* (primordial matter)—manifested from their unmanifested state. The interaction between these two created a fine material called *mahat,* or universal intelligence, and from mahat emerged the stuff of individual self-awareness and differentiation, *ahamkara,* or ego. All manifested objects are composed of three qualities, or *gunas: sattva* (clarity, purity), *rajas* (turbulence, activity), and *tamas* (inertia, ignorance). The three gunas also correspond to our states of mind. If we are in a sattvic state, we are peaceful, calm, compassionate, wise, and clear. If we are in a rajasic state, we are unsettled, agitated, and discontented. And when a state of tamas rules, we feel lazy, "foggy," and only slightly self-aware.

In terms of Sankhya cosmology, three products emerge from the vibration of sattva: the five senses (sight, sound, smell, taste, and touch), the five actions (speech, grasping, ambulation, procreation, and elimination), and mind. From tamas emerge the five *tanmatras,* the objects of the sense faculties: sound, touch, form, taste, and odor. From these tanmatras emerge the five elements: ether, air, fire, water, and earth. These are the building blocks of matter.

Yoga

Yoga, an ancient Indian Sanskrit word meaning "to yoke" or "to unite," is based largely upon Sankhya philosophy. Its preeminent text is called the Yoga Sutras of Patanjali, which presents a complete system of Yoga philosophy and psychology and a description of the stages of meditative practice. The Yoga Sutras describe the eight limbs (astanga) of yoga. These include *yamas* and *niyamas* (ethical and clean living disciplines), asana (ideal posture for meditation), *pranayama* (breathing to direct prana or life force), *pratyahara* (withdrawal of the senses from external objects), *dharana* (concentration), *dhyana* (meditation), and *samadhi* (enlightenment).

This philosophy plays a role in the foundational practices of Ayurveda. In order to be healthy, one must be living according to the yamas and niyamas. In addition, Charaka states that the primary purpose of Ayurveda is to create optimal health so beings may achieve enlightenment. Yoga postures, or asanas, prepare the body, particularly the nervous system, for long bouts of seated meditation. What many folks are practicing today is more a form of exercise than anything else. The cadence and intention behind the asanas are not necessarily as they once were but vary by instructor, yet that doesn't mean they are not beneficial.

Sitting for a long time and focusing on anything but the physical body or restless mind is impossible if the body's elements are not balanced and its mental and life force energies are not flowing optimally without blockage, constraint, or misdirection. In addition to the musculoskeletal benefits of our modern yoga practices, the attention to deep breathing helps to free connective tissue and nervous system obstructions and allows for greater assimilation of life force with minimal energy expenditure. The information that arises during the deep yoga practices of pratyahara, dharana, dhyana, and samadhi requires a lubricated and toned system of connective tissue and a strong body, nervous system, energy system, and mind.

Even if someone is not trying to achieve enlightenment, they may be drawn to yoga or Ayurveda because they just want to feel better. In this context, Ayurveda and yoga work marvelously together in a hands-on and practical manner. A physical practice derived from the yoga system and adjusted according to one's constitution is an invaluable resource for achieving and maintaining physical and mental/emotional health and balance.

Mimamsa

No, this is not vodka and orange juice. Mimamsa is a philosophy that places a heavy emphasis upon the scriptures, namely, the Vedas. These are the foundational written treatises of Indian philosophy. It is interesting to note that when speaking of religion in India, one is not only referring to a particular belief system in terms of personal predilections toward worship of one or more gods or deities, but of underlying philosophies as well. One of the earliest philosophies of India, Mimamsa is credited to the teachings of the Sage Jaimini. It teaches the importance of scripture and its correct interpretation in terms of belief, ritual practice, and the understanding of the Vedas.

This philosophy has greatly influenced Ayurveda largely because of its emphasis on *karma,* which means "action." A crude way of understanding karma at a very basic level parallels the rule in Newtonian physics that states that for every action there is an equal and opposite reaction. The idea of karma is that whatever we do generates a ripple in the fabric of time and space, which creates consequences in our lives and the lives of others, whether foreseen or unanticipated. These ripples create impressions in the fabric of our innermost being, called our *atman,* or "individual soul."

These ripples, or impressions, may be complete actions that are carried out to fruition and completion, or they can be like seeds of potential energy waiting for the right time and space to germinate. Karma is tied in with reincarnation. One of the explanations for the origin of some incurable diseases in Ayurveda is karma. Conscious or unconscious actions in the past, whether in this life or another, create our now, for better or worse, according to the law of karma. It is important to be aware that this is a system of cause and effect, not one of sin and punishment. Generally, karmic ailments must be experienced in order for the karma to be exhausted. This can mean that the person may or may not be cured. Either way, the only way to cure some of these diseases is through "spiritual or religious purification methods."[3] These methods must be followed clearly according to the proper performance of ritual as outlined in the Vedas. The emphasis on correct understanding and performance of these rituals is paramount to the teaching of Mimamsa.

Correctly interpreting the Vedas and carrying out their instruction in ritual is also important in Ayurveda. Practitioners can relate to the experience of being faced with a complex case and needing guidance. This guidance is often self-generated and comes from going back to the root of the medical teachings, regardless of what model one is using. We take our experience and what we learned from our teachers and ultimately draw from the simplest teachings of source texts to help us find our way through the most challenging, complex, and often confusing cases. This is in part why Mimamsa is so important to Ayurveda. If we clearly and correctly understand our source texts, we can confidently move forward through the jungle of signs, symptoms, presentations, diagnoses, and treatment strategies. It is of utmost importance to perceive source texts as they were intended because the misinterpretation of them may lead to faulty perception and decision-making and ultimately a wrong diagnosis and treatment.

Nyaya

The primary influence of the Nyaya philosophy on Ayurveda is its focus on logic for determining the truth of an object. Nyaya focuses on realizing the ultimate truth of a thing and checking oneself for cognitive errors surrounding any given topic. There are four main ways one can analyze a situation according to Nyaya: perception, inference, comparison, and testimony. These methods are of paramount importance to a practitioner in determining a correct diagnosis and treatment plan.

Vaisheshika

The Vaisheshika philosophy gained popularity around the second century BCE and is attributed to the sage Kanada. The theory of *pramanus* is a great contribution to the scientific understanding of the nature of matter. It is basically a preatomic theory. Pramanus are believed to be indivisible little particles that make up everything in existence. When an object is broken down as much as it possibly can be, an *anu* is what is left. *Anu* is translated to mean "atom." There are five fundamental atoms that make up material reality: earth, air, fire, water, and ether. They combine in a myriad of ways to form all material objects, gases, and so on.

Vaisheshika lists the following six categories of reality:

1. *Dravyas* (substances), of which pramanus are a part, along with time, space, spirit, and mind.
2. Gunas, or qualities, which are opposites along a spectrum, similar to the yin and yang of Taoist cosmology.
3. Karma, or action, which, along with the gunas, need dravyas to exist.
4. *Samanyas* are similarities between two or more objects that allow them to be grouped into the same class.
5. *Vishesha* is a special quality that makes an object stand out in a group.
6. *Samavaya* indicates that certain things are inextricably connected.

Samanya and vishesha are concepts that relate to the specific actions of herbs and how they are classified.

Vedanta

Vedanta is a philosophical system that has self-reflection as its main focus. It originated with the seventh-century sage Shankara. It teaches that there is an unmanifest, absolute reality called Brahman. It is unchanging, indescribable, and timeless. It manifests itself as *maya,* or illusion. This illusory world is constantly in flux and is a reflection of our mind. Tools for self-reflection include selfless service, study, devotion, meditation, and yoga practices. Vedanta holds that ultimate truth is one, yet may express itself in many ways, hence the many systems of belief. Vedanta is based on a group of writings called the Upanishads.

Vedantists believe that our individual soul, or atman, is part and parcel of the larger transcendent whole, or Brahman, and that by experientially realizing the truth of the soul, one becomes aware of the oneness of existence and their personal illusion of separation from it. According to Vedanta, it is our responsibility to broaden and raise our consciousness so that we may correctly perceive the ultimate truths of existence, which would include understanding reality and medicine in such a way as to correctly perceive, diagnose, and treat an individual. To do this we must have a desire for discipline, nonattachment, discernment, liberation from ignorance or nonknowing, and to use our inner tool of meditation.

The *Katha Upanishad* states, "For the soul, there is neither birth nor death at any time. It does not come into being at any time, it is unborn, eternal and primeval. It doesn't die when the body is put to death."[4] Ayurveda has adopted Vedanta into its foundational fold, and this concept is part of how a trained practitioner views life. Ayurveda is the science, wisdom, or knowledge of life and how it works. Since this knowledge is based in the Vedas, according to Vedanta, it would naturally follow that it is representative of the ultimate truth of life, one aspect of which is medicine. This medicine is universal, since it has at its foundation the ultimate truth of existence and came from the true, ultimate reality.

Karma, Reincarnation, and Ancestor Worship

Ayurveda has become a spiritual practice in and of itself for many practitioners. Good Ayurvedic doctors are revered as sages. I have seen people of all ages and backgrounds bow at their feet. This is a humble act for someone of Western origin and speaks to the wisdom associated with the medicine. That is not to say there is not an equal reverence for Chinese medicine doctors. However, the two medicines have evolved in very different ways in the West. Ayurveda comes across as more of a spiritual discipline that is often paired with yoga and used as a tool to feel good on many levels. Chinese medicine has evolved to be more of an adjunct to allopathic medicine, after which its practitioner training is modeled. Traditionally, Chinese medicine practitioners were well versed in internal martial arts, the Tao, and in living according to natural laws. Both systems traditionally included long apprenticeships with seasoned masters. If one wishes to do such training nowadays they must travel to Asia and approach the right teacher in the hope that they will be taken on as a student.

Reincarnation, karma, and ancestor worship have played a role in determining how each medicine is practiced and what its energetic focus is. Really, they both are doing very similar things, just in different ways. This can be seen in their approaches to the five elements. All of the elements of Chinese medicine are tangible and palpable. They can be directly perceived by the five senses. I believe that this can be traced to the Tao and to the emphasis the Chinese put on inherited cultural beliefs of the interconnectedness of man and nature, a relationship with their ancestors as if they are still with them, and the importance of the life they are currently living. There seems to be more of an earthly "here and now" that doesn't come through quite the same way in the Indian system.

In Ayurveda, the five elements cross over from gross physicality to the etheric plane of existence. An example of how this compares to the Chinese view of the five elements can be found in the concepts of wood and space. The wood element in Chinese medicine has many of the attributes of the space element in Ayurveda. They are both the most expansive, spacious elements. Yet wood is tangible; we can relate it directly to trees, which we can see and touch. Space we need to think about. It is vast, empty yet full, and relates to all the spaces in the body. We don't usually think of the body as having spaces. Space is also the substance *akasha,* which, according to Ayurveda, is the original element from which all others are derived. This is very different conceptually from the more common sense, here-and-now element of wood. At least at first glance.

In many Asian cultures, including those in China and India, there is some form of ancestor worship or ongoing veneration of those who have passed that honors the deceased and, in some instances, incorporates a belief that they continue to have an effect on the living. Many now believe that people inherit actual memories of their ancestors through DNA, that they inherit beliefs and emotional residues from generations of family members they may not have even known. People who believe this think that they may have an ancestor or ancestors who suffered experiences that have been handed down to them at a molecular or cellular level. These stored experiences or memories, usually of an emotional nature, can affect one's very DNA and translate into physical, mental, and emotional imbalance in this life. As a result, there is a growing movement, largely of alternative medicine practitioners and energy medicine providers, working to help clients release this stored information and heal. Perhaps on some level the ancients felt this influence, and this awareness is what led, at least in part, to the practice of ancestor worship.

The belief in reincarnation has influenced the Ayurvedic view of life and death. Rather than focusing on the importance of this current life as if there is no other, life and death are believed to be a continuum, where one continually flows to the next. In Ayurveda, while one's environment and one's ancestors do affect the makeup of a person at the moment of conception, so does individual karma. This is not the same in Chinese medicine. The Chinese focus is more on familial karma, as they place more value on the collective than on the individual. This is another reason, perhaps, why Westerners resonate more easily with Ayurveda and yoga than Far Eastern practices. The ideal of the individual is engrained in our cultural psyche.

Now for a thought experiment. Just sit for a moment and focus on how it feels in your body to see your health and well-being in the context of someone who believes that what you do and who you are now and maybe some way into the future and what you leave behind is all there is. Take a moment to do this.

Take a deep breath. Now reflect on your innermost self, your very deepest being beyond likes and dislikes, and imagine that it never dies. Imagine that you are actually eternal, that you carry something that is only you from the past into this current life and into your future lives that you will invariably have. Notice how it feels in your body to think that your health and well-being are part of this eternal self. Breathe into this.

These are two very different takes on life that have influenced how life is lived, how theories of existence have evolved, how we understand the meaning life on a personal level, how we perceive health and disease, what we believe about being healthy, and how medicine is practiced.

Ayurveda incorporates death into the medicine as part of the wheel of existence and as a part of one's potential healing journey. If there is a karma that creates an imbalance that cannot be cured, then the karma is being burned away, not to be repeated in our continued existence as our Self in another body. This is not to say that karma is an excuse for anything. Only a person ignorant of the definition and depth of karma would perceive it in such a way. Karma doesn't eliminate choice or free will.

COSMOLOGY

Cosmology can be understood as a foundational system of thought that is used to explain basically everything in existence. From ancient times to the present humans have valued one cosmology or another. Today our cosmology is based on science, namely physics. Newtonian physics is at the root of our cosmology, but we are on the cusp of a paradigm shift. Quantum physics is a very attractive new paradigm; when it is combined with Newtonian physics, it results in a cosmology that closely resembles that of the ancients.

It is probably because of the newfound acceptance of things like alternate realities and dimensions and nonlocal healing that we are now open to the old ways of seeing the world and to the associated techniques available to deal with its complexity. We tend to question the legitimacy of mystical or otherwise unexplained personal experience. Unless it is validated by an outside source of authority and communally accepted we tend to ignore or negate it. That authority, for many of us, is the scientific community. Through discoveries in quantum physics, science is catching up at a root level with what heart-based rational people have believed for millennia.

Truth tends to stand the test of time. If something is true, it may not always be comfortable or welcome, but it can be felt within us, and it is unchanging. Ancient medicine contains organizing principles and concepts that can be utilized in our current era, concurrent with Western medicine. All medicine can be referred to as both an art and a science. With new developments in medicine, such as genetic typing to gear treatment toward a specific individual, it is becoming increasingly likely that we can blend the ancient diagnostic theories with Western medicine.

Cosmology of the Ancients

Both Sankhya and Taoism view existence as having emerged from non-being, no-thingness, unmanifest being, limitlessness, void, or unity. From there came duality, from duality came multiplicity of qualities, from multiplicity of qualities came qi or prana, and from qi or prana came form. Both traditions teach that there was an undifferentiated whole of "nothingness that wasn't nothing" prior to the "big bang," or spark of creation. It differentiated into the duality known as yin and yang or purusha and prakriti. In Taoist art, it is depicted as an empty circle because we simply cannot describe it. Our brains just can't grasp what it was/is because we're utilizing what came after it, from it, and of it to understand what it was/is. This "not nothing no-thingness" is called Wu Chi in the pinyin pronunciation of Mandarin, and *avyakta* in Sanskrit.

Creation occurred as a result of some initial stirring within the Wu

Chi, no-thingness. Modern science states that in the beginning, space and time were undisturbed, and creation, regardless of whether you're talking "big bang" theory or "string" theory, is the result of the disturbance of this space/time equilibrium.

Taoist and Sankhyan cosmologies describe a similar beginning, caused by a disruption of Wu Chi/avyakta, from which space and time formed. Sankhya states that the three forces of sattva, rajas, and tamas were in balance. A distortion of the balance between these three primal qualities caused the differentiation of purusha and prakriti from the void. Similar to Taoism's yin/yang theory, purusha and prakriti are representative of the polar opposites in existence. One is not better than another, as they are interdependent and interchanging. One is only preferred to another in reference to particular objects or our beliefs about them.

You may be familiar with the Tai Chi symbol. It's that half-white, half-black circle with a dot of white in the black half and a dot of black in the white half (see fig. 2.1). The circle symbolizes the whole

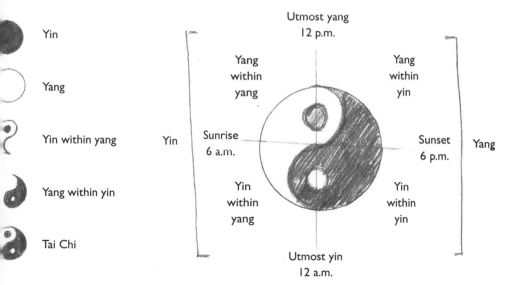

Fig. 2.1. The Tai Chi symbol

of existence. What is outside the circle and contains the circle is the Wu Chi, which represents emptiness, that which is unmanifest. The right side (black) is yin; the left side (white) is yang. Within yin there is yang, within yang there is yin. There is always a seed of the other in each one, as represented by the dots in the symbol. One way of understanding it is to say that the universe is made up of energy and matter, and they can transform into one another as described in modern physics theory.

Everything is seen as an interrelationship between yin and yang. A good visualization for yin and yang is to imagine the sunlight on a mountainside. During the day, when the Sun shines on a mountain, there is a shady side and a sunny side. The shady side is yin, which is described as cold, dark, moist, contracting like some flora, and accumulating and descending like dew. The sunny side is called yang, which is considered bright, hot, dry, ascending like evaporated dew or fog, and expansive like plants opening to receive the rays of the Sun. As the Sun moves through the afternoon and sets over the horizon, the mountain is more yin. As the Sun rises and moves toward noon, the mountain becomes more yang.

The Sun is yang and the Moon is yin. A cloudy or rainy day is more yin than yang. The desert is more yang than yin. Spaciousness is yang, density is yin. Energy is yang, matter is yin. But these are in relationship to each other; they are relative depending upon the context you are using. For example, matter may be more yin than energy, but fire is considered an element of matter, and it is more yang than say, water, which, when speaking in terms of the elements, is yin.

Men are more yang, women are more yin. Children are more yang energetically and adults are more yin. The expanse of infinite space is more yang, time and the hold it has upon us is more yin. Mind and spirit are more yang, the body is yin. Active people with high metabolisms who tend to run warm naturally are more yang. Those individuals with a slower metabolism and steady nature are more yin.

Similarly, in Sankhya philosophy purusha is male, prakriti is female. Purusha represents all the qualities of yang (energy or movement and consciousness) and prakriti of yin (stability, structure, stillness, and matter). Purusha is also considered the soul and consciousness itself. Prakriti is recognized as nature and creation. There are many synonyms in the Indian religion and culture for this interrelated duality: Shiva/Shakti, Narayan/Lakshmi, and Krishna/Radha to name a few. Indian cosmology has a divine, artistic, emotive nature. It is beautiful in its simplicity, but also in the way it beautifies and sanctifies potentially mundane, profane concepts with its careful use of language and metaphor.

QI AND PRANA

The two sides of the Tai Chi symbol are divided by a wavy line. This symbolizes movement: the two sides are constantly interacting with one another. The friction that is created by their interaction is called qi. Qi is one thing and everything. It is life-animating energy or vibration. It is what everything is made of and how everything functions, and it takes many forms. Indeed, it takes all forms. There are specific types of qi that are responsible for different functions in creation and in the body. Wind is *wind qi,* food qi is *gu qi,* the qi that repels pathogens is *wei qi,* and so on.

In Sankhya philosophy, the qi is called prana. After the emergence of cosmic intelligence (mahat) from purusha and prakriti and the development of the cosmic ego (ahamkara), the three gunas (cosmic qualities) further differentiated. From sattva (equanimity) came the quality of mind, from tamas (inertia) came the body, and from rajas (activity) came prana. Prana is not just form, it is not just function, it is not just vitality, and it is not just the communicator between cells and individual minds and bodies. It is all of the above. This book is prana, your seeing faculty is prana, your brain interpreting these words is prana, your mind digesting the concepts, integrating them, and coming up with new thoughts, judgments, and questions about them is prana. If you are sore from sitting too long or cold or hot as you read, that discomfort, cold, or heat is prana, as is your perception of it.

There is an old story about the importance of prana. It goes that five of our faculties were having an argument about which one was most important to the body: sight, hearing, speech, mind, or prana. Sight, hearing, speech, and mind left one at a time, and the body suffered each imbalance: it was blind, then deaf, then mute, and then unconscious, but it survived. However, when the prana left, something horrible began to happen. Not only did the body lose sight, hearing, speech, and mind, but it began to die. All the other faculties begged prana to return, and, as it did, vitality and power returned to them and the body.

Nadis and Meridians

All things are made of prana, even inanimate objects like dead bodies, but when prana circulates in its vital form, then a being is alive. This vital prana is said to travel along specific pathways in the body called *nadis*. In Chinese medicine, nadis are called "channels" or "meridians." Whether meridian or nadi, along these pathways there are intersection points, known as "acupoints" in Chinese medicine or marmani in Ayurveda. These points allow for multi-tissue communication within the body and communication between deeper parts of the body with the prana both inside and outside the body. Some of these intersection points can be manipulated through the placement of an acupuncture needle or through pressure to increase or dissipate the flow of qi/prana along its respective pathway. Sometimes the points work like railroad switches, releasing the flow of qi/prana to another pathway like trains changing tracks. Other times they are stimulated in order to restore flow to a particular meridian where a blockage to qi/prana flow exists, causing disharmony.

On other occasions the points along these pathways may be stimulated to effect change to internal organs and processes or to balance emotions and hormones. They can also be activated to gently persuade the body to take in more vital qi/prana from the outside world or to absorb it more effectively for distribution throughout the body and mind.

The nadis/meridians do not completely correlate to any systems in the body such as the circulatory, lymphatic, or nervous system, although they do overlap in some locations. They have instead been found to exist along known connective tissue pathways for electromagnetic energy in the body. The qi/prana travels along these pathways and circulates to the smallest places, like capillaries. Qi/prana is responsible for vitality in the organism and also for communication between bodily parts such as cells. According to Chinese acupuncture and Ayurvedic marma therapy theory, whenever there is a blockage or disruption in the communication of information between cells, organs, and tissues, there is disease. This disruption manifests as a distortion of qi/prana flow.

The smooth, optimal flow of qi/prana through the mind/body complex is the basis of a peaceful mind and healthy body. That is why it is important to have a strong, flexible body with smooth movement and good respiration and a positive mental attitude where thoughts and emotions flow instead of repeating like a broken record. Because the connective tissue is a good place for byproducts of cellular metabolism to accumulate during times of injury, sickness, or stress, Eastern types of exercise should be employed. Tai chi, qigong, and therapeutic styles of yoga are best. If the connective tissue is well hydrated and unobstructed, with good circulation, the qi/prana flows well, communication between and detoxification of tissues is optimized, and life is good.

Types of Qi and Prana

There are many functions and types of qi. Descriptions of these types can be similar from a clinical perspective, but the details concerning the number of types may differ depending on what you read or who you talk to. As mentioned earlier, in a general sense, everything is qi. In a specific sense, there are several primary types identified for the maintenance of life. From a Chinese perspective, qi performs several functions in the human body. These include communication, movement, transformation, stabilization, defense from external pathogens, and warming. In Ayurveda these roles are roughly associated with the functioning of the three doshas mentioned earlier: movement is vata, transformation and warming are pitta, and stabilization and protection are kapha.

In Chinese medicine there are two primary categories of qi: prenatal and postnatal. Prenatal, or *yuan*, qi is inherited from the parents and received by the fetus at conception. The amount received is set at birth and does not change. It is like our tank of fuel for life. All other forms of qi are postnatal. Once we run out of yuan qi, we are done. Therefore, instead of depleting and exhausting our essential prenatal qi, we need to use a renewable resource. We can supplement and protect our original source, or yuan, qi by enhancing the quality and quantity of our postnatal qi. We can do this by properly breathing good air, maintaining optimal circulation, keeping our transformative digestive functioning strong, and eating good food that resonates with our constitution. We can also practice qi-cultivation techniques designed to bring in, circulate, and store postnatal qi.

Yuan qi is responsible for fueling the transformation of the other types of qi. Clinically, in addition to yuan qi, we speak most often of *zong* qi, *ying* qi, *wei* qi, *zheng* qi, spleen qi, liver qi, lung qi, kidney qi, and *yang* qi. Zong qi is the qi of the chest. It facilitates respiration and is responsible for bringing in good *kong* (air) qi. Gu qi is the qi of our food. It is the qi produced from the spleen qi and when mixed with the kong qi becomes zheng, or "true," qi. This subdivides into yin and yang aspects. The yin of zheng qi is ying qi, or nourishment, and the yang of zheng qi is wei qi, an aspect of immunity or what we call "defensive qi." Yuan qi and kidney qi support and fuel these processes. We will further discuss kidney qi, as well as liver, spleen, and lung qi in the organ section.

Although Chinese medicine and Ayurveda are basically very similar, it is difficult to achieve an exact correlation between concepts and vocabulary. This is because they are organized differently. As mentioned, the Chinese use the word *qi* to describe many functions in the body: movement, warming, transformation, nourishment, stabilization, and protection. In Ayurveda, these functions are not discussed as the domain of qi, or prana, but are described as the specific activities of the three doshas and their subdoshas, along with other factors such as the seven *dhatus* (types of tissues). In the chapters to come these distinctions will be discussed in greater detail.

Basically, from an Ayurvedic perspective, cosmic prana takes the form of the three main physiological forces in existence: movement, transformation, and stability. In the human body, these forces are responsible for maintaining homeostasis. They are perceived to function in certain ways and govern specific processes, chemicals, and tissues and are concentrated in particular areas. Prana moves in five different ways in the body: inspiratory and forward (*prana* vayu), up (*udana* vayu), inward (*samana* vayu), down (*apana* vayu), and diffusing and spreading (*vyana* vayu). Its transformative function is divided into five categories: digestion, blood generation, emotion, vision, and temperature regulation. Its stabilizing function is differentiated into craving and early digestion, strength, taste, nourishment, and lubrication.

This triad of movement, transformation, and stability is in operation in the atom, in the cosmos, and in our bodies. We are a microcosm of the macrocosm of the cosmos; a hologram, so to speak. As above, so below. We are the ever-shifting interplay of yin and yang and of their expression through the form and function of the five elements via the vehicle of qi. Inside the body, most likely mirroring the origin of all things, the concepts of purusha and prakriti translate into the two main nadis that traverse the central axis of the body, which relate to the functioning of the right and left brain hemispheres, as we will explore in detail later.

Qi/Prana Resonance

There is a principle of resonance that goes with qi or prana: like increases like and, to some extent, opposites balance one another. This is qi/prana resonance. This resonance is a part of what people who preach or practice the Law of Attraction focus on. The Law of Attraction is basically the belief that what you put out mentally, emotionally, energetically, or physically directly affects the experiences you have in life and can influence material gains.

The way qi/prana resonance works is based upon vibration. Quantum physics posits that everything is basically vibratory. Oak trees have one unique vibratory frequency, house cats another. Inanimate objects also have vibration, as do thoughts and emotions. This vibration is qi/prana. The specific qualities of a thing each have a subtle vibration that creates a unique signature. We say like increases like, or same increases same. Not only do like vibrations resonate with each other, but they can also be naturally drawn to each other. This is how herbal medicine works to tonify or increase a substance or quality in the mind and body, for example.

All things have a vibration. Each person has their own individual vibration. This vibration is a combination of their DNA—which genes are turned on or off—the effect of the food they consume; their lifestyle choices; how they perceive reality and process experiences; their desires and aversions and the energetic residue accumulated from past actions; what's happening in their body; and what they think and feel. This thinking and feeling can be in the moment, about the future, or from the past, and it can be conscious, unconscious, or subconscious. Thinking in terms of vibration and using the Law of Attraction, let's look at how this works.

As we develop desires for things, say an inanimate object like a piece of jewelry, we vibrate or resonate the vibration of that thing. We both project and attach to it because we visualize it, feel what it represents or means to us, and vibrate that feeling, which incorporates the vibration of the object. We tune in to the vibration of the object and actually emanate it. Whatever it means to us personally is the resonance we project and the meaning we ascribe to the object. There is a natural resonance of sameness between the initial vibration of the desire with the object of the desire. In a sense, we actually vibrate that thing.

The vibration sets us on a path to interacting with the object. Let's say it's a diamond ring. We would think about it, desire it (emotionally charging our qi), then maybe find it a week or two later at a garage sale we never intended to pass by. Perhaps by spontaneously driving a different way that day we came across it. That perceived spontaneity is actually the following of the vibration we were resonating with. The resonance brought us together. It feels magical, and it is, if you still find wonder in the world around you or deep gratitude and awe for the processes of nature.

The same holds true for all desires. This is the way of resonance, the Tao of Resonance if you will. The Way or Tao indicates a natural pattern of existence and a pathway. The mind and ego can interfere with qi resonance, as it is a mechanism of free will, but it's free will being exercised at a low level. Say there is some goal you'd like to reach. It may be a number on a scale or a promotion at work. Perhaps you really want to achieve this goal, and you work hard to do so, but it just doesn't seem to be happening. Although you are visualizing it and emanating its vibration, at some level you may have an underlying vibration that doesn't allow for it. Maybe it's a belief that you can never do it or some other underlying pattern or vibration you are holding on to that is preventing you from manifesting the goal.

The universe, existence, whatever you choose to call all that is, doesn't necessarily care what we want or don't want, that's up to us to decide. Qi is a vibration and this law of resonance is impartial. This same process applies to healing. Specific herbal remedies are selected to achieve the vibration necessary to bring balance to the individual based upon what vibrations are present in the tissue. If there is a problem related to heat or inflammation, a more cooling substance will be prescribed. In fact, in Ayurveda and Chinese medicine, a slew of herbs are carefully chosen to heal the vibratory pattern in the patient. It's like using herbs slyly to trick pathogens or pathogenic processes. Instead of using a like substance that will increase the manifestation of the problem, we use something opposite to it. In addition to that, we use substances, oftentimes in the same formula, to increase the healthy vibrations in order to strengthen the person overall, so they will at some point no longer need the substances.

On a more subtle or less dense level of manifestation, using like to decrease like is also possible. Homeopathy is an example of this, as are some vaccinations. Homeopathy uses the energetic quality of a substance causing imbalance in the body or mind to treat the imbalance. A live vaccination is the substance the body wants to immunize itself against, in a form the body can handle. The introduction of the substance actually activates the immune system to fight it off and create a memory of it so if the body encounters it again, it will administer its own defense against the substance.

Auric Field

Prana extends out from each living entity into the air space around it. This fifth and higher dimensional glow is called the "aura." Some people, like the late twentieth-century American prophet Edgar Cayce, have a natural ability to perceive this with their eyes. It would be said of such a person that the acupoint, or marma, between their eyes is open, allowing for a more subtle perception, seemingly through their eyes, like a sixth sense.

This auric field is like a bioplasm that interacts with the environment. Its color, glow, and intensity is reflective of internal processes, both mental/emotional and physical, but also of the entity's interaction with the outside world. This world includes the attitudes and energies of other humans, as well as the weather and any other sensory stimuli. The aura can also be a diagnostic tool for a practitioner. Trained hands can feel disruptions in the flow of prana in this field that surrounds and permeates the body. External pathogens, colds for example, often first exist in this energy field before entering the body through one of its channels and settling in that channel or entering a deeper organ or pathway and causing disease. A skilled practitioner can actually move this out of the auric field before it goes deeper, preventing the illness or making it less intense.

Matrix of Prana

We are a matrix of prana and *of* a matrix of prana. We are a drop in the pranic ocean. Just as each water molecule is attached to the next, we are all connected to one another in this web. Everything in existence is connected to everything else. It might be zero degrees of connection or a million, but it is there. Look at distant healing. How fascinating that a human can focus his or her intention upon someone inches or miles away and effect a healing response. Prana knows where to go. A good illustration of this is based on a story of one of my first Reiki practitioner experiences, before I attended acupuncture school.

While working out of my friend Veronica's storeroom at her metaphysics shop, the Magic Moon, I encountered a woman who was interested in experiencing a Reiki healing. She looked thin, but not frail, and her skin was kind of ruddy. She was in her thirties and told me she had joint pain from systemic lupus. It was a small room, so I had to forego a treatment table for a regular folding chair. Mind you, this was in 1996 when most people were still calling yoga yogurt and had never even heard of Reiki, so there wasn't much along the lines of expectation when it came to the accommodations. She sat down and immediately my hands felt drawn to her neck.

Now, knowing what lupus was and that she had systemic pain, I was thinking she would feel like she wasn't being heard or that I didn't know what I was doing if I didn't do the hand positions on various places around her body. So I worked on some other areas, but still felt drawn to her neck. I finally surrendered to it and brought my hands there. I had them about six inches away from her body, one facing the front of her neck and one facing the nape of her neck. I started feeling a cold breeze coming into the palms of my hands. Being a pretty rational person with a healthy dose of skepticism, I thought that perhaps there was a breeze from the air conditioning coming in through a crack at the bottom of the door. I worked my hands down, remaining six inches from her in her aura, and slyly checked for a breeze under the door as I got down to her feet.

Nothing. Okay, back to the neck. Once I got there, the cold air intensified and it was all I could focus on. I didn't know what it was or what to do, so I just did what felt right and stayed in position. Within a minute or so, there was a loud crack! It was like the sound of a solid home run hit. And loud! We both jumped, and she stood up nervously, then sat back down. "I think you just cured my whiplash!" What? She said lupus, not whiplash! It turned out she had been in an accident six months earlier and had been seeing a chiropractor several times a month, sometimes several times a week, for that six months.

Needless to say, there are a few points to mention here. One is that I didn't cure anything. She was in the right place at the right time with the right circumstances, and her body was given the opportunity to do what it needed to or receive what it needed to heal itself. This is often the way these things happen. It wasn't as if all those chiropractic adjustments didn't matter. Perhaps without them she would still have had the whiplash. We just don't know. A clinic supervisor, Dr. Wang, said this during one of our shifts. We don't know what came before us. Just because someone is "cured" during or after a session, we can never take credit for it.

Another thing this points to is an experience of the clinical significance of cold. In Chinese medicine, we talk about how cold can actually lodge in the body and cause pathological changes. I honestly believe this was the case for her, and that I felt the cold actually leave her body. Think about what this means for people who have operations. It is freezing cold in the operating room, for good reason, yet the warmth inside the body is not protected from this.

Finally, you don't even need to touch someone in order to effect a healing response. The qi knows where to go and what to do, we just need to listen, like I needed to listen and act accordingly when receiving the guidance to go to her neck. The inner dialogue I had was an example of the mind almost getting in the way of a spontaneous healing response.

In another session I experienced removing a type of qi we call in Chinese medicine "plum pit qi," which is basically the experience of having a chronic lump in your throat. A friend of mine had the sensation of someone holding a hand to her throat for years. I did a couple of sessions on her, and the last one was rather profound. There's a technique in the energy healing field called psychic surgery. This is when the practitioner, sometimes with the aid of the participant, removes some subtle thing from the body. In this case, it was a dark lump at her throat about the size of a tennis ball. I can tell you, the phlegm that is spoken of in Chinese medicine and in Ayurveda is not only subtle but solid. I actually felt its weight and stickiness in my hands as I removed this lump from her throat. It felt like a round glob of sticky muck, but I couldn't see it, I could only feel it. And it had weight. I didn't know what to do with it. This had never happened before, and it was tangible. I couldn't just wipe it on my pants or throw it on the floor.

I looked around the room and saw a plant. The glob felt like it needed the earth to dissolve it and that it could nourish the plant like manure. I imagined placing it in the dirt and asked my friend not to tell the massage therapist, whose plant it was, that I had done this. It was so dark, heavy, and sticky that I thought it might stifle the plant's growth. A couple of weeks later I saw both women again. The friend hadn't felt the lump since our session, and the massage therapist said she liked having me use her room because it seemed that since I started there her plants were thriving!

This experience helped to prepare me for the discussion of phlegm, or dampness, in Chinese medicine school and kapha mucus or *ama* (toxin, dampness) in Ayurveda. These things exist in the energy or subtle-matter field as well as in the tangible three-dimensional world. It's only when they accumulate in the arteries or somewhere else that we pay attention, but I believe these forms of qi can be perceived and potentially treated well before they manifest as illness.

Prana/Qi as Communicator

Most of us have experienced the communication function of prana illustrated by the next story. It is not just a fluke when you think of someone and they call or email or text soon after. If you pay attention, you will recognize that when someone pops into your head you know you can expect to hear from them in the near future. There is a connection or a communication between the two of you on an energetic, thought, or qi/prana level that causes this phenomena to occur.

> One time in high school I was sitting in my room with my friend Jill. We decided to communicate with one another with our eyes closed. Each of us was to focus on a single thing and see if the other person could guess what it was. I remember that as I was concentrating I began to relax. I started to focus on the object it was my intention to transmit to Jill. As I did this I became more relaxed and saw nothing but darkness in my mind's eye. Just as I was about to fall asleep, I heard my name. It sounded pretty freaky, like when a cassette tape starts to warp or the battery starts to go on a tape deck (yep, I'm seriously dating myself here). It was like a demonic "brrrrriiiiiidgeeeeette." My eyes popped open as I was seriously freaked out. I don't remember what I sent to Jill, but when I asked her what she was thinking, she said, "Your name."

Someone's adolescent transpersonal experiments don't scientifically prove anything for anyone, of course. But when people have experiences that validate the existence of age-old concepts, it is more potent than any stamp of approval that one could receive from a professor or guru.

Prana as communicator and connector plays a role in distance healing and perception as well. I've been present for many distance sessions where the person was asked to set aside a few minutes, and a group of students would gather to send healing energy. Here's another example.

> *A group of energy healers that I was training for Reiki level 3 met to perform a distance healing practice on a friend. She was stationed at home, resting on her couch. The group and I were about twenty miles away in my office, sitting in a circle. We imagined her in the circle, on her couch. The thing is, none of us had ever been to her house, and we did not ask anything about the decor. We "worked" on her, pranically, for about ten or fifteen minutes. Toward the end of the session, although she seemed at peace in the visualization, I perceived a very dark cloud in the area where she had her physical ailment, which I didn't understand at the time. All I knew was that I was supposed to stay away from it. We finished the healing, and I saw her later that week. She reported sensations that confirmed several of the perceptions of other members in the group, as well as verified what everyone in the group saw: the colors of the clothes she had on, the room she was in, and what her couch looked like. Unfortunately, she also verified what the black cloud was. The disease was not gone, and it later took her. I think of her often and am less skeptical of what many would perceive as the more "woo woo" explanations for what can cause illness, like karma and spirits.*
>
> *As a clinically trained practitioner, you get a sense of the different things that are mentioned in the ancient texts. There are descriptions that hover on the precipice of what we would consider rational. This last experience was one of them. She didn't have an explainable illness, and she was very young. The best way I can describe the feeling associated with the perception of this dark cloud vibration was that of "evil qi." Chinese medicine and Ayurveda have many names for the ways qi manifests. Evil qi is one of them. It is a profound, strong, menacing qi that enters the body and wreaks havoc on many systems at once.*

These stories serve as experiential affirmations to me that the concepts of Ayurveda and Chinese medicine are not esoteric, otherworldly, folk tales. Qi/prana and its many forms are real things. Qi/prana is vibration, yet it also moves in a direction along a path within the living being. It is a communicator, a connector, and an animator. It is the mechanism that controls the rhythms of the respiratory system and the heart. It allows us to perceive information, and it is that information itself. It can take on qualities and, if it is deficient, has a perverted flow, or is blocked or stagnant, it can cause pain or illness, but when it is flowing at the right rate, in the right direction, in the right amount, and without what we would call negatively charged emotions, it can create health.

3

The Five Elements

Both Chinese medicine and Ayurveda view the five elements (FE) as a combination of a condensed periodic table and an explanation of how all the forces of nature manifest. The quantity and quality of their myriad combinations determines what objects form or how something operates or moves. Sometime long ago the two traditions probably had the same root knowledge of this topic but then veered off in slightly different directions, causing the differences between them that we see today. Their FE theories may not correlate exactly, but if we take into account where they overlap or that they really just differ in terminology and foundational context, they are basically saying the same thing. How couldn't they be? Ayurveda by its very name means "science" or "wisdom of life," and there is only this life we all share. Chinese medicine may not be called the science of life, but Taoism, from which it springs, is "the Way." It is *the* way, the same as Ayurveda is *the* wisdom of life. They are describing this same single existence, just with slight variations on how it is described and perceived by our limited minds.

In Chinese medicine and in Ayurveda, the term *five elements* doesn't quite capture their whole meaning. In Chinese medicine a more accurate term for the five elements is the Wu Xing, or *five phase,* theory. Speaking of five phases points to the fact that they are active processes, not just static entities. There is a slight difference in how the elements are viewed in the two systems. In the Chinese system, the elements are planetary based, as it is the planet's elements that make up the shell of the body. These elements are: wood, fire, earth, metal, and water.

To a large extent, the Chinese Wu Xing theory of the elements is more focused on what the element does than what it actually is. Of course there are associations between the elements and physical structures, as we will learn when we look at the organs. The Ayurvedic five element theory, which is derived from the Sankhya philosophy, describes the origin of the elements in succession and is focused equally on their form and function. Function is further developed in dosha theory, which is explained in the following chapter.

Ayurveda sees the elements as having emerged at the very beginning of existence, at the big bang, so to speak. This is why space is considered the first element. It shares many of the qualities of the wood element in Chinese medicine. The Ayurvedic *panchamahabhutas* (five great elements) are also not merely static principles but active forces busily working to bring balance to life. They are: space, air, fire, water, and earth.

The impact of a cultural worldview on the evolution of Chinese medicine and Ayurveda is particularly evident in their five element theories. Because the Chinese have a different view and emphasis surrounding the continuation of life after this life, they have a tendency to focus on the here and now and what they can perceive with the five senses. Contrary to this is the Indian foundational belief in reincarnation and the role of karma. A lot of Indian philosophy is not only focused on going with the flow but also with transcending it. This naturally equates to very different perspectives on life and creates a rift between the ideological foundations of the two systems.

To a large extent, each of the elements can be tangibly experienced. Earth, fire, and water share many of the same qualities in both systems, but the language for and the take on the other two elements are slightly different. The elements with different names between the two systems are wood and metal in Chinese medicine and space and air in Ayurveda. It is very tempting to say that wood is space and metal is somehow air and be done with it. While it is true that wood and space share many attributes, as do metal and air, they do not correlate exactly.

WU XING: FIVE PHASES

The Chinese five phase theory involves the five elements of wood, fire, earth, metal, and water and how they interact. The interactions involve two cycles that maintain homeostasis in the universe and in the body: a controlling cycle that keeps the elements in check and a generating cycle that supports and nourishes the elements. These two cycles are the root of five element acupuncture diagnosis and treatment. Although there are other patterns of interaction involved in imbalance, for the purposes of this discussion we will focus on these two. The Chinese describe the elements in terms of their individual qualities but also in relationship to one another, similar to the descriptive style of yin and yang. The Chinese elements are the end category so to speak in the differentiation of matter as they are spoken of in terms of constitutional attributes in and of themselves. This differs from Ayurveda in that the energetics of the five elements are further differentiated into three doshas in the Ayurvedic system. This will be explained in the following chapter.

One of my final projects in Chinese medicine school was a research paper on the breath and its usefulness as a tool for healing and transformation in ancient medicine. I interviewed Paul Karsten, one of the school founders, head instructors, and a longtime Zen practitioner, who helped me understand his work with the breath cycle in terms of the five elements (see fig. 3.1). As he explained it, each phase of the breath cycle is a phase in five element theory. He explored a platform from which meditation students can understand their own breathing abnormalities using the breath cycle and five element theory. This five element diagnostic model is useful for people interested in their own healing process and for medical and bodywork practitioners working

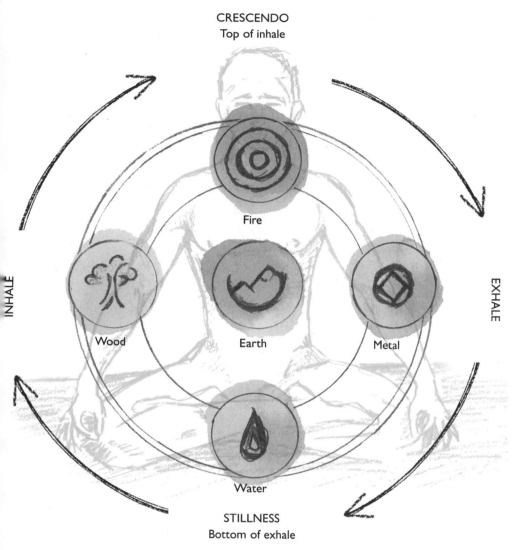

CRESCENDO
Top of inhale

INHALE

EXHALE

Fire

Wood   Earth   Metal

Water

STILLNESS
Bottom of exhale

Fig. 3.1. The breath cycle and the corresponding elements

with clients. Meditation on this model can help to clear the energetic, emotional, and physical bodies of built-up toxins, blockages, and stuck emotional patterning. He described a cycle of breathing that I had been working with for over a decade in my yoga study, in a way I had never before conceived of. Yet it was entirely natural. Something clicked.

It may serve you to read through this paragraph once and then reread it slowly, allowing the information to sit with you as you breathe it. There are four phases of the breath cycle, and there are five elements. The earth element is you in the breath cycle, at the center of it. The breather is earth, and the other elements flow around and through it. The inhalation is related to beginning, birth and growth. If you pay attention to the in-breath there is a newness to it every time. This is wood. The transition at the top of the inhalation feels like and represents ultimate expansion, expression, crescendo, or peak. This is fire. During exhalation is a letting go. This is metal. The pause between the end of the exhalation and the beginning of the next inhalation is the stillness of being, the void. It is the death of the breath cycle, the ultimate end before the birth of the new in-breath. This is water. Let's go a little deeper into the soul of the elements.

Wood

Wood is the quality of growth. It is like a germinating seed sprouting. It is the anticipant pregnant mother and the growing fetus. It is the energy of the plant breaking through the earth toward the sun. It is the dawn of a new day and is related to the process of awakening. Wood is strong and flexible; it stretches and spreads and strives. It is also expansive and spacious. Think of the space in hollow bamboo or the porous wood of any tree. This relates to akasha (ether, space) in Ayurveda. There is air in the wood that pushes it or makes it move. This is why wood is also associated with vayu (air) in the Indian system. In the breath cycle it is associated with the beginning of the in-breath—initiating, opening, and reaching toward the top of the inhale, as the diaphragm descends to compress the liver.

The liver is associated with the wood element in Chinese medicine. It is responsible for the smooth flow of qi and blood, and in certain contexts, we know it can partially regenerate. It has a spreading function, and its energy tends to rise upward or across the body, like branches of a tree or a vine reaching up and out. The liver is further associated with wind and the spring season. Spring is when everything is sprouting, emerging, birthing, and there is a sense of anticipation and newness in the air and a looking forward. These are all qualities of wood. In addition, the green color that spring denotes is associated with wood and the liver. Many people are drawn to liver cleanses in the spring and use spring herbs like dandelion to cleanse.

In the body, there should be a spacious unhindered sensation associated with wood stretching, reaching, and moving forward. If there is a sense of desperation or frustration in striving, the function of wood is out of balance. If obstacles block the growth of wood, it becomes very frustrated, irritable, unhappy, and angry. These emotions and feelings disrupt the smooth flow of qi and blood and are said to injure the liver if intense and sustained. In fact, unexamined, suppressed, or chronic anger is the primary emotion said to harm the liver. It is frustrated or blocked wood energy that continues to have stretching, expansive momentum that builds up behind the blockage. This stagnated energy can wreak havoc on the qi flow and the mind and, according to Chinese medicine, can not only create imbalance, but also disease.

Fire

Fire is the crescendo in any pattern, situation, or life cycle. It is peak experience, and life in its prime. It is the full blossoming of a flower, the explosive power at the height of a volcanic eruption, and the manifestation of creative expression. It has an upward moving nature, like the rising of smoke and heat. It is combustion and is associated with any combustive process in nature or the body. It is midday, when the Sun is at its highest point in the sky, and represents wakefulness. In the breath cycle it is the peak of the inhalation and the transition between the inhale and the exhale, before the exhale occurs. It is associated with warmth, heat, enthusiasm, creativity, and dynamism. There is a sense of joy in life when fire is at its prime.

When it's out of balance, fire burns. It leads to inflammatory conditions caused by displaced or excess heat in the body and nervousness of the mind. It can cause insomnia and heart palpitations. The fire element is associated with the heart and small intestine, blood vessels, tongue, and complexion. It is also associated with the *shen,* or spirit, one of the Three Treasures in Chinese medicine. Of course, fire is associated with red, the color that fire types are most comfortable being around or wearing. The taste associated with fire is bitter, and its season is summertime. In the summer, the qi is weak and the digestion is sluggish. An invasion of cold or wind in the body is actually more likely to occur in the summer, so it is best to avoid cold food and drink and drafty places. Because the body and its digestion process are weakest in the summer, frequent small, easy-to-absorb meals are most appropriate at this time.

Earth

One way to conceptualize earth is as the center, the fulcrum, the transition time and space between the change from one phase to the next. It is the exact moment of balance between two phases. It is the medium in which a plant exists and where it derives its nourishment and stability. In acupuncture, there is a point on the Stomach channel adjacent to the navel called the "celestial pivot." It represents the balance between the upper and lower aspects of the body, and it corresponds to earth with regard to its function of regulating the spleen and stomach. Earth is yin. It is dense, heavy, and moist and because of its relationship to the spleen and stomach has much to do with digestion.

Oftentimes, when stress and worry are abundant, wood, or the liver, can overact on earth, negatively impacting digestion. A deficiency of earth corresponds to an inability to take in, break down, and absorb food, fluids, and information. According to modern science there is a connection between the brain and the gut. This connection is quite literal in terms of nerve impulses in Western science and digestive and intellectual capacity and performance in eastern medicine.

Earth is the stabilizing principle in the five phase theory. It's related to late afternoon and the humid transition time between summer and fall. It is more yin than yang due to its solid, stable, constant, wet, nourishing qualities. Without nourishment from earth, the rest of the elements cannot fulfill their physiological functions and yang will separate from yin. This separation eventually leads to the death of the organism, when the spirit (yang) leaves the flesh (yin).

Metal

Metal is associated with dusk, the time of the setting sun. It is the time of waning, degeneration, and letting go. It is detachment and the quieting of life's activities, the exhale and the release. It is related to autumn and the leaves falling from the trees. There is a beauty in their transition. There is a bittersweet feeling associated with many aspects of the process of letting go.

In Chinese medicine metal is related to the lungs and large intestine. The lungs are responsible for processing grief, yet are damaged by excessive, stored, or unresolved grief. It is not uncommon for us to end up with a cough, cold, or pneumonia in the process of dealing with the death of someone we love. Oftentimes when we contract these ailments there is a corresponding disturbance to large intestine function as well.

Water

Water is the element of stillness. It is representative of the emptiness from which we emerge and to which we eventually return. It is the height of midnight, dark and cool, the ultimate yin. It is associated with winter and hibernation as well as very old age and death. Some also consider it to be the yin time of gestation, the potential contained within the seed. It is the pause at the bottom of the exhale, representative of complete stillness, emptiness, no-thingness, the void.

Water balances fire. Without it, the fire of the heart would rage out of control. Water is associated with the kidneys and bladder. There is an introspective energy associated with water and not enough of it can lead to inflammatory thinking and tissues as well as insomnia, irritability, overheating, nervousness, and anxiety. Waning kidney yin is also caused by a depletion of the water element. In the case of menopause, water would be associated with female hormonal balance. As the hormones that promote lubrication wane, heat symptoms abound. Hot flashes are a good example of this. As smoke and heat rise in nature, so too do they in the body.

THE FIVE ELEMENTS
IN AYURVEDIC MEDICINE

To reiterate, Sankhya cosmology is at the root of five-element manifestation in Ayurvedic medicine. From the more static vein of the cosmic consciousness of inertia (tamas) emerged the tanmatras, or objects of the senses, and from those objects the five elements emerged in order, from the most subtle to the most gross. First emanated the subtle sense object of sound, and from that the more material element of space. From touch came air. From light or something to see came fire, and from something that has taste came something you can taste and need in order to taste, water. From space, air, fire, and water came the subtle thing of smell and the matter to fulfill that, earth.

Each succeeding element contains the elements that came before it, and each increases in density in comparison to the elements before it. For example, as space becomes air, it becomes more dense. One can say that air is the element of space at a greater density. It is what happens to space as it becomes more gross or descends from the subtle toward a more gross state of solid matter. As Nikola Tesla once wrote, "All perceptible matter comes from a primary substance, or tenuity beyond conception, filling all space, the akasha or luminiferous ether, which is acted upon by the life giving Prana or creative force, calling into existence, in never-ending cycles all things and phenomena."[1]

Space/Akasha/Ether

Space is the first element to form. Remember, the elements are the building blocks of matter and have functional qualities as well as static, material qualities. The proportion of each element in a given thing makes up its physical form. Each element has specific qualities, or gunas, associated with it. These differ from the three gunas, sattva, rajas, and tamas. Sattva, rajas, and tamas are qualities of the mind. The gunas referred to here, although used by some to metaphorically refer to mental or emotional states, or personality traits, are actually meant to refer to qualities of material nature, of physicality. These gunas are the physical element's personality, so to speak. Space is also called ether or akasha. You may have heard the term *akashic records.* Twentieth-century American prophet Edgar Cayce used this term to describe the place on which he would focus his awareness while in trance to make his predictions. He believed that there is a plane of existence that stores everything that has ever happened, ever will happen, and is happening right now. According to the Edgar Cayce readings, this place is like a grand library containing the lives of every individual, the history of the cosmos, including the Earth, and potential futures given the current circumstances and society's choices. Akasha, being space, is infinite. Something holding such vast knowledge, including unspoken thoughts, must surely be vast and infinite. This is a good sense of what space is elementally.

Space is present in the body as the substratum of the mind, upon and through which thoughts fluctuate. Remember also that the atom is primarily composed of space, with very little matter present. Science has proven that solidity is illusory at the root of things, at the atomic level. Space is also in all the open places and empty spaces in the body like the alveolar space, the intestines, and porous bone. Space is necessary for the other elements to exist, yet an overabundance of it causes a degradation of necessary tissue and a lack of nourishment to the organism. Like all the other elements, space has gunas, but those gunas can be largely seen as an absence of the opposing guna. For example, space is subtle because it has absolutely no density. It is cold because it completely lacks any semblance of heat. It is inert because it lacks the movement of air.

Shabda, or sound, is associated with space. This is why it is said at the beginning there was the sound of OM and from it all things in creation manifest. It is the sound of the universe. It is the sound of space. Sound waves move through space. The ripple and its movement are due to the presence of air.

Air/Vayu

Air is the second element to manifest in Ayurveda's Sankhya cosmology. In the fabric of vibrational space, a contact of some kind arises. It is a slight differentiation, a relationship between vibrations, a contraction or an expansion. This movement is the origin of air.

Air is dry, rough, subtle, mobile, clear, cool, and light. All movement in existence is due to the presence of air. Air is called vayu in Sanskrit; it is space and air in combination. The particular force the attributes of these elements combine to form is the vata dosha. This will be explained in the following chapter.

Tejas/Fire

The friction created by the movement of air against itself and space generates heat, or fire. The fire element is associated with vision and the eyes. Because of the subtle potential for sight, fire was made manifest. Fire's attributes are: hot, sharp, dry, non-slimy, and light. We know that fire requires air, or oxygen, to survive. Therefore, we could say fire is nourished or flourishes because of the presence or existence of air. Remember that wood in the Chinese system is the most spacious of elements, and has many similarities to the qualities of air in the Indian system. In Chinese medicine, we say that wood nourishes fire. If we were to personify this relationship, we could say wood is the mother of fire. In Ayurveda, space and air are present in the makeup of fire.

Fire is responsible for all transformation in the cosmos. It is considered radiant heat and nuclear reaction. In a sense, fire acts as a bridge between the more subtle elements of space and air and the grosser elements of water and earth. It is like a turning point in creation. Fire can turn the grosser elements into subtler elements, and in that sense it is inherently present in the denser elements of metal, earth, and water. It turns earth to ash. The qualities of this ash are close to that of air. It becomes more like air as air itself acts upon it, degrading to the finest dust and then to just molecules present in the wind. Its action on water causes water's evaporation and transition back to air.

The manifestation of fire in the body is called *agni* in Sanskrit. Agni is present in the digestive tract and cellular metabolism and is responsible for transforming raw materials into nourishment and nutrition. If the agni, or metabolic fire, is low, a myriad of ailments ranging from a lack of appetite to a lack of enthusiasm for life can result. If agni is out of balance, burning acid reflux may occur, and if it is damaged it can become a major contributor to many disease processes. Agni encompasses all acids, enzymes, and bile. Notice that this fire is not just dry; it also has a liquid quality. Think of bile for example. It is a hot, penetrating liquid. In terms of doshic theory, this is in alignment with the pitta dosha, which is a combination of fire and water, the fourth element to come into existence.

Water/Jala

As fire becomes more dense it liquefies, and from this liquid water manifests. As it gains density, it also begins to cool. The attributes of water are: liquid, soft, mobile, cold, heavy, viscous, dull, and dense. We need water to survive and flourish. Water, or *jala* in Sanskrit, is associated with taste, and therefore with the tongue. Without water, taste does not arise. Without taste, there is no nourishment and earth cannot be maintained. The word for "taste" in Sanskrit is *rasa*. Rasa also means "enjoyment" and "connection."

In Chinese medicine, water is associated with flow, or the primary action of air: movement. But it also has a holding, nurturing quality to it and a sense of stillness like a deep, undisturbed pool. In Ayurveda, connection is a primary principle of the water element, specifically through the process of cohesion. Two droplets of water placed close together will naturally try to connect and merge with one another. This is cohesion. German scientists have recently discovered that water takes on the vibration of what it comes into contact with. This includes form. They found when a flower was placed in a vat of water, each individual droplet displayed the form of the flower when viewed under a microscope.[2] In Ayurveda this retentive quality is associated with water to some degree, but more specifically with the kapha dosha.

Zen recommends that we be like water and go with the flow. Water also happily assumes the shape of any vessel it is placed into. Given the information in the German study, we can also say we are like water in that we naturally become what is placed within us. We become the food we eat and the thoughts we think, and we associate who we are with what we feel.

Memory is a form of cohesion, and the German study indicates the presence of memory in water droplets. In Japan Dr. Masaru Emoto did a study of water at the molecular level. He found that water charged with emotions exhibited varying crystalline forms when viewed under the microscope. In fact, water placed in receptacles that were labeled with words such as "love," and "fool" did so as well. The water molecules in the containers labeled with pleasant, uplifting words displayed the symmetry and beauty of perfect snowflakes. The water molecules subjected to negative-feeling words displayed crystalline structures that looked like distorted, deformed, melting snowflakes.[3]

The correlation here between either of these experiments and the cohesive, memory-containing nature of water is that since we are made up of so much water, what we think, feel, see, and experience is remembered at a deep elemental water place within us. This memory can further generate like experiences, creating a state of balance or dis-ease. Therefore, what we think, say, read, write, paint, draw, sculpt, feel, and do all contribute to our wellness, or a lack of it, at a molecular level. We can easily imagine how water became such an important symbol in religious ritual—in some traditions even deemed powerful enough to purify the intangible soul.

A good meditative technique to try is to consciously drink water. Instead of just unconsciously gulping it down, know that you can affect the water within you by bringing in water with life-enhancing intention in its molecular structure. Think of the positive qualities of water as you drink. Think of it as being charged with the power to heal. Feel its coolness washing away impurities. Feel its liquidity accessing even the densest reaches of bodily tissue. If you heat it, imagine its warmth transforming phlegm and cleansing negative emotional states from your mind and body.

Earth/Prithvi

Earth is the final element to emerge. It is a combination of the other four elements, plus itself. Earth, called *prithvi* in Sanskrit, arises as water congeals or increases in density, and it is the material substance necessary for something to have a smell. The element of earth is associated with nurturing, solidity, and form. Its qualities are: heavy, gross, dense, static, dull, and cloudy. It is the most dense compound of matter and in the human body is represented by anything solid or structural, such as bones, muscles, and teeth. It is also associated with the organs of digestion. Earth is the element that resonates with the root chakra, and its organ of action is the anus. It is responsible not only for stability but also for elimination. There cannot be stability in the system if proper elimination is not maintained.

When bacteria are present, or there is tissue or cellular degradation, an odor is emitted from the body. Usually, healthy people do not exude a foul odor. Ancient physicians were trained to use their sense of smell, made possible by the presence of small particles of the earth element suspended in the air, to detect illness and make a diagnosis. Just like we know today that sweet-smelling urine is indicative of diabetes, the ancients knew that there were more than a dozen urine smells that indicated different patterns of metabolic imbalance.

Ayurveda's Five Elements in Modern Scientific Terms

Modern science recognizes four elements in chemistry as the building blocks of life. They are: carbon (C), hydrogen (H), oxygen (O), and nitrogen (N). Several authors have varying opinions when comparing and contrasting Ayurveda's five elements as the basis of matter with science's basis of living matter. One of those authors is Dr. H. S. Palep. In his book, *Scientific Foundation of Ayurveda,* Dr. Palep explains that hydrogen is synonymous with the fire element because of its association with fusion reactions, solar radiation, and the intensity of energy's release and potential for transmutation. He categorizes fire specifically as solar radiation.

He goes on to say that no smell can exist without carbon, and therefore he equates carbon with the earth element. Water, of course, is H_2O, and air is a combination of N and O. Interestingly, NO is responsible for muscle contraction. When it is disrupted, involuntary movement results. This is a symptom of deranged air or vata in the body. Dr. Palep equates sound to space because of resonance. Resonance, he says, is essential for life, and therefore equates space to sound waves. Sound waves are vibration, and all things vibrate. Dr. Palep also explains how earth and water combine to form fats and carbohydrates, and from there, air is added to form amino acids and proteins.[4]

This seems like a reasonable explanation and is wonderful food for thought. Whether he is correct is not relevant for our discussion. It is merely mentioned here because it is interesting to point out the amount of thought that goes into the correlations between all these theories. I encourage the reader to suspend a need for scientific explanation, however, as it always seems to pop up and validate Eastern thought. Or maybe we should see it the other way around.

GENERATING AND CONTROLLING CYCLES

In Chinese medicine, there is a natural self-regulation among the elements. The elements are constantly in flux, and they work with and against each other in an effort to maintain the body's homeostasis. This balance is maintained according to particular patterns. By understanding these patterns and cycles and how they change when functioning well or when exhibiting pathological presentations, a practitioner can help to balance the pattern. The practitioner does this by dispersing energy or tonifying it where needed, typically by using acupuncture.

One way in which the elements work is to nourish and nurture one another. Nourishing, supporting, and nurturing functions happen in a predictable way, according to what's called the generating (*sheng*) cycle (see fig. 3.2). Let's start with water. Water is like the ground of existence from which all things—often referred to as the "ten thousand things"—emerge and to which they return. Water is responsible for nourishing wood. In the terminology of the generation cycle, water would then be considered the mother, and wood the child. The mother always nourishes the child in the generating cycle.

Water nourishes wood in the same way rain nourishes a tree. Wood generates fire as is evidenced when you light it in your fireplace. Fire generates earth by creating ash. Earth generates the metal that is mined from it. Metal generates water. The ancients observed that as metal is heated or cooled it develops condensation and that this water goes on to nourish wood.

The controlling (*ke*) cycle has a very different dynamic. It's like checks and balances. Each element has a power that helps to balance one other element. Sometimes an element can get a little too rambunctious. When this happens, its energy needs to be dispersed or brought

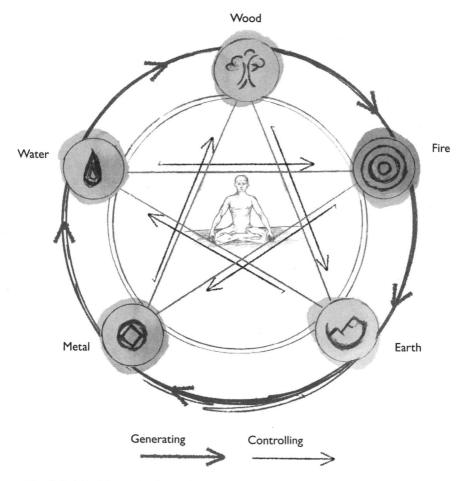

Fig. 3.2. Wu Xing, the five phases or elements in Chinese medicine, with the generating and controlling cycles

back into balance to keep it from going out of control and destabilizing the whole system. If this excess control is needed, the element that is out of balance is said to be overactive on another element in the group. If the element it is acting against is the particular element that's meant to control it, it is insulting that element.

One example of the way in which the controlling cycle works is when water controls fire. Too much water can diminish or dull fire, or, if it is overacting, water can put out fire. There is an important balance that occurs in the body between fire and water. They are the yang and yin, respectively, constantly working to keep the balance. If there is too much water, the fire in the body suffers. For example, when the warmth and circulation that aids in transforming and transporting water is lacking, fluid can build up. If water is predominant, kidney yang is suppressed or diminished and heart fire may flare. If fire is predominant, ailments such as menopausal symptoms and inflammatory conditions may arise.

Just as water controls fire and can overact on it, fire controls and can overact on metal. An example of this would be fire melting metal. When this occurs in the body, we experience it as the heart energy dominating the lung energy. This manifests as a drying and heating of the lung mucosa and results in conditions like dry cough and thirst.

Metal controls and can overact on wood—for example, when a tree is chopped down by an axe. In the body, metal can restrict the spreading, growing aspect of wood by supplying insufficient bodily qi and inhibiting the functioning of the liver, causing liver deficiency. Since the liver regulates the smooth flow of qi through the body, this can have systemic consequences. It can cause stagnation that eventually leads to a buildup of heat and inflammation. The person may experience skin problems, shallow breathing, and a host of associated ailments, including physical and mental tension, insomnia, and vivid, draining dreams.

Wood controls and can overact on earth, as when the roots of a tree crack through rock. Since wood energy can spread sideways across the torso, as does the shape of the liver, its qi can encroach upon and inhibit the functioning of the stomach and spleen. This can lead to repressed appetite, abdominal bloating, nausea, acid reflux, indigestion, malabsorption, and worry.

Earth controls water, as when the pressure in the Earth regulates how much water is released from the mantle or how the banks of a river contain its flow. Too much food can disrupt the body's ability to process it properly and lead to the accumulation of wastes and fluid, or damp-ness, in the body. The kidneys' function of processing fluids becomes impaired and, in addition to damp conditions in other regions of the system, lower-body edema may emerge. The person may feel lethargic, and elimination may become sluggish. When this happens, even more dampness builds up, kidney yang function decreases, and earth may end up getting depleted in the long run.

CHECKS AND BALANCES IN AYURVEDA

It is so fascinating how each of the elements has the ability, so logically, to balance the others. It is science's concept of homeostasis, but from the ancient's perspective. This concept manifests in Ayurveda in terms of the doshas, or constitutional tendencies, being able to regulate one another.

Vata accumulates en masse in the lower portion of the torso. Although vata is present in every cell, this lower area of the body is largely governed by the vata dosha because force is needed to act against gravity in order to move blood and fluids up from below. Pitta's primary location is in the middle of the body. It is the transform-ational pivot between the light airy vata below and the heavy, dense, wet kapha above. Kapha occupies the space in the torso above the diaphragm. The kapha dosha is crucial for lubrication, which mani-fests as mucosal moistening and the fluids necessary for the proper functioning and protection of all bodily tissues, particularly the lungs, pleura, pericardium, and heart.

The placement of the doshas in the body, in their respective *jiaos,* as we might say in Chinese medicine, not only serves as the equivalent of a controlling cycle, but also of a generating cycle. A jiao is a region in the body that is often translated to mean "burner" but may more accurately be defined as "environment." The diaphragm is considered the dynamic heat exchanger between the upper and middle jiao. Heat builds in the middle jiao area due to pitta, and the diaphragmatic movement is pivotal in moving this heat up and out instead of allowing it to accumulate and create imbalance. The kapha dosha is cooling and mostly made of water. This water is required to not only protect the upper body from the rising effects of heat but to create a substrate that fire can burn and transform without damaging the tissues. The air of vata from the lower jiao rises up and stokes the fire of pitta in the middle jiao (see fig. 3.3). Without warmth, there is no movement,

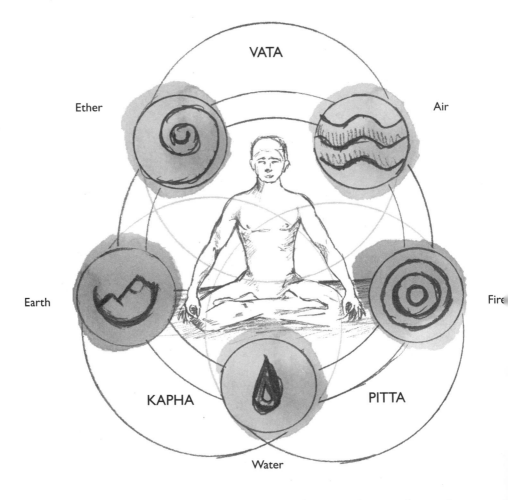

Fig. 3.3. The five elements and their doshic equivalents in Ayurveda

even in the lower jiao. This is in part how fire helps air. This fire also heats the cool kapha in the upper jiao, keeping it thinned and lique-fied so it doesn't congeal. Pitta fire, or agni, also steams the kapha, allowing it to rise like a mist to moisten and nourish the orifices such as the nasal mucosa and sinus cavities.

The Chinese describe this phenomenon as being like a rice cooker, with the rice representing what we ingest. The flame (pitta agni) is stoked by air in the lower jiao and heats the food in the pot of the middle jiao, creating steam—the qi—above. This process is qi transformation. Air, earth (in this case, rice), fire, and water are required to generate qi in the body, and the pictogram character for qi represents this. We know that there is a generating cycle inherent in the elements in Ayurveda because of how they initially form. Ether came first and generated air, whose fric-tion generated the heat of fire, which generated water, providing the sub-stratum for earth, which is a combination of all five elements.

We can visualize the elements not just in their own process of cre-ation but also in the creation of a living being. We will look first at the creation of a person and then at the life cycle of a flower. The womb in the woman's body is a space that allows for the movement, merging, and growth of an egg and sperm, which combine to form an embryo. The potential of who this being will be is dormant in these seeds before they merge. The two seeds touch and a spark is released. The connec-tion and movement and touch is air; the spark of spirit is fire. Water is responsible for carrying the electrical charge of air, and the presence of earth defines the four directions and the stability of the embryo in the womb. Air causes the cells to go in the direction they need to after they differentiate. The combined presence of water and earth gives nutrition and form to the growing being.

Each element has an inherent intelligence that guides it to proper action within the framework of its given attributes and natural ten-dencies. I love the way Dr. Sunil Joshi, in his book *Ayurveda and Panchakarma: The Science of Healing and Rejuvenation* describes the life cycle of a plant to illustrate the presence of the five elements in action. In a seed lies the potential for an entire plant and the spaciousness for movement to arise. The right conditions—the moist earth and access to sunlight—allow for the life process to ripen. The seed, once sprouted, becomes less and less dense as it expands in every direction. This expansion is space. Space is necessary for any further growth to happen.

As the process continues, the air element allows for cellular differentiation and enables the cells to "know" where to place themselves. Then heat, or the fire element, within the seed increases so that the sprout has enough energy to break down the shell and burst forth through the earth toward the surface. The water element then emerges in response to a need for nutrient uptake and transport. Finally, the earth element is represented by the plant form that the seed manifests into and the nutrients that feed it.[5]

Using Gunas to Understand Checks and Balances

In the Ayurvedic system, each of the elements possesses exact qualities, or gunas, that constitute their form and function. There are ten pairs of gunas that are most useful in Ayurveda for bringing imbalance to the individual. They are also applicable to the polarities in the natural world and help better define and describe material existence. They are as follows:

1. Weight: heavy–light
2. Intensity: slow/dull–sharp/quick
3. Temperature: cold–hot
4. Emolliency: oily–dry
5. Texture: smooth–rough
6. Viscosity: solid–liquid
7. Compressibility: soft–hard
8. Fluidity: static–mobile
9. Density: subtle–gross
10. Adhesion: sticky/cloudy–transparent/clear

Applying the gunas to the Chinese elements offers insights into how and why the generating and controlling cycles work. Some attributes, or gunas, are more pronounced than others. Gunas in one element are more predominant than in the one they are influencing. It is the relative nature of each guna's category—for example, compressibility or weight—and its association with each element that influences the element's nature. In Chinese medicine, the guna theory is less definite than in Ayurveda in terms of describing the elements' inherent qualities, the generating and controlling cycles, and the way that elements contrast with each other.

In Ayurveda, each quality seems more fixed. Even if a quality lies along a spectrum, it is well defined. For example, coolness is attributed to kapha in Ayurveda, but it is not at either end of the guna category of temperature—it is not cold or hot but somewhere in between. However, we don't typically say kapha is not as cold as vata or is more cold than pitta, we say vata is cold, pitta is hot, and kapha is cool.

Chinese medicine, however, is less definitive. Things are described more in terms of their relativity to one another, as in yin/yang theory. In using the gunas to describe the Chinese elements, we might say the elements are in relationship to one another along a spectrum in each category. For instance, wood isn't completely dense, but it's not subtle either. It lies somewhere along the spectrum between subtle and dense. Its subtlety is overpowered by the density of metal, which helps metal keep wood restrained in the controlling cycle. The basic qualities of wood in the Chinese system are: dry, rough, soft (compressibility), light (compared to all elements but fire), subtle in density (compared to metal and earth), and mobile (but not as mobile as fire or water). If you think about the dry quality of wood, you can see how it must be nourished by water. Chinese water qualities are: liquid, smooth, soft, cool, clear, and mobile. The liquid is necessary to nourish the wood, which needs to be moist in order to flourish but not completely wet all the time. Wood can be controlled by metal as metal has strong opposing qualities to those of wood. It is heavy, dull, cold, solid, hard, static, and gross. Metal's heavy, dull, hard, and gross qualities possess the natural ability to control the growth of wood.

Fire is light, sharp or quick, hot, mobile, clear, and subtle. It is nourished mostly by wood's dryness (a primary quality of air in wood). Fire is controlled by the same quality that nourishes wood—liquid—but also by water's greater density and its coolness. A combination of these qualities best serves to control fire.

Earth is heavy, dull, cool, moist, smooth, solid, soft, static, gross, and cloudy or sticky. It is nourished by the ash that fire creates. This ash is dry, light, cloudy, static, and soft. Earth being nourished by fire is easier to understand in terms of how agni, or the digestive fire, works in the body. It has an oily (water) quality that helps to keep it from raging out of control, yet it is necessary for breaking down raw material into something the body can use to build or regenerate, thus supporting and increasing earth.

Earth is controlled by wood. The moist, dense stability of earth is counteracted by wood's drying, subtle, mobile, and rough qualities. When wood overacts on earth in the body, it is the movement aspect that pushes and disempowers the softer, static earth, along with the drying aspect that can encourage a buildup of heat that disrupts the digestive functioning and creates worry in the mind. Metal is generated by earth, which houses it within its depths. Earth provides the minerals metal uses to build itself. It encourages metal's heavy, dull, hard, and gross qualities. Metal is acted upon by fire to create balance.

Fire's heat transforms the metal thereby keeping it from overexerting its activity upon another element. Water's generation from metal comes from heat or cold acting upon the metal, thereby generating water from it in the form of condensation. Scientists have recently recognized that water is trapped within minerals under enormous pressure deep within the Earth. As Earth's pressure increases upon these minerals, water is released and it moves toward the surface.[6] Water's fluidity and mobility are well controlled by Earth's static nature.

The elements are used in both systems for diagnosis and treatment. While the doshas are the functional mechanisms that are emphasized in Ayurveda, at their root are the five elements. To properly treat a patient it is sometimes easier to look at the roots of the dosha which are the elements that comprise it, than to just focus on the dosha itself. In Chinese medicine diagnosis and treatment, the five elements are utilized mostly by five-element and Japanese acupuncturists. In Chinese herbal treatment, the gunas play a significant role, particularly in customizing formulas. Although they are not called the gunas in this system, they are still understood as qualities that are necessary for bringing balance to the mind and body. In terms of gunas in therapies, like increases like, and opposites balance each other. This is very important when prescribing herbs and recommending foods.

4

Constitution

Constitution is a magical concept. It is the theory that there are categories of body, mind, and personality. By going through a checklist of characteristics, we are able to gain insight into what constitutional type we are and then tailor our choices to better suit our type. Most of us are fascinated with some form of self-classification. It may be through astrology, numerology, psychology, blood type, or some other system that tells us who we are. Constitution theory makes us feel that somewhere, in the grand scheme of it all, we, as individuals, completely fit in. We belong, we are known, and we are heard by some unseen, ancient knowing. Our traits and tendencies are accepted as they are because after all, they Are. Not only are we known, but we can modify everything in our world to enhance the attributes of our constitution like food, exercise, diet, sleep, color, sound . . . everything.

Someone, or many someones, in antiquity were able to identify the categories of mind/body tendencies, and what they discovered is still relevant today. Think about this. If you knew your individual constitution, things you never understood about yourself might make sense for the first time ever. The reasons behind the unconscious reactions you had to life or the impressions they left upon you might become clear. The same goes for the likes and dislikes of things as simple as food, colors, and temperatures. Self-judgment might subside and make room for self-acceptance. You might get a sense that you are not alone or that you are connected at a real, tangible level to thousands, no, millions of other souls and the world around you.

Fitting our bodies and minds into a category of attributes can help us understand ourselves better as an individual, a family member, and a friend and figure out where we fit in nature. Constitutional theory can also help us better understand our children, friends, parents, siblings, coworkers, bosses, employees, and so on. In understanding, connection, acceptance, compassion, and forgiveness are possible. Interactions between constitutional types are also fairly predictable. Familial quarrels can be seen in a new light, potential hazards can be avoided, and parents can have a keener insight into their children's differences and how to raise them more comfortably. In work environments, interpersonal interactions as well as health and productivity can improve.

Ayurveda and Chinese medicine both have well-thought-out, foolproof constitutional theories. There are five primary constitutional types in Chinese medicine and three in Ayurveda. As we have seen, the five elements in Chinese medicine very closely relate to those in Ayurveda. The elemental constitutional types are also very similar. Both systems recognize that each of us is a combination of all five elements. Chinese medicine uses the five elements directly in meridian therapy and constitutional assessment, and Ayurveda uses the doshas (vata, pitta, and kapha), which are based upon the five elements, to describe constitutional attributes, tendencies, and imbalances. The types tend to relate to how the elements behave. The flicker of a flame, the flow of water, the stretch of wood are all related to vata, for example. The intensity of pitta can be found mostly in wood, fire, and metal, and the stillness of kapha in earth, metal, and water.

In both systems there is a primary constitution related to the person's genetic makeup which, and there is debate about this, doesn't change. Then there are the constitutional factors a person presents with that are out of balance or not in harmony with their primary, unchanging constitution. In both systems, a straying from the primary constitution indicates an acquired issue that is throwing the mind/body out of balance. It can be a pathogen, seasonal change, trauma, lifestyle issue, or any other cause of imbalance.

In Ayurveda, our original constitution (*prakruti*) is basically our genetic blueprint. An acquired constitution is how one has strayed from one's original state or how one has gone out of balance (*vikruti*). One is in balance when there is no vikruti, no difference between the constitution at birth and the constitution now. Balance is recognized when our constitution stays the same as when we were conceived. We measure this in pulse diagnosis and it is when the pulse at the prakruti level matches that of the vikruti level. Original constitution cannot be changed. Genes can be turned on and off, but that is part of the process of vikruti. Vikruti can, however, be so strong that it encroaches on the prakruti and almost masks the correct prakruti in the pulse. In constitutional theory, we can be balanced, but by nature we all have innate tendencies toward certain modes of imbalance.

DOSHA THEORY: CONSTITUTIONAL TYPES IN AYURVEDA

As we have seen, each of the three doshas—vata, pitta, and kapha—is associated with a fundamental principle of reality: vata with movement, pitta with transformation, and kapha with stability and sustainability. Vata includes subtle movement like that of prana, thoughts, and emotions. Pitta refers to the transformation of food and fluid into energy and nutrition but also to how we process and digest experiences, thoughts, and emotions. Kapha is the physical structure of our being. It is our muscle and bone as well as our ability to be present and comfortable in the body. It deals with holding, both form and energy, and it is associated with memory.

Without movement there is no breeze, no flow of rivers, no tide, no pollination, no circulation, no respiration, no ambulation. Without transformation there is no heat, no digestion, and no chemical reaction. Without stability there is no medium for these processes to occur, a vessel for them to occur within, or a cohesive force that holds the space for them to function.

Each of the three doshas is a combination of two of the five elements: a dynamic or more yang element, which is the element primarily responsible for the functioning of the constitutional aspect or dosha, and a more yin, static, or passive element, responsible for being the vehicle or substratum through which the dosha operates. This is a major reason that the Chinese and Indian systems aren't completely aligned in terms of the elements and constitutional factors.

Vata is a combination of space and air. Pitta is composed of fire and water. Kapha is water and earth. Space is inert, and vata moves through space. Think of air moving through the space of the sky or through the space in the intestines. Protective prana, or wei qi, moves through the *cou li*, the space beneath the skin. Because the more active element, air, best connotes the function of vata, it is sometimes considered the most accurate word to use when referring to the vata dosha. It is important to note, however, that what we normally think of as air is not all of what vata is, and the word is far too limited to express vata completely. Still, it is the best word we have in modern common vernacular, although people also use the terms *wind* and *breath*.

In terms of the pitta dosha, fire is controlled by water, yet utilizes it as a medium to protect the tissues from excess heat or inflammation. Without water, pitta is dry fire raging out of control. With too much water, transformative processes are dulled or inhibited. One quality of pitta, or agni, is its ability to spread. The consistency of pitta is more oily than watery. *Fire* is the word most often used interchangeably with pitta.

The kapha dosha is considered more water than earth in Ayurveda because water carves its way through the earth, and so earth is the vessel for water. Water is naturally cohesive, and because this concept of cohesion is a great descriptor for kapha, water is the element most often used to describe it.

In Ayurveda, there are three single type constitutions—vata dosha, pitta dosha, kapha dosha (see fig. 4.1 on page 84)—which are the predominant types, six dual type, or dual dosha, constitutions, and one type of constitution where the three factors are in equal proportion called the tridoshic constitution. Again, all the elements, and therefore all the constitutional factors are present in every person, but in different quantities and qualities.

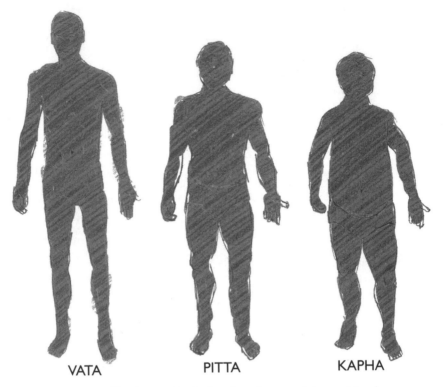

Fig. 4.1. The basic physical traits of vata, pitta, and kapha

Vata Dosha

The vata dosha is movement, and it designates how and where things move. It is responsible for the smooth flow of qi and blood through-out the mind/body complex, and it initiates the heartbeat, the breathing rhythm, and the blinking of the eyes. It also governs the nervous system, circulation, respiration, elimination, energy movement, pranic pulsation through the bodily and mental channels, and transportation and exchange of information. This information exchange can be in any context. It can be information flowing between the brain and body, between people, between cells, or at cell walls. Any time something moves or is transported from one place to another, it is governed by the vata dosha.

In Ayurveda, vata is a combination of air and space. The vata dosha can be said to be elemental air flowing through elemental space. This could be electrons flowing around an atom, nerve impulses streaming through synaptic space, weather patterns traveling through the Earth's atmosphere, electromagnetic energy surging through the connective tissue, a football flying through the air from the quarterback to the receiver, and gas being passed through the large intestine. Any context in which something travels or moves through or to something else is a situation where vata is present. If you associate movement in your life with vata on a regular basis, you will internalize and clearly comprehend what vata is, and you will perceive ever subtler implications of vata in your body, mind, and in the world.

Remember the twenty gunas, or attributes, of nature? These attributes do not exist separately from the matter they are associated with. The attributes for vata are: mobile, cold, light, dry, rough, subtle, flowing, hard, and clear. These attributes may manifest at times in some ways and not in others, and in some ways more than others. For example, not all vata types will have dry hair or rough skin. Just like a substance of primarily one or two elements may not exhibit all of the attributes of those elements, the same is true for how the doshas may manifest in an individual. Also, like increases like. This means that if there is an increase in any of the attributes of vata in diet, mentality, or environment, the vata dosha will increase in the individual.

Vata individuals tend to be tall and thin (see fig. 4.1), with a fine bone structure, and they are inclined to have dry skin, hair, and nails. Their skin may be rough as well as dry, their hands and feet may be cold, and their joints tend to be flexible. Their energy usually comes in bursts, with alternating periods of fatigue. Vata types are creative and like to be on the go; they love change and movement. They are also creative, airy, social, empathic, and forgiving. A stereotypical vata-predominant individual would be a professional ballet dancer. They are long, light, lean, flexible, agile, and always moving.

Vata folks tend toward changeable moods, cracking joints, and darker complexions. Their faces are usually thin, bony, and elongated, and their eyes are usually small and can be bulging or deep set with thin, scanty lashes and lids that blink frequently. Their teeth tend to come in crooked or protruding, and they tend to have thin, coarse, brittle, or wiry hair that's dark in color. They may have prominent veins close to the surface of the skin. Vatas have little perspiration. Compared to the other doshas, they tend to have a lower libido and to walk and speak quickly. They are typically light sleepers and usually get only five to six hours of sleep a night. Their dreams often consist of fears, flying, falling, climbing, running, and jumping.

When in balance there is a sense of going with the flow; bowel movements are regular, and digestion is good. Thoughts and emotions come and go with ease, and the body is limber. When out of balance, vata can manifest as muscle tightness or tension, mobility issues, pain, gas, constipation, twitching, spasming, nervousness, fear, anxiety, sleep disturbances, scattered thoughts, a lack of concentration, follow-through, or grounding, and dry hair, skin, nails, and mucous membranes.

Because like increases like, aspects of our environment may increase or decrease the vata dosha. For example, desert environments will increase vata because deserts are dry, rough, and even in warmer climates have an aspect of coldness at night. Likewise, certain times of the year will increase the vata dosha. Doshas accumulate, aggravate, then stabilize at a subtle, yet deep level with the Earth's journey around the Sun and the change of seasons. Vata begins to accumulate in early summer, from May to July, when the sun's rays dry spring's dampness. The body is naturally weakening, and the digestive power has waned considerably compared to its strength in the winter. Vata then fully aggravates in late summer, from July to September. Vata naturally begins to balance back out in the fall from September to November, which is the beginning of the hydration period in the yearly cycle[1] (see "Ritucharya: Seasonal Routine" in chapter 10).

This may not make much sense at first glance because the leaves dry out and fall to the ground in autumn, while summer is more associated with warmth and humidity. One may think of vata as aggravating in the fall instead of calming. This is not the case, however, according to what is prevalent at that time of year at the clinic. The Earth itself is hydrated from late summer to late winter and is dehydrated from late winter to late summer. This hydration/dehydration cycle forms the foundation for the accumulation, aggravation, and balancing of the doshas. From mid-January to mid-July, the sun's rays and the wind's sharp velocity and dryness absorb the moisture from the earth. The Earth itself, whether through winds or solar radiation, progressively dries through the late winter, spring, and summer. This dryness creates more weakness.

In terms of the time of year from the Earth's perspective, a gradual drying begins and the days get shorter leading to a decreased sun exposure. Dryness increases vata, as does decreased sunlight. Many factors can cause vata aggravation in other seasons, but in a healthy individual living a balanced life according to the seasons, late summer is the worst time for vata aggravation. Winter's stillness, naturally occurring tendency toward introspection, moisture, heavy foods, and increased internal fire and appetite help to balance vata at a deep cellular level.

The times of life are also attributed to each dosha, and vata's time is later in life. Beginning around age fifty, sometimes earlier, vata qualities increase in our bodies. Our hair, skin, nails, and mucous membranes begin to thin and dry. Our muscles, joints, and skin begin to lose their elasticity. Sleep disturbances increase, and the older we get the more varied and feeble our appetites become. Our bones become brittle with the onset of osteopenia, and later with osteoporosis, our memory fades, and we become slower mentally and physically. We lose muscle tone and weight, becoming lighter, and we feel the cold more markedly, another indication of high vata.

As this vata-dosha-predominant drying, decaying process continues, our movements may become involuntary, and we may shake from some type of tremor disorder. High vata in the joints creates pain and cracking, and anxiety, also a vata predominant condition, increases. Later in life we naturally withdraw our senses from the external world to focus on the internal world. It is traditionally a time of self-reflection, awareness, and realization in Ayurveda and in India as a whole. As we age past the childrearing years there is a natural progression toward thinking less about what we can achieve or attain and more about what we are leaving behind as we look toward our own mortality. This can be a difficult process, but if we learn to embrace it, it can provide a great deal of freedom.

We cannot stop this process from occurring, but we may be able to slow or mitigate its effects so that our quality of life is better. Treatments for vata balancing are located in the second part of this book. It is important to note that whichever doshas are predominant in you are the ones most likely to go out of balance. And those that are out of balance are more likely to be more heavily disturbed at those times in life that are dominated by that dosha. For example, the vata time of life will most likely be more uncomfortable for someone of a predominantly vata constitution or with a chronic vata derangement than for someone who is primarily of a kapha or pitta constitution.

The body has a daily clock, and in four-hour increments, twice a day, one of the doshas is predominant. Vata times are 2 a.m. to 6 a.m. and 2 p.m. to 6 p.m. From 2 a.m. to 6 a.m., the nervous system begins to stir. It is the best time to wake up and to tone the nerves and the mind through meditation, yoga, or a good walk in nature. From 2 p.m. to 6 p.m., vata is again dominant, and you are more mentally alert as the nervous system is at its most active. Abundant creative energy flows and is more easily accessible. This is a good time to write, paint, sculpt, and problem solve.

Vata and Chinese Elemental Constitutional Analysis

In terms of the five elements and Chinese constitutional diagnosis, vata qualities are included in the descriptions of wood, fire, metal, and water. Wood is the most spacious (space) of the Chinese elements. It stretches into form, and this movement (air) and the space it stretches into are governed by the vata dosha. Flames flicker, and this movement is vata. Fire types can be more fickle, and they are prone to starting projects they unintentionally don't finish. This is also true of vata types. Water either flows or stagnates, and this movement is also governed by vata. Like vata-predominant individuals, water types are creative, have difficulty sitting still, and may be prone to anxiety and fear. The aspect of flow in Chinese medicine is vata, but the chemical makeup and natural tendencies of water as it behaves when it isn't moving is more kapha.

Pitta Dosha

Pitta is the universal law of transformation in Ayurveda. Pitta governs the transformation of food into energy and nourishment, the transformation of thoughts and ideas into knowledge, and the transformation of emotional energy into clarity and inner peace. The gunas, or qualities, that amplify pitta are: hot, light, oily, sharp, spreading, and liquid. Pitta is a combination of fire and water in Ayurveda. The right balance of fire and water needs to be maintained or problems could result. Without enough water, fire can rage out of control and consume bodily tissues. Too much water can put a damper on fire and cause issues like diluting digestive enzymes, which causes malabsorption.

Mentally, pitta types are fiercely intellectual, and they love learning. They have a tendency toward short tempers, frustration, anger, and irritability. They are usually drawn to athletic pursuits, and are the type A kind of personality. Whatever they do, they strive for perfection. They always have a goal and are not shy about moving toward it, regardless of who or what they need to plow through on their way. They are witty and extroverted with a keen intellect and well-formed opinions. Their sharpness can translate into a sharp tongue, meaning they can be overly critical and judgmental. This judgment turned inward fuels their type A tendencies.

Pittas have a medium build compared to vata (thin boned) and kapha (larger boned and sturdier). They tend to have heart-shaped faces and sharp facial features with ruddy complexions. Their noses and tongues tend to be pointy, and their voices tend to be loud and sharp. Their hair is thin, and they tend to go gray or lose their hair early in life. They are prone to skin ailments like psoriasis, acne, rashes, oily skin, and eczema. They can also have an inclination to develop mouth sores and bleeding issues. Pitta types usually have lighter hair and eyes. They also have strong appetites and digestion. Don't get in their way in the buffet line if it's past their meal time! They can get pretty cranky if they haven't eaten.

Due to their fiery nature, pitta types tend to run warm and be prone to any kind of burning disorder, such as heartburn or acid reflux.

Any inflammation in the body, including tendonitis, bursitis, colitis, or any other "itis," can have a pitta imbalance or displacement as a primary causative factor. Other burning sensations can be brought on by their love of all things hot. They aren't just lovers of spice, but of spicy hot. They may sweat easily and if they do, it may be smelly. Because of their tendency to feel a good deal of stress they may be drawn to alcohol or overexercising to release the pent-up tension. They are passionate people and may also be interested in adrenaline-junky activities to calm their minds and fulfill their desire for a challenge.

Pitta's seat in the physical body is mainly in the small intestine. This is indicative of its relationship to digestion. Hydrochloric acid balance in the stomach, bile secretions from the liver and gallbladder, and enzymatic activity in the intestines are all governed by the pitta dosha. These are strong, sharp, penetrating substances necessary for cutting through, dissolving, and transforming the food and drink we consume. Pitta types' strong intellect is just as cutting, clear, and discerning.

In terms of seasonal cycles, the pitta dosha accumulates in late summer, from July to September. It gets aggravated in autumn, roughly from mid-September through mid-November, and calms down in early winter, from mid-November through mid-January. As the watery aspect of the yearly Sun, wind, and Moon cycle increases, so too does the watery aspect of pitta. This can affect digestion negatively leading to the poor breakdown of food and poorer assimilation of nutrients.

Many people teach that summertime is when pitta aggravates, but this is only true if people engage in unbalanced, pitta-aggravating lifestyle activities. The sunlight is strongest at this time, and traditionally people exercised or did outdoor activities very early in the morning to avoid being active in the hot sun. This is not so in our culture these days. Pitta is related to the blood, and sunbathing or exercising in the sun, which we are prone to do to in the West, can aggravate the blood. Also, the digestive power is weaker in the summer than in the winter, and if any meals are eaten improperly in the summertime, it can more easily affect agni.

Proper food combining is largely ignored, and foods that are difficult to digest or that should be eaten alone are often combined during the summer, further taxing the digestion. Being in the sun alone can tap a lot of the body's strength and cause exhaustion and throwing enzyme-inhibiting iced products on top of a naturally diminished digestive capacity only exacerbates the effect. Smoothies, shakes, ice cream, sugar, iced coffee, iced tea, melon mixed with other fruit, fruit mixed with yogurt, alcohol, late nights, early mornings, and being out in the sun all day are all things that aggravate pitta in the summertime. But that doesn't mean summer is the time of year that pitta aggravates according to *ritucharya,* or seasonal cycles. Pitta aggravates naturally in late fall and early winter. There are a lot of inflammatory and autoimmune disorders in our culture that seem to peak in the autumn and early winter. It makes one wonder how much of it could be alleviated if we lived in accordance with nature instead of doing the opposite of what we "should" be doing seasonally.

The pitta time of life is roughly puberty to menopause. This hormonal time brings with it many issues related to heat in the body, including anger, frustration, an explosive temper, premenstrual syndrome (PMS), heavy menstrual bleeding, hormonal headaches, sweating, acne, a lack of impulse control, and a strong libido. It is the time of life when we are most driven—learning, working, providing for a family, and setting oneself up for the vata time of life: retirement. People who are of a strongly pitta constitution will have a greater tendency for disturbance and discomfort in the pitta time of life.

Pitta times of day are 10 a.m. to 2 p.m. and 10 p.m. to 2 a.m. The best time to eat the largest meal of the day is between 10 a.m. and 2 p.m. because digestion is the strongest when the Sun is highest in the sky. The nighttime pitta cycle is a great time to be asleep. It is the time the liver is most active in its role of purification and detoxification. Bodily energy is better used for this purpose at this time of night than for anything else.

Pitta in Chinese Elemental Constitutional Analysis

The pitta dosha most closely resembles the elemental Chinese types of wood and fire, with a touch of metal. While vata is the spacious, stretchy aspect of wood, pitta is the determined force of wood pressing forward. Wood can reach deep into the ground, even cracking through boulders to reach its goal of hydration. Pitta types are much like this, plowing through obstacles in their path without regard for who or what is in the way or how intense the challenge is. In fact, they love challenge, and tend to be competitive. Pitta types are driven, determined, intelligent, athletic, and ambitious. They can push themselves hard and you harder if you let them.

Their fiery aspects can be found in transformation, their intelligent witty intellect, and to some extent, their appearance. They can be highly critical and judgmental of both themselves and others. Like fire, they consume and transform. They consume knowledge and can either regurgitate it or make it their own. Fiery types have pointy physical attributes like a flickering flame, which is very pitta. They love learning and intellectual pursuits and make great college professors or passionate leaders. Pitta qualities that most reflect metal are a tendency toward loud speech, a potential for being short-tempered, and a strong digestive system. Like metal types, they can be predisposed to some of the inflammatory disorders mentioned above.

Kapha Dosha

Kapha is a combination of earth and water in Ayurveda. Because earth is inert, kapha is mostly associated with the quality of water. Water lubricates, moistens, contains information, and carries the vata dosha's electrical impulses. At a molecular level, water's primary quality is cohesion. Similarly, kapha's watery influence is about holding or drawing together to itself, and the presence of the earth element creates stability. The attributes, or qualities, of kapha are: stable, cool, oily, heavy, cloudy, gross, dull, slow, and smooth. Remember that these qualities in the environment or one's dietary intake will increase the kapha dosha.

Kapha types tend to be short, curvy, and attractive. They have large, beautiful eyes and lustrous thick hair. Their skin tends to be fair and smooth, and they may have strong white teeth. They have hardy constitutions and a large bone structure. They like order and routine, and are regular in eating habits and elimination. Kapha-dominant people exude peace and stability. They tend to be good, patient listeners, although they can get a little aggravated with someone whose vata is very unbalanced. Their stoic, strong nature makes them solid, loyal friends and trustworthy individuals others feel are "always there for them."

The stable, heavy, dull, slow nature of kapha can cause laziness, sluggishness, and weight gain. Kaphas love sweets and crave baked goods, breads, and pastas. Unfortunately, they don't quite have the metabolism to process these things without easily putting on weight or becoming mucusy. They are prone to mucus build up in the head and chest. Kapha's main seat in the body is the lungs, and they are therefore prone to upper respiratory infections including coughs and colds, as well as seasonal allergies and breathing issues like asthma.

The kapha time of year begins in late winter, from January to March, when it starts to accumulate. It aggravates in the spring, between March and May, and begins to calm as drying vata accumulates in the summer, from May through June. While kapha is accumulating we become more mucusy and may start craving lighter foods. When kapha aggravates, it's the optimal time to do a cleanse. This is because the toxins that built up all year internally are being pushed out through the mucus membranes along with the increased mucus. If one is properly guided, one can detoxify harmoniously without damaging any doshas or dhatus. This is important as improper attempts at detoxification, fasting, or dieting can unbalance the doshas. Kapha calms down in the hot, dry summer, from mid-May to July.

The kapha time of life is from birth to about age twenty-five. It overlaps with pitta time during puberty. Early life is kapha time because it is a time of growth and development when nourishment is most important. Kapha is viscous, heavy, smooth, soft, and slow. Think of a baby with all that chubby baby fat and all the mucus secretions. Little children are always getting sick with coughs and colds. The focus at this time of life is on nourishment, enjoyment, play, and sleep. Themes that occupy this time of life are contentment, possessiveness, and dependency, and issues may include obesity and difficulty getting up in the morning. Remember kapha's heavy, slow, dull aspects. At the kapha time of life these are all helpful for nourishing and developing, but they have a flip side if play isn't active and diet and movement aren't balanced.

The kapha time of day falls between 6 and 10 a.m. and 6 and 10 p.m. In the morning, it is best to wake before kapha time. Otherwise, because of kapha's heavy, dull, slow nature, it may be difficult to wake up. If we don't wake before 6 a.m. we may keep hitting snooze button and feel groggy and crave caffeine when we do wake up. Between 6 and 10 p.m. we should be taking advantage of the qualities of kapha and begin to settle for bedtime. Interestingly, cortisol levels start dropping at this time of day so it is also considered a good time to settle down from the perspective of Western science.

Kapha and Chinese Elemental Constitutional Analysis

Kapha is most equivalent to the earth, water, and metal types in Chinese elemental constitutional analysis. Earth is completely kapha in nature in Chinese medicine. Kapha types are naturally compassionate and nurturing with a good solid physique, strong bones and musculature, and an organized, disciplined, reliable, steady way of being. They are built like Chinese earth types and prone to the same ailments.

The water type is akin to the vata/kapha dual doshic constitution in Ayurveda. The watery attributes affiliated with kapha in this case are the tendency to be laid back and exude an inner peace and the water metabolism issues suffer when kapha is out of balance. Water types also share kapha's body-shape characteristics, such as a round face, broad cheeks, and round belly. They also tend to have an aversion to spring and summer, when kapha and vata are most prevalent and go easily out of balance.

In Ayurveda, metal types would be considered predominantly kapha, with the kapha qualities of stoicism, discipline, organization, inner strength, stillness, and leadership. Like kapha, they have a tendency to internalize their emotions. Metal types make strong leaders or managers due to their reliability, solid thinking, and steady nature. These are all kapha attributes as well. Metal is cold, dry, and hard and can be ungrounded and spacey, a tendency that can also be found in out-of-balance kaphas. Metal types can also be rigid, and if this rigidity is due to the inertia of earth, kapha is at the root of the issue. Like metal types, kapha is associated with a strong physique, round face, and pale complexion. Kaphas are quiet, calm, honest, and stable.

CONSTITUTIONAL TYPES IN CHINESE MEDICINE

In Chinese medicine, there are several camps of thought when dealing with constitutional types. Some say there are five, six, nine, or more types. It just depends on what school of thought you're coming from or who you study with. To keep things simple, we will talk about one school of thought on constitutional typing: the five elements (see fig. 4.2). The Chinese, Japanese, and a branch of Chinese acupuncturists from the Worsley school all use the five elements in diagnosis and treatment (although Worsley himself didn't believe in constitutional typing). All five elements are present in each individual in unique proportions, similar to how constitutions form in Ayurveda, with their basis in elemental qualitative and quantitative makeup. Chinese

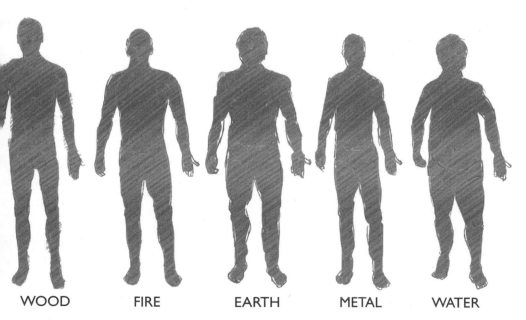

WOOD   FIRE   EARTH   METAL   WATER

Fig. 4.2. The five physical constitutional types according to five element typing

medicine views a part of this makeup as inherently flawed, and this is where disease processes have their root. This perspective is akin to how Ayurveda views the doshas. In fact, the word *dosha* actually represents the concept of a flaw. In five element constitutional diagnosis in Chinese medicine, there is a strong mental and emotional focus. All of the elements relate to environmental forces and bodily tissues and organs but also to personality.

Wood Type

The wood type displays many of the characteristics of a dual doshic vata/pitta (movement/transformation) constitutional type in Ayurveda. Wood types' tall, lean, sinewy bodies tend to look and behave more like those of vata types, and their will, functional and physiological predispositions for imbalance, and personality are more like pittas. Their faces tend to be bony and chiseled, with deep-set eyes, long thin noses, slender cheeks, and high foreheads. Wood types may have broad shoulders and a straight back[2] and bony fingers with knotted joints.

Wood types tend to be ambitious and determined and will forge ahead to achieve their goals regardless of who or what may be injured as a result, including themselves. They are smart and drawn to intellectual work and may be travelers and explorers. They are easily frustrated and can succumb to the need for caffeine to stay focused and alcohol to relax. They have the standard type A personality: driven, motivated, and good at motivating others. Wood people are known for getting easily frustrated and angry and may be prone to thinking too much.

Health issues typically attributed to wood types are muscle and tendon spasms and injuries, joint problems, restlessness, and involuntary movements. They are prone to insomnia, migraines, blood pressure issues, sensitive eyes, herpes, varicose veins, hemorrhoids, and hernias. If they have an allergy, it will most likely be seasonal, but they may also have problems with topical substances, the sun, insect bites, and chocolate. Menstrual cycles in women can include a lot of pain, PMS, and breast tenderness, and they may be prone to fibroid cysts.

Wood types benefit from moderate exercise, stretching, breathing, and mindfulness meditation. Regular walks in nature, especially among trees, are also beneficial. Wood types benefit from a mindfulness practice because they are prone to thinking about the future. This takes them away from the present, which can feed the stress, overthinking, and worry they are disposed to. Although it may cause them frustration and resistance, they should focus on slowing down when they are young so that as they age they may appreciate life and experience gratitude for what is, as opposed to what could be. With a predisposition for looking ahead, the wood type's driven nature can be uncomfortable and difficult to manage as they move into old age. This is why incorporating presence practices earlier in life is beneficial for balancing wood.

Fire Type

The fire type in Chinese medicine is also a combination of pitta and vata, with pitta being the more physical aspect this time, and vata relating more to the personality and how the nervous system handles and the mind processes information. Fire types have small hands and feet with long flexible fingers and pointy fingertips. They have ruddy or reddish complexions with an oval or heart shaped face and narrow forehead. Their cheekbones may make them appear cat- or wolf-like, and they have catlike eyes. In essence they resemble a flame with tall and/or pointy heads and either curly or scanty hair.[3] They are sometimes redheads or gingers and may or may not have freckles.

Fire types are talkative and charismatic, eloquent and expressive. They are friendly and warm and easily make others feel comfortable. They can also be fickle like the movement of a flickering flame, never in one place for long mentally, emotionally, or physically. This may make them seem untrustworthy to others who are close to them. They can be prone to selfishness, but the flip side of that is their drive for connection and love. When balanced, they tend to be lighthearted and joyous, but out of balance they can be anxious and experience insomnia and palpitations. Although they are quick to anger, it doesn't usually last long.

Health problems associated with a fire imbalance are: anxiety, nervousness, insomnia, bipolar disorder, depression, nervous laughter, blood pressure issues, memory loss, mitral valve prolapse, heart murmur, scarlet fever, cardiac insufficiency, angina, pericarditis, adrenal burnout, low libido, urinary tract issues, acne, rashes, dry skin, and heart palpitations.

Because of their social nature, they may benefit from taking a little alone time to settle. Not too much, as their craving for intimacy and connection is a necessary need to fulfill, but enough to keep their energy levels, restless nature, and emotional outpouring in balance. Good breathwork practices for overheated fire types are *sitali* pranayama and alternate nostril breathing. Of course, meditation is great for all types, but fires may really resonate with some kind of visualization practice to keep their busy minds focused but active. Journaling can also be beneficial for fire types, and regularly scheduled activities such as mealtimes, sleep, and exercise can help keep them on a consistent, even keel.

Earth Type

The earth type is most closely and almost exclusively associated with the kapha type in Ayurveda. Words that describe earth are *roundness* and *stability*. They tend to have round heads and faces and round or full bodies. Generally well proportioned, they are solid, thick, and short with a well-developed overall physique and musculature. They have a yellowish skin tone and a steady gait, and they are trustworthy, likable, peaceful, and compassionate. Like the kapha type, they can be described as a Rock of Gibraltar when it comes to friendship. They are loyal and stable and good listeners. They are the type of person one feels drawn to in order to feel safe and secure in times of illness, turmoil, or crisis.

Earth types are natural nurturers and love to garden and to do crafts like knitting, quilting, or cooking. They love food and tend to crave carbs, which can cause them to gain a little too much excess weight. They are prone to excessive worry, but their type of worry is due to attachment. The earth type tends to accumulate things, and their tendency to want to possess may make them vulnerable to codependent relationships. Predispositions tend to be toward digestive issues, especially since their worry can damage the digestive system. Stomach ulcers, hiatal hernia, low blood sugar, diabetes, and lymph disorders are also common.

Metal Type

Metal types tend to be a mix of vata or pitta with strongly internal kapha attributes. The kapha/vata or kapha/pitta dual type has a physique that tends to be more lean than a typical kapha. They are also more predisposed to movement and putting themselves out there energetically than the stereotypically reserved and stoic kapha. Remember that all people are a combination of all five elements. This means that whether kapha/vata or kapha/pitta, these types will still have attributes of all three doshas, as is true with all of the five Chinese types. They have strong, muscular bodies and a fast metabolism and oblong or oval faces with wide-set cheekbones and soft, smooth, firm, pale skin. People who have a dominant metal element have strong voices, and although they can be short-tempered and fierce,[4] they are generally quiet and calm. They make effective officials[5] or leaders, and they are organized and tend to err on the side of perfectionism.

Metal types are prone to bottling up emotions and can seem cold and aloof. They have a good sense of boundaries and are masters at keeping their personal and professional lives separate. They also have good minds and decision-making prowess. When imbalanced, they can tend toward diseases of the lung and large intestine, as these are the organs/meridians associated with the metal element. This also includes the skin since it is in the domain of the lung system in Chinese medicine. Examples of metal imbalances are frequent colds, asthma, emphysema, diverticulitis, colitis, hemorrhoids, gastritis, eczema, psoriasis, and lymphatic congestion. They may also be prone to tendonitis, arthritis, and rheumatism. Due to the dry nature of metal, they have a tendency to crave oily and moisture-producing products like milk, which may add to phlegm accumulation and the frequency of colds.

Water Type

Water types in Chinese medicine are similar to vata/kapha types in Ayurveda. Their heads tend to be on the larger side, and they have round faces with broad cheeks, narrow shoulders, and large, long abdomens.[6] They move around a lot because they have difficulty being still. When in balance, water people can easily go with the flow. They are introspective and peaceful. Although determined, they focus on moving forward along the path of least resistance.

When out of balance, water types can succumb to fear. Their tendency to be introspective can lead to emotional turmoil and stuck patterns of negative thought. Connection with others is important for their emotional well-being, and although they may not realize it or care when they get wrapped up in their own heads, it is important for them to remain social to stay balanced. Being around water is good for them, as is being still for meditative practices. As the kidney and bladder organs and meridians are water element associations, water types are prone to issues resulting from fluid metabolism imbalance. Puffiness, dark circles under the eyes, edema, and urinary tract infections are common. Other ailments may include kidney stones, vertigo due to inner ear fluid imbalance, blood pressure issues, and adrenal depletion.

FINDING YOUR TYPE

When you compare the Chinese elemental types with the Ayurveda doshas you can see that they are quite similar, just organized differently. You probably have a good idea of where you fall with regard to the types and constitutions just from this little bit of information. It is natural to be confused about the details here and there or have trouble deciding which of your traits are dominant. Over a lifetime things change, and it's sometimes difficult to discern which category fits you the best. This is partly because of vikruti, or imbalance, and partly because we are a combination of all the types, and it's difficult to diagnose oneself. In order to organize your thoughts in terms of constitution, I've included a quiz for you (see table on pages 102–103). For each category in the left column, circle the quality in one of the other three columns that best describes you. I recommend using a pencil and taking the quiz twice. The first time you take it, circle those qualities that most fit who you are today. The second time you take it, circle the ones that better fit who you were at the youngest age you can remember. This is a rough way to discern your vikruti (first test) from your prakruti (second test). In the next section of the book we will discuss how to bring balance to the constitutions.

AYURVEDIC DOSHA CONSTITUTION QUIZ

Category	Vata	Pitta	Kapha
Build	Thin	Athletic	Stocky/solid
Height	Tall or very short	Average	Shortish
Eye shape	Deep/sunken, small	Average/thin brows	Large, attractive
Eye color	Dark brown	Green, hazel, gray, light blue	Soft blue or light brown
Eye movement	Darting, nervous	Penetrating, sharp	Soft, calming
Nose	Crooked/uneven, possible deviated septum	Long, pointed	Short, rounded
Teeth	Protruding	Medium size, yellowish	Strong, white
Mouth	Small	Medium size	Large
Lips	Dry, cracked	Red	Full, smooth
Face shape	Narrow, long	Heart shaped	Round, full
Hair color	Dark brown, black	Fair, blond, red tones	Brown
Hair texture	Coarse, brittle, easily knotted	Fine, straight, soft, gray, bald	Thick, lustrous, wavy
Skin texture/temperature	Thin, dry, rough, cool to touch	Warm to touch, sweats easily	Smooth, thick, cool to touch
Complexion	Dark	Rosy, freckles, easily irritated, burns easily	Pale
Weight	Difficult to gain	Easily gain or lose	Easily gain, difficult to lose
Joints	Protruding, crack a lot, hyperflexible	Medium, fairly flexible	Strong, dense
Nails	Dry, rough, brittle, breaking	Sharp, flexible, healthy	Thick, smooth, shiny

Belly button	Irregularly shaped, may bulge in places	Oval, superficial	Deep, round
Bowel movements	Irregular, prone to constipation	Regular, prone to loose	Regular, formed
Diet/appetite	Can forget to eat, skips meals, grazes	Strong appetite, gets cranky fast if hungry	Tendency to overeat, can feel heavy after eating
Temperature	Cold, cold hands and feet, sensitive to wind, prefers warmth	Warm, runs warm, likes cool weather	Cool, dislikes cold and damp weather and humidity
Sleep	Irregular, light, easily wakened	Less than 8 hours but sound	Likes to sleep, sleeps deeply, slow to wake
Speech	Rapid, quick	Penetrating, sharp	Slow, deliberate
In conversation	Changes topics	Intellectual/teaching	Supportive, listens
Movement	Quick	Intentional	Take your time
Financial	Spends frivolously	Pampers self	Saves
Negative emotions go to	Fear, anxiety, nervousness	Anger, jealousy	Sadness, clinging, attachment
Reaction to confrontation	Flight	Fight	Freeze
Intellect/memory	Quick to learn and to forget	Intellectual, loves learning and knowledge	Good memory
Natural state	Free spirit/creative	Keen intellect, motivated, determined	Calm, serene, homebody
Totals			

5

Anatomy

Nuts and (Lightning) Bolts

Another fascinating subject common to both Ayurveda and Chinese medicine is anatomy and physiology. In addition to covering structures and functions, such as bodily tissues and organs, this topic also gives us insight into our energetic makeup. It includes knowledge of the energy bodies, or *koshas,* energy circulation through specific channels, or meridians/nadis, intersections along those pathways called acupoints or marmani, and major areas of energy and information exchange called *tan tiens* or chakras. Another concept that falls under the heading of anatomy and physiology is that of the three Chinese treasures *jing,* qi, and shen and their Ayurvedic correspondences *ojas,* prana, and tejas.

Interestingly, subtle anatomy has a lot to do with consciousness. This is because there is no true differentiation between what happens between the mind and the body in these two medicines. There is body consciousness, and there is a consciousness attributed to the mind and beyond the body. Consciousness envelops awareness and information. Therefore, a consciousness of some sort underlies all of existence. In terms of therapeutics, because the mind and body are so connected it is not only difficult to completely distinguish between the two, it is also discouraged or unnecessary. There is overlap, information exchange, or communication between them. This chapter will focus primarily on body consciousness and gross anatomy and subtle anatomy, and the next chapter will concentrate primarily on the mind and consciousness as it operates through the mind.

Acupuncture is a fascinating and increasingly popular field of study. More people are training in it and trying it out than ever before. It involves treatment of tiny energy centers along the lines of transport that supply qi to all the organs and tissues of the body. Modern science continues to attempt to isolate and map these pathways. Although they are found to partially equate with the nervous system, the circulatory system, and the lymphatic system, none of these is an exact match. Modern science has also been able to pinpoint electrical pathways in the connective tissue. These pathways are tracts of higher electrical conductivity than the surrounding tissue and correlate precisely with the layout of acupuncture meridians.

Another theory that corresponds to acupuncture channels is that of "Bonghan ducts." Bonghan, a North Korean scientist, and other researchers over the past 50 years located a network of microscopic threadlike channels that carry fluid. They seem to overlap with the location of acupuncture meridians and correspond somewhat to the circulatory and lymphatic systems. They also wrap around organs.[1] There is a subtler network of channels in acupuncture theory that supplies the tissues directly with qi and nutrition (ying qi) that is called the microcirculation channels.

It's interesting to note that modern science is concerned with the structures that carry the life-giving energy and fluids, while the ancients determined their location primarily by focusing on function. They paid attention to what was happening in the mind/body complex, to the result, and from there determined that these structures must exist. It seems the meridians do indeed correlate with these gross anatomical pathways and systems, yet it does not really matter that they do. The theory behind how a person is treated will not change as a result, nor will it be more refined. It is perfect as it is; science is merely catching up (probably by accident in many cases) and trying to put unfamiliar terminology into common language. There is great wisdom in these ancient traditions; perhaps as a society we ought to take a bigger leap of faith in trusting them, or base our research on the foresight of the ancients.

The subtle energy lines that carry qi to the tissues and organs are called jing and *luo* (collaterals) in Chinese medicine. They are also called meridians. In Ayurveda they are known as nadis, which is Sanskrit for "flow," "motion," "channel," and "vibration." It is also used synonymously with "nerve." This may be because the nervous system and the nadi system are both under the domain of vata dosha, particularly, prana vayu.

There are innumerable channel pathways, from the extraordinary vessels, to the twelve primaries, to the sinew channels, to the collaterals and microchannels. In acupuncture theory we regularly use twelve primary meridians (see fig. 5.1) for diagnosis and treatment. The strength, weakness, and quality of flow of these channels can be assessed through

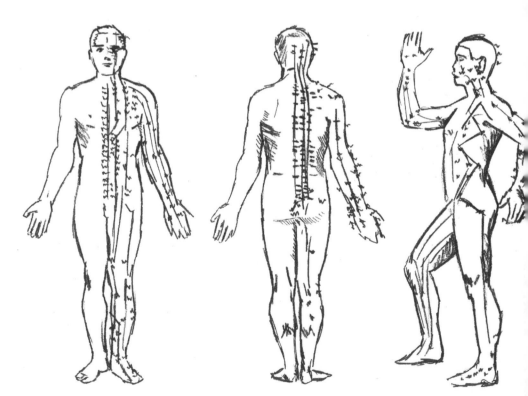

Fig. 5.1. The acupuncture meridians

the pulse, and points along them can be needled or stimulated to effect healing. In addition to these twelve, there are what we call the "eight extraordinary vessels." These are sometimes viewed as deeper, more subtle, and perhaps more diffuse channels that formed prior to the twelve primary channels.

We access the thousands of other pathways through the twelve primary meridians and two of the eight extraordinary vessels. The other channels are divergent channels and luo channels, which connect the twelve primaries, and minute collaterals, which are smaller and smaller branches of the major channels. These branches go deep and supply qi to every cell. This is similar to how the circulatory system branches from large arteries to small capillaries. There are also sinew channels that influence tendinous muscular pathways under the control of the twelve primaries.

The channels serve the purpose of forming, protecting, nourishing, and vitalizing the body, storing energy, and exchanging information internally and with the environment. They open to the surface and contain access points that affect the deeper organs and tissues. They also have branches that connect with parts of the body that may not seem intuitively linked, like the Urinary Bladder channel having branches in the brain for example. These branches allow for the exchange of information and energy between the internal organs and other structures of the body. They are like energy and information highways.

The twelve primary channels or meridians are: Lung (LU), Large Intestine (LI), Stomach (ST), Spleen (SP), Heart (HT), Small Intestine (SI), Urinary Bladder (UB), Kidney (KD), Pericardium (PC), San Jiao or Triple Burner (TB), Gall Bladder (GB), and Liver (LV). The eight extraordinary vessels are: Ren, Du, Chong, Yin Qiao, Yang Qiao, Yin Wei, Yang Wei, and Dai Mai.

There is no part of the body that goes untouched by qi from the meridians unless it is completely blocked or sealed off from the rest of the body by trauma or disease. Along these pathways are points that are like little springs that arise from the surface of the body and exchange information superficially with the outside world and at a deep level between internal structures. Some believe that the deep reservoirs where the acupuncture points are located contain greater concentrations of minerals than do the surrounding tissues. An astute practitioner can focus on a point with the gentlest touch of a fingertip and read the energy at the point. This means that they can ascertain if there is an energy and/or information blockage or an excess or a lack of energy at the point and in the meridian. If the point is a source point to an internal organ it may actually give information about the organ it is associated with it. The same is true for pulse diagnosis.

PULSE DIAGNOSIS

In either Chinese or Ayurvedic medicine, bodily strength or weakness or the presence of a pathogen can be perceived from reading the radial pulse on the wrist. There is a point on each wrist for each of the twelve primary channels and their associated organs. It is by feeling this pulse with well-trained fingers that one can decide the health and strength of a given organ or channel supplying the organ.

In Ayurveda, the original and acquired constitutions are diagnosed by a skilled practitioner by taking the pulse. There are seven layers at which the pulse can be taken that begin at the surface of the skin and descend to the bone. There are also three pulse positions. This means that the practitioner will place his or her index, middle, and ring fingers on the wrist, equally spaced apart, to perceive or read the pulse. Usually the most superficial pulse is read first so the client's mind/body can acclimate to the presence, touch, and intention of the practitioner before deeper aspects of the pulse are explored. The deeper the intrusion into the pulse, the more sensitive the client becomes, and a reaction can trigger a change in the pulse.

Other factors that can shift the pulse reading are: what the client did or didn't eat or drink the night before, if they slept well or not, if they moved around just before the pulse was taken, and if they feel anxious or threatened while it's being taken. Food eaten the night before, like a spicy meal for example, can temporarily change the pulse the next morning. Having sex the night before can do the same. It's important, when having a constitutional pulse diagnosis, to refrain from sex, spicy foods, alcohol, or caffeine for twelve hours before the consultation. In addition, any distraction due to poor diet or lifestyle can adversely affect the perceptive skill of the practitioner. Usually, pulses are taken in the morning on an empty stomach. This prerequisite may vary from practitioner to practitioner based upon their skill, training, strong meditation practice, sattvic, clear mindedness, or gifted pulse-taking acumen.

EMBRYOLOGY

Embryological development is a good place to start when discussing the origin of energetic anatomy. It was known to the ancients and includes a quite detailed scientific explanation. In addition to the observable scientific fetal development, the Chinese and Indians describe what happens at the unseeable, subtle energetic level. The Charaka Samhita, a text written well before the discovery of the cell or microscope, describes in detail the seed from the mother and the seed from the father merging. It also describes each stage of embryonic development and how the various tissues are guided into being by the soul and each of the three doshas.[2] The Ayurvedic version of embryology focuses on consciousness, the five elements, the mind, karma, the health of the parents, and the doshas' role in the formation of the fetus. It's actually in quite precise alignment with modern science.

Chinese medicine embryological development begins with the yang of the father, the yin of the mother, and the jing of both parents merging. A polarity forms, and then the extraordinary vessels, which define the spatial planes, arise. Clinically speaking, it is probably fair to say that more has been written about the eight extraordinary vessels in the past fifty years than in the preceding thousand years. Classically in Chinese medicine, the eight extraordinary vessels have to do with providing the proper balance of fluids in the lymph, interstitially, and in the connective tissue. Although they cannot be cited from classical sources as being primary in the process of embryogenesis, the Ren Mai (Conception Vessel) and Du Mai (Governing

Vessel) channels are said to spring from prenatal essence. The origination of these vessels is followed by the genesis of the twelve primary meridians. These meridians form the blueprint for the cellular differentiation and organization of the bodily structures, tissues, and organs. The eight extraordinary vessels and twelve meridians share the responsibilities of maintaining the form and function of the body, as well as the communication between bodily tissues and structures.

In Ayurveda, embryogenesis begins with the karma, or tendencies due to past actions, attached to the incoming soul. The soul, or atman, is a transcendental, unchanging, untarnished entity that is a drop from the ocean of pure cosmic consciousness. Without it, a living being cannot exist. This soul has passed in and out of various forms and has picked up little "clingers" along the way in, through, and out of those forms of life. We can say these little clingers are karma. This particular karma draws the individual soul to a particular set of parents as a result of the parents' physical, mental, environmental, societal, spiritual, and emotional tendencies and physical location on the Earth, i.e., their karma. The five elements and dosha tendencies are present in each of the parent's seeds. Upon conception, the prakruti is determined, and the *jivatma* or individual soul can enter. It is the intelligence of the soul that directs the growth of the embryo.

In Ayurveda, in addition to nadis there are channels called *srotas.* These are more gross physical channels that guide the passage of food and fluid through the system. The combination of gross and subtle energy lines work to regulate prana/qi flow, provide nutrition, stimulate growth, regulate fluids, transport qi and blood, ensure proper immunity and oxygenation, process information, clear toxins from the system, regulate yin and yang functions, provide protection, and manage animation, movement, support, strength, insulation, lubrication, memory, luster, and communication.

SUBTLE PATHWAYS/NADIS AND YOGA

It is difficult to speak of nadis without getting into Yoga theory, as they have a stronger focus in Yoga than in Ayurveda. Charaka talks about the vessels that originate from the heart, but he is speaking in terms of gross physical channels, or srotas, such as the arteries in the circulatory system or the gastrointestinal tube. These types of channels are emphasized in Ayurveda because they are observable and more readily treatable with herbs, diet, and so on. The nadis are more emphasized in Yoga theory and practice as they are more subtle and more perceptible in meditation.

In Yoga, the nadis are subtle pathways that transport life force energy (power or shakti) and information. There are three primary nadis: *ida, pingala,* and *sushumna.* Basically speaking, ida nadi runs along the left side of the spine and relates to the right side of the brain. Therefore, its function is associated with the yin and the feminine, creativity, coolness, and relaxation. It is the rest-and-digest nadi. On the other side is the pingala nadi. It is related to the yang and the masculine, warmth, activity, analysis, and the left side of the brain. It is the balance-your-checkbook nadi. Often, the ida and pingala nadis are illustrated as crisscrossing through the spinal cord on their journey through the body. Their path looks like the caduceus emblem of intertwined snakes used as the symbol for Western medicine. Derived from the staff of Aesclepius, this symbol also has its roots in esoteric anatomy. The ida and pingala nadis intersect at the energy centers called chakras, which are described below.

In the center of the spinal cord lies the sushumna nadi. It is responsible for consciousness awakening to the true nature of itself and existence and is connected to a power source that lies at the base of the spine called *kundalini shakti.* This kundalini lies dormant in most individuals, according to Yoga, until it is awakened through force, karma, or cultivation. It is like poking a sleeping cobra with a stick. You can imagine it springing to life and rising up at you fully aware as if it were never resting. This is similar to the nature of kundalini rising or awakening. I would imagine that the kundalini is akin to the primary tan tien and the storage of essence and power, and its awakening is similar to turning the light around in the third eye meditation practice called "the golden flower" in the Chinese system.

There are also nadis in the head that connect regions of energy and information potential associated with higher or more developed states of awareness. Moving the energy along these nadis to switch on or awaken those regions is *hiranyagarbhaya* yoga, and it is an advanced cultivation/meditation, self/cosmic-consciousness tool for becoming fully enlightened. There are also prana pathways that directly connect the brain and heart. In fact, there are tens of thousands of pathways. The goal of Yoga is to clear them of obstruction and strengthen them so that they can handle the increased pranic voltage of a kundalini awakening. It's like exercising a muscle so it can endure the challenge of more work. If the pathways and the regions along them that collect and store information and energy are not first cleared of obstruction, a person can short out their nadis. The effects of this are mental, emotional, spiritual, and physical and are seldom temporary.

In the process of clearing the nadis, one must cleanse the srotas of the physical and mental bodies in order to free up the body's energy circulation so that the energy can then go to clearing out the tiny, more subtle nadis. There are many processes capable of doing this including Ayurveda, panchakarma, exercise, breathing practices, detoxification, concentration, visualization, color and gem therapy, vastu (feng shui), bodywork, yoga asana (poses), and Vedic astrological (jyotish) advice.

CHAKRAS

The chakras in Yoga and the tan tiens in Taoist internal martial arts practices such as qigong or tai chi are places in the etheric and physical body that affect the physiology, mental/emotional states, and access to greater dimensions of awareness. They are responsible for storing information and energy as well as transforming that energy. There are seven primary chakras (see fig. 5.2) and three primary tan tiens.

The nadis are fueled by the energy and information stored and processed by the chakras. The word *chakra* means "wheel" in Sanskrit. This is because the chakras are said to spin like wheels or vortices. I visualize the chakras to be like major hubs in a busy city. The chakra

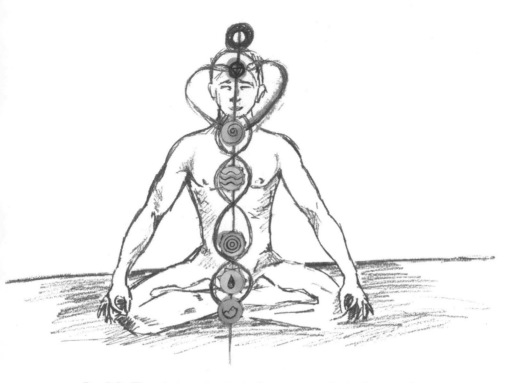

Fig. 5.2. The chakras in the Indian system, their elemental
associations, and the three primary nadis

would be the center square, and all the cars that drive around it and radiate out in all directions are the prana. The center square/chakra is like a pranic generator or telecommunications hub, and the roads are the nadis. The chakras are not actually part of Ayurveda, traditionally, but they have become a modern day obsession among Yoga and New Age enthusiasts. This may be due in large part to our modern day comfort with chakra theory due to its linear categorization and the associations modern psychologists have drawn between them and the mind.

Historically, the chakras were very difficult to access. One needed to disassociate with daily living and become a hermit who focused on the chakras 24/7. Today, we talk about and work with them as if they are easily accessed. I believe they can be easily accessed at a superficial level with our focused awareness, but that there is a depth to them we don't often put ourselves in a position to really know or experience. Working with this powerful aspect of self is a deeply mystical, life-altering journey.

Who isn't drawn to the allure of the chakras when they first learn of their existence? They are beautifully colored vortices of light, common to us all, that emerge from deep within and expand into a magnificent rainbow cloud of light around us called an aura. Besides a specific color, each chakra has a musical note, seed sound, syllable, deity, and various other characteristics associated with it. Each is in a specific part of the body that corresponds to a major nerve plexus or endocrine gland. Many of the endocrine functions in the modern scientific model are associated with their respective chakras.

The chakras exchange information with the outside world. Each has a specific set of functions that governs the physical body and the mind and is associated with the information they give and receive. For example, joy and love would be processed by the heart chakra. The energies of joy and love would enter the body through the heart chakra and emanate from the heart chakra. Any issues with joy or love could hinder the functioning of the heart chakra and the deeper tissues if left to fester.

Whatever we send our energy to greatly affects how we feel and function in life. For example, if you have any unclear issues regarding something in your life, even if you are not conscious of them, your energy goes there at a subtle level. It can be anything, and it doesn't have to be something you focus on consciously or try to heal. Healing sometimes happens in layers, and we peel away at the layers like we peel away at an onion. We may not know what lies at the heart of an issue or disease state until sometime late into its exploration, if ever. Whenever there is a root, vital energy will go to it.

If someone has an issue with a quality pertaining to a particular chakra, this chakra becomes the reactive, dominant chakra force guiding the life choices of the individual. In kundalini-awakening practices like the various forms of yoga, the issues governed by and perhaps damaging the chakras and their associated tissues and body parts must be healed before we can proceed. This is because there are layers to every issue, and if a light is suddenly turned on something that should be given time to emerge and process, it can be too much for us to handle. This is a real phenomenon and can result in long-standing consequences if not handled properly.

Some of the information stored in the chakra centers pertains to what some believe are past-life and deep present-life issues. This is why the guidance of a well-trained somatic therapist, yogi, or seer—someone that specializes in bearing witness to their clients' processing of intense issues on a regular basis—is best suited for someone wanting to work at this level. There are many resources on the chakras and if it is a topic of interest, I encourage you to investigate it further.

I mention chakras here because they are part of the energetic makeup of a person and have a direct relationship to physical, mental, emotional, and spiritual well-being. Some people liken chakras to marmani and acupuncture points, which function in a similar way in that they directly affect the physical body as we will see in the next section. However, the chakras are more subtle as their primary access is through the mind.

MARMANI

The vital points on the body described in the Ayurvedic texts, particularly by Sushruta, are called *marmani*, or marma points. Marma points are usually located at the intersection of tissues, such as blood vessels, muscle, bone, and nerves. They are useful in the diagnosis and treatment of a variety of conditions—most notably nowadays, pain. Practitioners apply differing levels of pressure, oils, herbal preparations, and poultices on these points to effect healing on the surface and in deeper tissues and structures of the body. Because these points are so essential to the well-being of the individual, an injury that would otherwise be harmless any place else on the body may cause chronic issues if it falls on a marma point. Sushruta warns against cutting these areas during surgical procedures as any trauma or injury to them can create a dire situation for the patient that ranges anywhere from chronic health issues to death. There are detailed descriptions in both the Astanga Hridayam and the Sushruta Samhita of what will occur if particular points are injured or cut. In the Astanga Hridayam, Vagbhata calls the marmani the "vital spots," speaking to their great importance.[3]

In Ayurveda, the psychospiritual and esoteric aspects of marmani aren't as present in the ancient texts are they are in modern teachings. They document the nuts and bolts, leaving the important details beyond the physical to be purveyed by the master teacher. Traditionally, the slokas were memorized and written in verse form for easy memory. Then the student would apprentice for years and learn the finer points and subtleties of the medicine and of life as it pertains to the medicine. This means there is a vast sea of knowledge in Ayurveda that is passed on in a lineage, as it is in martial arts or yoga and in Chinese medicine. It is important for students of either form of medicine to have a good teacher and mentor to turn to so that they may truly understand the life force of these medical arts. Only then can they gain a deep, complete knowledge of any of these practices, including marma therapy.

The primary source of traditional teaching on marma therapy is in the south of India, where this knowledge was well-preserved. In places like Kerala, martial artists are the experts. Kerala's martial art, which focuses on striking marma points to overcome a threat, is called *kalaripayattu,* or *kalari.* Many believe it is the source of kung fu. Those trained in kalari know marma point locations and how to injure any opponent by harming the marmani. The flip side of this is that they are also trained to use the points for healing injuries sustained in training and battle. This knowledge can be applied to therapeutics in the general population, and the elder lineage holders and practitioners are known to be the greatest sources of information on marma therapy.

Marmani can be useful not only for treatment, but for diagnosis. The tenderness a person feels at a marma point, as well as what the practitioner perceives when focusing on it, are both helpful pieces of information that lead to a greater understanding of what's happening in the body. Marma points can tell of the quality or flow of prana in a given tissue or internal organ for example, or the status of the doshas governing the point.

> *I was once in a marma workshop led by Dr. Vasant Lad. I watched as he palpated the abdomen of one of the other workshop participants. She had volunteered to be the case study in his abdominal marma point palpation demonstration. By touching gently and listening to a few points on her belly he was able to diagnose that she had a history of mono from her teenage years, the residue of which was still present in a liver marma near her ribs. In addition to this, he asked about her digestion because he was able to perceive she had recently been abroad and contracted a parasite. She confirmed she had recently returned from a trip to Mexico and that she was having bloating and elimination issues. He then looked at her tongue, named the parasite, told her some foods to avoid, and wrote her an herbal formula. Since Dr. Lad was only visiting our city to teach, she followed up with my teacher, mentor, and friend, Kumudini Shoba. Between the initial formula Dr. Lad prescribed and Kumudini's guidance, she not only received immediate relief but was completely recovered in a matter of weeks.*

ACUPOINTS

While many of the marma points are usually in an area of extreme tissue concentration, right on a bone for example, the acupuncture points, or acupoints, are usually in the space between tissues. There is a Chinese story about how the best butcher doesn't need to force his way through a carcass, he instinctively knows where to place the knife, and the cut happens effortlessly. The Zen of Butchery, however off-putting, is an appropriate metaphor for the needling done by a masterful acupuncturist. Someone well trained and intuitive will instinctively know where to place the needle.

According to Chinese medicine practitioner Jason Robertson, acupoints are sites where "there is transformation and transportation of information, regulation of channel and organ function, irrigation of surrounding tissues, and connectivity to the channel system as a whole."[4] He goes on to describe the connection between the channels and points, how they collectively and individually play an active role in the physiology of the organ systems, and how the channels connect the internal organs to the limbs. One needle affects an entire channel, organ, and indirectly, the whole body.

Each regular channel has the same name as the organ it is associated with. Remember, there is a difference between what we refer to as the organs today and what was meant by them originally in the East. The ancients saw the five yin organs as seats of consciousness, with their own unique energetic qualities and responsibilities. They not only possessed gross physical mechanisms of action, but also subtle, intangible effects that far exceeded the responsibilities of the organs as science has defined them for us today.

In his text *Applied Channel Theory in Chinese Medicine*, Robertson includes his translation of the Divine Pivot in describing the points. "[Among] the intersections of [these] articulations, there are 365 meetings. The knowledge of their importance can be spoken in [just] a few words. [Nevertheless,] to be ignorant of their importance is to invite endless confusion. These articulations . . . are where the spirit qi moves, exits, and enters. They are not [the same as] skin, flesh, sinews, and bones."[5] The spirit qi, or shen, is in one sense the organizing intelligence of the body, akin to the mahat, or universal intellect, in Sankhya. To the Chinese, spirit qi is described as "something that cannot normally be seen or felt."[6] Robertson also indicates that the points are places of interchange, not merely empty or hollow places: "Acupuncture thus creates movement through the open spaces along the course of the channel to initiate a cascade of physiological change throughout the organs."[7]

There is usually a depression in the tissue, a groove, or a puffiness (if the point is full) at a point location. The word for a particular acupoint in Chinese describes its physicality as an opening, as well as its nature as a place of movement. While marma points may help to regulate the srotas, they are not described as lying on a channel or nadi. Acupoints are defined in part by the meridians they lie upon but also by what they access or balance in the body, how they direct the flow of qi through the meridian, and any special qualities they may have. They may be chosen for treatment based upon the location of a blockage somewhere else along the meridian, how they have been documented as being used in the past, or how their use has been passed down from teacher to student.

Acupoints are part of the interconnected meridian network. How the ancients were able to map this network and figure out how it worked is unfathomable. Somehow, they managed to lay out exactly where these pathways were, both internally and externally, where the major points were located along them, and what they affected mentally and physically. Because of the connections between the points and their homes along their respective meridians, it is only part of the story to speak of the points without also discussing their pathways. The ancients used the flow of water as a metaphor to describe just how energy or qi moves through the body. This is a beautiful descriptor for visualizing qi flow along the meridian pathways.

There are two main ways energy circulates through the body: as a circuit with qi moving from channel to channel or as an inward flow from the fingers and toes to the interior of the body. There are several types of points along the channels where the energy of underlying structures and processes can be accessed and manipulated to achieve healing and homeostasis. Source points, for example, are points where a meridian's organ qi can be accessed. There are also points on the meridians through which the information regarding underlying structures, tissues, organs, spirit, and physiology as a whole can be obtained.

There are five transport points—the jing well, the ying spring, the shu stream, the jing river, and the he sea—that lie along their respective channels from the tips of the fingers to the elbows and from the toes to the knees. Consider a river then imagine its source and follow its flow as it grows and travels to its destination, and you have a good idea of channel flow at the transport points. Each point along the route—beginning at a source deep within the Earth and traveling along the flow route to the sea—represents the momentum of channel flow. It starts with that deep well-like source at the tips of the extremities which are the jing well points. The well then springs forth at the ying spring point a little further up the channel. This flow builds from a small spring to a stream at the shu stream point. Qi flow accelerates and builds to the force of a river at the jing river point, and opens into a grand sea at the he sea point by the elbow or knee.

The qi bubbles and starts to flow at the jing well points. These points are used for treating fullness below the heart and dispelling stagnation and obstruction along the channel. The qi begins to gush or flow at the ying spring points, which are good for clearing heat from the body and nourishing yin. At the shu stream points the qi flourishes or pours. These points are good for supplementing qi, warming yang, transforming dampness, and treating the joints. The qi picks up force at the jing river points, which are good for regulating channel qi movement. Finally, the qi dives deep into the body at the he sea points, which are used to regulate organ qi and change the direction of qi when it's moving in the opposite direction of where it should be going.

The imagery the Chinese use to describe the flow of qi through the body is helpful when visualizing what it must actually be and feel like. The saying "go with the flow" is quite apropos in this context. The smooth flow of qi, blood, and fluids through the body is usually indicative of excellent health, both mentally and physically. One can see how the Chinese saw the water element as being analogous to qi and how similar this is to the Vedic seers describing the qualities of air, prana or life force energy, and therefore some aspects of vata dosha or prana vata.

If you've ever been to a spring that bubbles up out of the earth or seen an eddy, you can imagine how the energy must surface at the channel points. The water flows around obstacles like rocks, but if it becomes dammed, its flow is obstructed and it backs up and becomes stagnant. This is a great way to think of a blockage along a channel. There may be some kind of obstruction, and it may take time to emerge, like a chronic obstruction, or it may be an immediate trauma, say from an injury. When the qi flow is blocked, there is discomfort or pain. A block creates stagnation in the channel up to the blockage and can cause a buildup of toxins and maybe even a deficiency of flow beyond the blockage. This is a context in which points can be used to not only access deeper sites of influence but also to heal channel flow abnormalities. Points can be used to remove blockages, correct eddies and restore flow, reduce stagnation, transform or release toxins, and tonify deficiencies.

ORGANS

In Chinese medicine, and to a lesser degree in Ayurveda, each of the organs is described as its own entity that functions as a part of a whole system. Each has a wider range of actions, characteristics, predispositions, and functions than we assign to them in Western biomedicine. In terms of Chinese medicine, the organs have a life or an intelligence of their own. They are categorized as either yin or yang. The yin organs are solid like the heart, lungs, spleen, liver, and kidneys. The yang organs are hollow. They are the small intestine, large intestine, stomach, gallbladder, and urinary bladder. In addition to these are the pericardium, or heart protector, and the san jiao, or triple burner.

The yin, or solid, organs house the five spirits, which the ancients referred to as aspects of the mind. The heart houses the main spirit of the person, the lungs house the energetics of the body, the spleen houses rational thinking, the liver houses transcendental awareness, and the kidneys house the will. This means that if the body is out of balance in any of these organ systems or in the fluids and meridians connected to them, then there will be an imbalanced state in any one of those five aspects of mind. This will be explained more in depth in the next chapter on consciousness.

While the yin organs are located at deep levels in the body, the yang, or hollow, organs all have openings to the outside world. Each set of yin/yang paired organs are related the way they are because their corresponding meridians are directly connected, and the organs themselves are connected via internal meridian branches. Each of the organs' meridians has a point that directly accesses the qi of the organ. The meridians also have points that are like railroad switches that can be shifted to move the flow of qi in the direction of the meridian of the paired organ like trains switching tracks. This might be useful, for example, if a meridian is showing a deficiency. The point on its paired meridian can be needled to move more qi into it and tonify the deficiency. When speaking in terms of the functions of a pair of organs, it is usually the yin organ that is emphasized.

Lungs and Large Intestine

We usually speak about the organs in the order of how the energy flows through the meridians. Energy flow starts at the Lung meridian, so the lung organ system is the first we will discuss. The lungs, along with the spleen and stomach, are responsible for bringing in and maintaining the quantity of qi available for circulation to vitalize the body. The lungs are paired with the Spleen meridian into an energy pathway called the Tai Yin, or great yin. The Tai Yin channel serves as the meridian that regulates dampness in the body.

To a large extent, the lungs help control the flow of qi through the body. They do this partially in tandem with the heart. The relationship between the two can be felt in the pulse when there is a sinus arrhythmia. As the person inhales, the pulse speeds up, and as they exhale it slows down. The qi moves the blood, and the heart pumps the blood. When there is a disordered qi flow, it can affect the blood circulation.

In terms of specific movement of qi through the body, the lungs move qi downward. In Ayurveda, this would partially be the function of apana vayu, the downward movement of the vata dosha. This is particularly important in water movement through the body, as it sends water to the bladder for elimination. The lungs are also connected to wei qi, or the immune defense of the body. Although delicate and in need of protection themselves from external pathogens and internal imbalance, the lungs help regulate the skin's first line of defense to pathogens by opening and closing the pores and sending qi outward to warm the muscles.

Part of the immune responsibility of the lungs begins in the nose. The nasal and sinus passages and the throat are all the domain of the lungs in Chinese medicine. This is part of the upper burner in the triple burner organ, or the region of the kapha dosha in Ayurveda. Like kapha, the lungs should be moist with ongoing secretions that serve to moisturize, humidify, and expel pathogens from their midst. The nose acts as a first line of defense for the lungs in that the nasal hairs and mucosal lining extract pathogens such as microbes, viruses, pollens, and dust from the air that enters them.

Of all the organs the lungs are the most adversely affected by grief, whether recent or longstanding. Have you ever experienced a loved one passing and ended up with some kind of upper respiratory infection or cough? Or perhaps you've seen this in a friend or colleague. It is not uncommon.

The lungs have a symbiotic relationship with the large intestine. When the large intestine doesn't function well, it can cause issues with qi counterflow in the lungs, i.e., the qi does not descend as it should. This can result in coughing, shortness of breath, and wheezing. When the lungs are attacked, heat can result and not only mess up the descending action of the lungs but also affect the function of the large intestine. Oftentimes with bronchitis, pneumonia, or some other ailment of the lungs, there is also constipation. Practitioners will often treat the lungs by draining heat through the intestines using purgative herbal formulas.

In Chinese medicine, the large intestine is paired with the lung system. The lung system takes in nutrition in the form of gasses and qi, filters toxins, and then releases gaseous nutrition and qi to the circulation. It also releases gaseous toxins and wastes from the body. The large intestine receives nutrition and semiprocessed foodstuffs and byproducts of digestion from the small intestine, absorbs more nutrition, and separates out wastes to be released from the body. The large intestine may not be considered the most glamorous or valued of the internal organs, but think of how you feel if you are constipated for any length of time, or how far you will get from your house if you are hit with diarrhea. The large intestine is part of the Yang Ming, or yang brightness, meridian system, which is the Large Intestine meridian paired with the Stomach meridian. This network is responsible for processing heat in the body. This is similar to how the Tai Yin processes dampness.

In Ayurveda, the large intestine is the home of the vata dosha. The vata dosha is the movement principle, but is also very closely related to the nervous system. In the fight-or-flight response, the nervous system makes the bowel empty. Chronic anxiety, nervousness, or fear will adversely affect the large intestine. Yes, it is affected by grief, given its direct connection with its paired organ system, the lungs, but it is also affected by fear and all of its manifestations. Does fear create tension or holding or keep you from letting go? If so, constipation may result. If fear manifests as acute nervousness, acute anxiety, or panic, it may have quite the opposite effect. Perhaps the fear is masking underlying grief. When confronted with large intestine issues like colitis, IBS, and the like, it is important to investigate the presence of fear and/or grief and to contemplate what would be in one's highest good to let go of, either emotionally or in one's life.

The lungs and large intestine organs are also related to the skin—the skin breathes, as we know from Western biomedicine. Like the lungs and large intestine, it takes in nutrition and qi and it releases toxins and wastes. Aloe is a wonderful tonic for the skin and can be used both internally and externally. It can also regulate the bowel. I usually recommend using an internal aloe that does not contain aloin for regulating large intestine heat and dryness. Most of the aloe vera juice on the market has the aloin extracted from it because it is a strong purgative.

Finally, the organ of opening for the lungs is the nose, which is in charge of breathing and smell. The nasal passages and sinuses are extensions of, and are governed by, the lung system. If lung qi is weak, the voice may be feeble or hoarse. The state of the voice is a direct representation of qi quality, quantity, and circulation. If the lungs are weak, there is weakness in the voice. If they are obstructed by phlegm, the voice will reflect this.

Spleen and Stomach

The spleen in Chinese medicine is responsible for the transformation and transportation of food and fluids throughout the body. Whoa, that's quite a task! It is similar to many aspects of pitta (transformation) and vata (transportation) in Ayurveda. When we look at the spleen in Chinese medicine, we see it in terms of the Western medical functions that the spleen, pancreas, small intestine, and to some extent the liver are responsible for. The ancients chose to attribute this massive amount of functioning largely to the spleen. In Ayurveda the transformation function of the spleen qi can be likened to the agni, or digestive fire.

It is important to mention that all of the processes that are carried out at the gross physical level, in this case by the spleen, are also occurring at a cellular level. Just as the spleen is responsible for transformation of food for the body as a whole, and specifically in its role as part of the digestive system, this function is also occurring in the lungs, for example. The air sacs in the lungs contain enzymes that are responsible for breaking down nutrient material that oozes out into the alveolar space during the inhale. These enzymes help to break down tiny particles of protein, carbs, and fats. Upon exhalation, these "digested" foodstuffs reenter the general circulation. Interestingly, the fourth difficulty of the Nan Jing, a Chinese medicine classic, states that between the inhale and exhale, the spleen receives grains and flavors. If there is dysfunction associated with the spleen, it can occur anyplace in the body that there is metabolic activity, from the muscles to the brain. In fact, the spleen and stomach system govern the health of muscle, and the spleen houses the aspect of mind responsible for thinking and memory.

As spleen qi governs any process that is involved with the breakdown of food and drink into nutrition, its function roughly correlates in Western biomedicine to the action of acids, enzymes, and bile in the digestive tract. The bioavailable nutrition that results from the digestive process is called the gu qi, or nutritive qi. It emerges and circulates as a result of the transformation of food and fluids by the spleen.

When we are stressed, constantly thinking in loops, worrying, studying too much, or just overly pensive, the spleen's transformative function is inhibited. This can result in poor digestion and malabsorption of nutrients. In Chinese medicine and Ayurveda, teeth marks at the edges of the tongue that look like a scalloped shell are an indication that this is happening. In Ayurveda, we might say there is a decrease in enzymatic function in the small intestine resulting in malabsorption. This would be due to diminished agni caused by worry. In Chinese medicine we call it spleen qi deficiency.

When spleen qi deficiency occurs due to excessive stress or worry, it may be diagnosed as the liver harassing the spleen and stomach. A well-functioning liver makes us feel like we are in sync with life, like we can just go with the flow. When that is inhibited due to overthinking or stress, the liver energy builds up and becomes like a bully. It moves transversely across the abdomen and invades the spleen and stomach area, thereby disrupting their functioning. This can result in a number of abnormalities like loose bowel movements, hiccups, burping, acid reflux, nausea, and lack of appetite.

The stomach is the vessel for grains (food) and fluids. It has an intelligence that subtly alerts us to what is needed for the body to function optimally. You feel it when you are not following this intuition. Not following it consistently for any length of time enables you to completely ignore its impulses, totally confusing the information the body is trying to send your mind so that you can take appropriate action with food choices. Just as the information a mother's body receives from a baby's saliva tells it what the infant needs from the breast milk, there is a communication from your body to your mind telling you what it does and doesn't need. This is the intelligence of the stomach. In Ayurveda, it is the *kledaka kapha* in the stomach.

When the stomach and spleen are in harmony, the person is listening to and following the body's guidance on optimal food choices. The spleen then has the best raw material to work with based upon what enzymes it is mostly producing and what the body needs. When this happens, there is great efficiency in processing and absorption of foodstuffs. There is no reflux, bloating, pain, discomfort, loose bowel movement, or undigested food in the stools.

The spleen and stomach have a symbiotic relationship in that the spleen tends to become damp and the stomach to become dry. They rely on each other to keep a balance so that this doesn't happen. The spleen moves qi upward, and the stomach moves it downward. In Ayurveda, the upward movement of qi in the body is governed by udana and prana vayus, while the downward movement by guided by apana vayu. This up/down movement must be balanced, and that is a function of the spleen/stomach qi dynamic.

In addition to digestive functioning, the spleen is responsible for holding. This holding is not only akin to the stomach's holding of food and fluid but also an actual healthy force in the blood vessels that holds in the blood. It is also found in the basic lifting function of the spleen qi. It holds bodily structures in place. When it is weakened in this capacity, there can be bleeding, as in the blood vessels, and prolapse, as with organs and hernias.

The spleen helps not only to produce qi and hold blood but to produce blood as well. This is because it is at the root of the transformation of food into qi and blood. The spleen and stomach govern the muscles. If there is an issue with the muscles, such as a weakness or lack of tone, there is an issue with the spleen/stomach. Since the spleen's opening to the outside world is through the mouth, its condition manifests in the lips. Dry, cracked lips may indicate a spleen qi abnormality.

Heart and Small Intestine

In every tradition, the heart plays a key role. When we think of the heart, things that come to mind are courage, love, strength, heartstrings, and heartbreak. When we are overwhelmed with positivity we may say our heart is overflowing. At the depth of despair, it is broken. When we refer to ourselves, we touch our chest, an indication that the self resides in the heart. The heart is recognized in many ancient cultures as the seat of consciousness. It is the place where the pristine, refined essence of qi transformation resides. In Ayurveda we call this ojas. In Chinese medicine it is recognized as the seat of the mind, or shen spirit. Among organs, even in modern biomedicine, the heart is on a pedestal.

The heart is considered the commander of the other organ systems. In fact, it is so important that the ancients recognized the pericardium as the "heart protector." The pericardium is the first line of defense when a pathogen may be on trajectory for the heart. When people are sick with a microbial infection, acupuncturists will not treat the Heart or the Pericardium channel because we don't want to open the pathway to either organ.

The heart is associated with the fire element. Fire, as we know, is transformative. In the cycle of the five elements it is also the main quality associated with peak experience. As a fire organ, its energy needs to be balanced with water, the domain of the kidneys, to which it has a close relationship. Fire/water imbalances are the leading causes of disease in the body and mind. Because they can be brought on by so many of the things we encounter, it is important to stay aware and take care of ourselves properly before things progress.

The heart is in charge of circulation and is related to the blood and the blood vessels. The qi of the heart pumps the blood, which is warm, an aspect of the fire element. From the blood, sweat is produced. Excessive sweating can very easily deplete the body fluids, thereby injuring the blood and also the qi. This all directly affects the heart system since the heart is in charge of the blood, and the blood nourishes the heart. The heart and heart blood also house the spirit or shen. It is the yin blood in the heart that tethers or holds the yang spirit in the body, in the appropriate way. When the blood, qi, or fluids are disrupted anywhere in the body it is difficult not to notice it. This is because the consciousness is tied into the body through the heart organ and the blood supplied to it and that it supplies to the body. There is a very strong connection between the mind and the body via the heart. When the heart is disrupted for any reason it is very noticeable, unsettling, and difficult to ignore.

Too much fire from the heart will disrupt the mind and emotions. Anyone who's ever had a hot flash, trouble sleeping due to mental activity, or an anxiety attack can attest to this. Going through menopause causes heat and heart symptoms. These may manifest as upper body heat sensations, sweating, insomnia or disturbed sleep, mental fluctuations, feeling unsettled, and nervousness. It can disturb the moisture balance of the lungs and inflame the ministerial fire of the liver, resulting in digestive dysfunction. If left unchecked long enough, it can manifest in autoimmune disorders.

Excessive heat and sweating can easily deplete the qi and blood and injure the heart. Good examples of this range anywhere from slight dehydration to heat stroke. Anyone can become dehydrated at any time of year, regardless of their activity. The general rule of thumb is to drink half your body weight in ounces of water a day to stay hydrated. Electrolytes are also important. These carry the pranic currents through the body and help to regulate water balance and metabolism.

If you are exercising or working out in the hot summer sun, it's probably in the forefront of your mind to stay hydrated, which includes not only water but some kind of electrolyte-replenishing beverage. Many people are also exercising inside in really hot rooms or overindulging in saunas at their local gym. The rise in the popularity of hot yoga is also an issue. People pass out in hot yoga classes every day. This is because the heart qi and blood is damaged. Passing out in hot yoga may seem like an extreme and rare scenario, but it's pretty common nowadays. What practitioners often see in the clinic, aside from physical injuries from overdoing it in yoga class, are people coming in with conditions potentially brought on or exacerbated by an overindulgence in hot yoga. These include skin rashes, palpitations, anxiety, hot flashes, difficulty getting pregnant, sleep disturbances, irritability, mental restlessness, and fatigue. One person with an autoimmune condition even told me she thought that although she may have ended up with it anyway at some point, it was accelerated by her addiction to hot yoga.

Because the body's fire is sensitive to external heat sources or overgeneration of internal heat, yoga is traditionally practiced before the Sun rises. In fact, in Ayurveda, steaming the head is not recommended. An Ayurvedic steam sauna isn't a room in which you enter and shut the door, it is a chair you sit in that is enclosed in a structure that allows your head to be outside to avoid heating it. Traditionally, yoga was never practiced outdoors in the sun. If people did practice outside it was very early in the morning or indoors. They also kept the windows closed to guard the body from any breeze that might upset the life airs. When you do yoga, you are opening yourself up to the elements at a deep level. You are inviting deep circulation of qi and blood through breathing practices and stretching of not only muscle but of tendons, nerves, and connective tissues. And you are oftentimes overexerting to do it, which can injure the qi and blood of the heart, which leads to the symptoms already mentioned.

It is recommended in Chinese medicine and in Ayurveda to only exercise until you induce a mild sweat. This is a glisten on the brow in the ancient texts, not sweat pouring off your body for ninety minutes a day. There is a pop culture belief in the power of sweat in detoxification. Although there is some detox that occurs when you sweat, you're also sweating out nutrients. A little known or emphasized truth is that 70 percent of the body's detoxification happens through the breath, if the person is breathing healthily. That's more than the rest of the body's detox mechanisms, including sweat, combined.

Keep these things in mind before engaging in overheating activities. Water is depleted first and most as we age. It is important to protect it. An overabundance of fire can result in dryness, thirst, constipation, insomnia, palpitations, irritability, nervousness, panic and anxiety attacks, heartburn, skin rashes and irruptions, malabsorption of nutrients, racing thoughts, and disturbed speech. When heat has unsettled the mind, the heart, which opens to the tongue, cannot express itself properly. Heart pathologies are very closely related to issues with vata dosha in Ayurveda, particularly issues with the qi, dryness, and movement. Its paired organ, the small intestine, as well as the blood have a strong relationship to the pitta dosha.

Major transformation, a fire quality and therefore associated with the activity of the heart and small intestine, occurs in the small intestine. We know that enzymes and bile transform what we ingest. We know that molecules increase in speed in the presence of heat. If there is too much heat in the small intestine, the speed by which the foodstuffs move through it increases resulting in possible undigested food in the stool, loose bowel movements, and sometimes diarrhea. These are also signs of malabsorption. If this is happening in the body, and the heat in the small intestine is not dealt with, food and fluids, including expensive shakes and vitamins, may not be getting assimilated.

Since there is a direct connection between the heart and small intestine, when there is excessive heart heat it is often cleared by needling the Small Intestine meridian. The heart was traditionally considered so easily influenced because of its fiery, unstable nature, the importance it held in governing all other bodily functions, and the fact that it is the main abode of the spirit, that its meridian was not needled. Some practitioners will only needle certain points on the Heart channel to this day, and many don't use it at all. Instead, the energy of the heart is often accessed through the Pericardium and Small Intestine channels. A branch of the Heart meridian travels internally to the small intestine, and it terminates at the inner tip of the little finger, connecting to the beginning of the Small Intestine channel.

Kidney and Urinary Bladder

The kidneys support the functioning of the entire rest of the body. Once the kidney system is damaged or depleted everything else will suffer. When fire and water become imbalanced, inflammatory conditions potentially result. Digestion weakens, mental peace is disturbed, the body is fatigued, and the quality of life wanes. The kidneys are the deepest and best-protected of the yin organs, indicating their importance to our vitality. They are the root of both yin and yang in the body. As a physical and energetic system they are responsible for storing essence, and they carry our ancestral memory. They are responsible for the creation of all other organs and tissues and for procreation.

The kidney system consists of the right yang kidney, the left yin kidney, and the adrenals. The adrenals can also be interpreted as the yang and the kidneys proper as the kidney yin. Another interpretation is that the bladder is yang and the kidneys are yin. The *ming men,* or source fire in the body, resides between the kidneys. Kidney yang is related to fire, transformation, and internal heat and combustion.

Kidney yin is related to water, cooling, balance, and calm. Water is cohesive and holding, like a hug or reassuring hand on the shoulder. If water is weak, fire can rage as there is nothing to contain it. It rises up unchecked, harasses the heart, and causes premature depletion of the body's deepest resources, resulting in fatigue. If fire is weak, water is too abundant and there may be edema, congestion of lymph and fluids, and a lack of a zest for life.

There is a saying that the kidneys are like two feet on our back pushing us through life. This is yang qi. The kidneys are the seat of will in the body. Not just the will that says, "because of will power I avoid sweets," but a deep will, the deepest one. At the root of kidney energy is the will to exist and to push your existence into creation. Kidney energy taps directly into the limitless void. It has the power to bring energy into matter and to keep it there. Kidney will propels the fetal development. In qigong, the tan tien is related to the kidneys, and it is where we store our life force. In Taoism, it is the root of us and houses our essence, the jing.

I think if you've ever gone through childbirth, you have experienced the power of your kidney energy. It gives you the will to endure, it causes the baby to move through the birth canal, it connects you to aspects of reality you may not have consciously known existed. It is like the bridge or the tether to the unknown. The importance and depletion of kidney energy is clear after birthing, while in recovery from the exhaustion and in processing the experience of the new being who, through the combined effort of his and your kidney energy, was able to manifest himself in this life. How amazing it is that this can happen!

The kidneys have an awesome power. They connect us to the Earth and stabilize us in the presence of the unknown. Yet they can be so fragile if their great strength is overused or compromised. They can be injured by various consumed toxins, lack of water, and fear. There cannot be a discussion about the kidneys without talking about fear. Prolonged, excessive fear is detrimental to our will, our well-being, and ultimately our survival. It is a normal, healthy emotion in moderation and at appropriate times. There are books written about the power of our fear, and how it can be utilized to heal. Sustained fear, however, wreaks havoc on the entire mind/body system and ultimately the kidney energy.

Issues with the mind channels are the main cause of imbalance I see clinically, most having their root in sustained fear, whether conscious or unconscious. Fear triggers many reactions in people, survival mechanisms like anger, depression, clinging to grief, and shame. It is often lingering under the surface slowly draining our kidney energy and unsettling our minds. The unsettled mind often grasps for a myriad of distractions, further disrupting or inhibiting the energy flow within the body. This eventually drains the kidneys and causes conditions that lead to the depletion of kidney vitality. Insomnia is a biggie. It is closely related to the energy of the heart spirit, and the heart and kidney axis is a special relationship between organ systems in the energetic and physical bodies.

Fear has a cold, numbing quality to it. It creeps and seeps. Fear's creation of cold in the body is antagonistic to the warmth we are supposed to have. Coldness damages the fire and dulls the transformative processes and internal flow of information. Think about the nature of cold vs. the nature of heat. Cold is congealing; it blocks movement and slows or stops transformation. Stress creates the fight, flight, or freeze response. Hence, the expression "frozen with fear." Over time fear and cold damage the kidney yang, or warming function of the body, or can injure the kidney yin, or the deep lubricating, grounding, sustaining fluids.

When there is systemic inflammation, the fluids are often consumed by fire, and the kidney yin may be damaged. Remember fluids have the qualities of the water element, and water has an inherent property of cohesion, connection. Once this sense of connection, whether to mind/body or to self/other is lost, a host of other issues may arise. Unchecked heat rises in the body like a fire in a building. This manifests in a myriad of signs and symptoms including cold/heat regulation issues, blood pressure imbalances, dizziness and vertigo, hot flashes, night sweats, exhaustion, and shen disturbances like insomnia, anxiety, and chronic irritability.

Fear keeps us from being able to feel safe in our bodies and our lives. This lack of safety creates misperception, influences our thinking adversely, and affects the decisions we make on a day-to-day basis. Many self-help gurus talk about making choices out of love vs. fear and that when we make our choices based upon fear, we may be blocking our growth and our ability to live to our true potential, missing out on beneficial life experiences. When making decisions, it is not a bad idea to reflect on whether our choices for ourselves and our families are based on trust and love or on some kind of fear. Sometimes fear is valid, and certain issues may need to be taken into consideration when making choices, but as in everything else, there is a natural inclination toward balance that is best not to ignore.

The kidney's paired yang organ is the urinary bladder. Kidney deficiencies are often recognizable by urinary symptoms. Kidney deficiency symptomatology often manifests in incontinence, frequent urination, waking up at night to pee, and poor or weak flow. The kidney energy opens to the ears, so its imbalance may manifest in hearing problems, but it is open to the outside world through the pathway of the urinary bladder. In this way the bladder is a line of defense for the kidneys. Thus, it is very important not to ignore potential urinary bladder infection symptoms. Due to their close connection, an overgrowth of untreated bacteria in the bladder may travel to the kidneys and cause a kidney infection. This is a much more serious issue.

By the process of qi transformation, the bladder removes water and waste from the body. Without a healthy bladder, wastes could back up in the kidneys. In Ayurveda, urine is called *mutra,* and it is a *mala,* or waste. Traditionally trained Ayurvedic practitioners, as well as other types of traditional medicine practitioners, are educated in diagnosing a problem based upon the observation of urine. This is called "urine diagnosis" and involves recognizing the presence of doshas in the urine and identifying any malodor. It can even involve tasting it to check for sugar.

If there is a blockage in urine flow, a start and stop, or an inability to urinate completely for any reason then there is qi stagnation, and this can be coupled with a kidney qi or yang deficiency. From an Ayurvedic perspective, there is a defect in the functioning of apana vayu, which has as part of its function the releasing of waste products from the body. For men, any urinary flow issues, as we know, may be prostate related. The prostate is part of the kidney bladder system in traditional Chinese medicine.

Pericardium and San Jiao or Triple Burner

The pericardium in Chinese medicine is the heart's protector. It is known as *da bao* or "great wrapping." We do not needle the Pericardium channel when one is sick with a cold or flu because we don't want to send the pathogen there and risk it going into the pericardium or heart. Pericarditis would be an example of the pericardium taking on a pathogen and becoming inflamed as the last ditch effort to keep the heart from being invaded. It is interesting that the lung pleura is not seen in the same way, which could possibly be an indication of the great importance the heart holds in the Chinese medical model, as it is the king of the whole system.

The pericardium, like the heart, is considered a yin fire "organ." Due to its association with the fire element, points along the Pericardium channel can be used to clear excess heat from the body. The most used point on the Pericardium channel is PC 6, which counteracts "rebellious qi." This is usually stomach qi or a full Chong Vessel during pregnancy that results in nausea and/or vomiting. Wristlets with acupressure magnets that activate this point and are marketed to treat nausea associated with travel/motion sickness can be purchased in most drugstores.

Interestingly, the pericardium is coupled in Chinese medicine with the san jiao, or triple burner organ. Books are written on the triple burner. It is an organ in Chinese medicine unlike any other. It is considered a yang organ and is associated in Ayurveda with the principle of dosha, corresponding most directly with the location of the primary seats of vata, pitta, and kapha. It is an amorphous organ that is responsible for regulating the dispersion of heat and circulation of fluids throughout the body. There are three "burners" in the body: the upper burner is located in the chest and corresponds to root of kapha, the middle burner is below the diaphragm and corresponds to pitta, and the lower burner is beneath the navel and corresponds to vata.

The three burners are in charge of qi transformation and heat generation, which allows for transformation, or metabolism, to occur in the body. The upper burner is responsible for metabolic activity in the chest. This can be seen as transformation in the alveoli in the lungs. The middle burner governs metabolic activity of the liver, pancreas, stomach, spleen, and small intestine. The lower burner may correlate to the manufacture of vitamins in the large intestine, as well as to some metabolic activity associated with the kidneys. Although it is somewhat common to see musculotendinous issues or bumpy areas representative of dampness in the Triple Burner channel, with the exception of a couple of points for regulating heat or local points for pain, it is typically only focused upon for diagnosis and treatment in the Warm Disease, or Wen Bing, triple burner theory of pathogenesis, which centers on the location of an illness as it pertains to the triple burner. This does not make it unimportant, however, as the triple burner has direct functional ties with the connective tissue of the entire body, the communication pathways along it, the lymphatic system, and the mesentery lining in the abdominal cavity.

Recently, Western science has identified the interstitium as an organ that sounds a lot like the san jiao and has classified the mesentery as an organ. I suspect this is what the Chinese were talking about when they discussed another body part—the elusive *mo yuan,* or membrane source. Until now, this, like the triple burner, has not been widely looked at in terms of disease etiology. Historically, the mesentery was considered to be mostly structural, but I think they are going to find it has numerous functional responsibilities as well. These will most likely have roles dealing with spleen qi, as blood supply passes between the mesentery and the intestines. I believe they will also find it has ties to wei qi, or immunity, as this communication between the mesentery and intestines may have something to do with probiotic strains. It is also a great area for lurking pathogens to hide out in. In addition, the mesentery, if it is the mo yuan, may be the fat tissue discussed in Ayurveda as the foundational fat that generates other bodily tissues, including bone.

It is interesting to speculate about what the ancients meant when they discussed the mo yuan, which I believe includes the mesentery and perhaps some functions of the other organs it has direct contact with. This is located in the middle burner and the lower burner. In terms of channels, it is paired with the Gall Bladder meridian. This means that there is a path of qi that travels continuously along the Triple Burner and Gall Bladder channels. Traditionally, all channels were paired and considered one continuous meridian, not separate entities. Triple Burner 5 is paired with Gall Bladder 41 to open the transverse extraordinary channel that wraps around the lower waist and to clear heat. The most commonly used point on the Triple Burner channel tends to be TB 5. Diagnostically, we usually only emphasize the triple burner organ as a primary cause for disharmony or focus of treatment in the case of wen bing pathogenesis. Rather, we focus on the organ pathology that lies within it.

Liver and Gallbladder

The liver has a hand in pretty much everything that happens in the body. It is responsible for the free flow of qi and blood throughout the system, and any blockage in flow involves the liver either directly or indirectly. One of the most commonly diagnosed pathologies in Chinese medicine is liver qi stagnation. A comprehensive examination of its manifestation lies in the example of PMS. Moodiness and irritability are associated with liver qi stagnation. Because the Liver channel runs right through the breast and nipple, breast distention and tenderness are also due to liver qi stagnation, as is lower abdominal cramping. Depending upon its severity, PMS can also be attributed to blood stasis.

The most commonly used formula in the Chinese pharmacopeia for mild moodiness, depression, tension, anxiety, and the above-mentioned symptoms is called "Free and Easy Wanderer," a name that describes the formula's purpose and is an affirmation for the person taking it. If you aren't feeling free and easy, like you are flowing in the stream of life without going against the current, you have liver qi stagnation. Frustration, repressed or recurrent unhealthy anger, depression, anxiety—all the things we associate with stress—are manifestations of liver qi stagnation.

The liver can also be deficient, usually in blood (red blood cells, specifically) or yin (fluids and plasma). The liver is a wood organ. Wood has a tendency toward dryness; therefore, fluids and blood are imperative to its optimal functioning. Oftentimes we say we need to soften the liver because it becomes either dry or hard. We use moistening and sour herbs and foods in order to nourish and soften this dry, hard tendency. When wood presents with patterns of blood or yin deficiency, there is also qi stagnation. This is because at a root level, the liver does not have the sustenance it needs to remain in balance, which can affect the menstrual cycle, digestion, metabolism, detoxification, sufficiency of red blood cells, immunity, libido, sleep, fertility, hormones, and ultimately peace of mind.

The liver has a close relationship with kidney energy. The kidney is a water system, and in the Chinese generation cycle, water is the mother of wood. Therefore, in order to maintain healthy liver functioning, one must have healthy kidneys. If the liver is deficient, practitioners will tonify the kidneys as well as the liver. In addition, the liver/kidney relationship is responsible for menopause and menopausal symptoms. One primary symptom is sleep disturbance. It is said the liver houses the *hun,* or the aspect of the shen spirit or consciousness associated with our understanding of who we are as spiritual beings. Hun is the aspect of shen or the spirit of the mind/body that we would most likely equate to the soul. In Indian thought, this would equate to the jivatma or individual soul. It is associated with movement, or the vata principle, and becomes unsettled when the liver blood is deficient. This causes dream-disturbed sleep (the mind wandering or moving), as the hun is yang or ethereal in nature, and requires the holding of yin liver blood to remain anchored in the body, especially at night.

The liver's energy is very strong and can manifest outwardly to others quite clearly. This is particularly the case when someone is projecting negatively, usually with some variation of anger. Anger is said to damage the liver. This does not mean that anger is a negative emotion, but that, like any repressed or habitually revisited feeling that doesn't arise naturally as part of maintaining homeostasis, it can upset the physiological balance. Any repressed emotional energy causes imbalance, and anger is related to frustration, irritation, short temper, rage, criticism, judgment, and narrow-mindedness. There is a general lack of acceptance of life as it is and anger that it's not as one wants it to be.

Over time, these habitual mental/emotional states can lead to inflammation, shallow breathing, fatigue, depression, anxiety, high blood pressure, bleeding issues, acid reflux, and gallbladder issues. The gallbladder is the organ that is paired with the liver. It is responsible for holding bile salts for excretion in the small intestine so the body can digest lipids. When the bile duct becomes blocked or stones build up in the gallbladder there is epigastric pain and possibly nausea, vomiting, and loose bowels.

The liver is injured by anger, and in Ayurveda it is said the gallbladder is injured by these states. One may say that gallstones are the physical manifestation of hatred. Luckily, if caught early enough, this condition may be ameliorated with a combination of mindfulness meditation, bodywork such as acupuncture, and herbal therapy. Some people do a "cleanse" that involves drinking a lot of oil in order to "flush" the liver and gallbladder of stones. Though this may work for some, it is suggested that a skilled, trained practitioner be consulted before attempting this sort of process. The body can be thrown out of whack rather easily, especially if there is already an imbalance present. It is sometimes more important to do nothing and do no harm than it is to shock the system into doing something that may complicate the problem more.

BODILY TISSUES

The Chinese and Indian traditional systems of medicine both have theories for how disease manifests. Both recognize that certain parts of the body are more vulnerable that others, and if they are imbalanced or attacked by pathogenic factors, the person may be seriously injured, impaired, or even die. As mentioned in the last section, some organs are more critical to the organism's survival than others. For example, an acute imbalance of the heart will be more devastating to the person than an acute imbalance of the large intestine. For this reason, the Chinese focus on layers or levels of an organ's importance to the organism's survival in terms of pathology and pathogenesis. Generally speaking, the deeper or more yin the organ, the greater its critical importance to the survival of the organism. The more superficial or yang the organ, the closer it is to the first line of defense in protecting the deeper levels of the body.

There are several frameworks in which the Chinese perceive the origin and journey through the body of various pathogenic influences. These may be internally or externally derived. They look at six stages of disease, four levels, three burners, or any of the above, depending upon a practitioner's training and philosophical slant. The six stages emphasize the channel and organ systems. The four levels look more at the qi and fluids and how they are affected. The triple burner considers placement in terms of the vertical decent of a pathogen through the body.

In Chinese medicine the internal organs are closely linked to and govern the various tissues of the body; the fluids stand on their own. For example, blood is blood, a tissue in both Western medicine and Ayurveda, yet in Chinese medicine it is categorized as a vital substance. However, there are still various players involved in the blood process in Chinese medicine. The spleen, with help from the heart, lungs, and kidneys, produces the blood, and the liver stores it. Liver blood is responsible for the nourishment and proper functioning of the sinews (tendons). In this sense, the liver system is closely related to the tissue of blood, but the tissue type the liver governs is the tendons. The other vital substances are qi, jing (essence), and jin-ye, or body fluids. These include interstitial fluid, synovial fluid, cerebrospinal fluid, plasma, sweat, tears, breast milk, saliva, secretions, and excretions.

In Chinese medicine, blood is considered a yin fluid overall, but also has yang qualities. Plasma is considered blood's yin aspect and is more of a fluid, while the red blood cells are considered blood's yang aspect. Blood quality, quantity, and flow, or lack thereof, are all important diagnostic criteria in Chinese medicine. Blood should be plentiful, balanced in constituents, not flow too slowly or too quickly, not be too watery or too viscous, and not be blocked. Blood is warm and is believed to house the spirit. Blood nourishes, and if it is unable to do so for some reason, the body, and indeed the consciousness, can suffer. If a person has a blood imbalance, particularly a blood deficiency, he or she may experience mental fog, poor memory, nervousness, sleep disorders, easy bruising, fatigue, shortness of breath, and dryness of the skin/hair/nails/membranes. If someone suffers from blood stasis, a common symptom is stabbing pain.

To summarize, the liver, spleen, and heart generate and distribute blood and plasma. The liver is in charge of the healthy functioning of the tendons, the spleen is responsible for healthy muscle, the heart is responsible for the vessels, the lungs govern the skin, and the kidneys are related to bone health. Bone marrow is the end product of kidney essence and includes the nervous system and brain in Chinese medicine. Let's now look at the Ayurvedic model of bodily tissues called the dhatus.

Dhatus

In Ayurveda the seven tissues are called dhatus and are as follows: *rasa* (plasma), *rakta* (blood), *mamsa* (muscle), *medas* (fat/adipose), *asthi* (bone), *majja* (nerves/marrow), and *shukra/artava* (male and female, respectively, reproductive tissue and fluids). There is a fascinating model that the Indians created to explain the generation, preservation, and nourishment of the tissues.

There are two ways in which the tissues are nourished. One is that when food is eaten, it is first processed by the rasa dhatu, which takes what it needs for nourishment and passes the rest on to the rakta dhatu. Rakta then takes what it needs and passes the rest on to mamsa. This continues on until the shukra and artava are nourished. The second avenue for tissue nourishment is that each dhatu just picks out what it needs from the digested foodstuff that is circulated to it and then passes on what it doesn't need. This is what the other tissues need so it works out pretty well.

Disease can manifest in any dhatu for a variety of reasons. Usually, it begins with a dosha imbalance, which if left unchecked, progresses to an organ or dhatu level. For example, a kapha (mucus) imbalance in the kapha part of the body (lungs/stomach) can be cleared through vomiting therapy. It is when more than one dosha is involved and the imbalance settles into multiple or deeper tissues that diseases become difficult to treat.

The Three Treasures

The crown jewels of the human body are called the "Three Treasures" in Chinese medicine. They are jing or essence, qi or vital energy, and shen or spirit. We have discussed jing and qi, and will now elaborate more on shen. The term *shen* is usually translated as "spirit" and is correlated with the mind and consciousness. People today expand its meaning to encompass the emotional and higher spiritual awareness as well.

The Three Treasures are the most subtle, refined substances circulating in the human mind and body. Their quality and quantity is a gauge of the overall health and well-being of the individual, and they affect the consciousness as well as the physical body. These three substances are prized in Chinese metaphysical or internal martial art practices and are what Taoist practitioners attempt to purify the body for and to connect with consciously to cultivate, circulate, and replenish their body and mind.

The Three Treasures correlate well with the Ayurvedic subtle vital substances: qi corresponds to prana/vital energy, shen loosely parallels tejas/vital spark, and jing relates to ojas/vital essence. In Ayurveda, these three vital treasures are considered the super fine essences of the doshas. Prana in this sense is the subtle ground of existence for the vata dosha, or the foundational principle of movement associated with the qualities of ether and air. Tejas is the twinkle in the eyes, the spark of vitality associated with the pitta dosha, or the law of transformation containing the qualities of water and fire. It is the essence of agni, or transformational fire, and it promotes cellular metabolism and gives luster to the skin and eyes. When someone has bright, clear, twinkly eyes we say they have good shen, or a healthy spirit or mind, which is a quality of balanced tejas. Ojas is the refined ground of being for the kapha dosha, or the law of sustainability and stability associated with the water and earth elements.

There are two types of essence in the human body: prenatal and postnatal. Prenatal essence is finite, and its presence can be seen in the strength of the bones, teeth, hair, and body in general. Once it is used up, the body dies. Postnatal essence can be supplemented by good living habits like appropriate diet, breathing, meditation, energy cultivation practices, and a balanced exercise regime.

Cellular ojas is deeply nourishing. The highly refined end product of all digestion is ojas and the beginning point of all bodily activity is due to ojas. Cellular prana is vibration. Prana is vitality, energy, vibration, pulsation. Cellular tejas is cellular intelligence, and cellular ojas is often equated to cellular memory.

In Chinese medicine, the kidneys store and retain the essence, or jing. At the most tangible, gross physical level, the essence is the ova and sperm or, in Ayurveda, the artava and shukra, respectively, which get their qualities from essence, or ojas. Less tangibly but just as importantly, essence is a nectar in the body that very subtly nourishes the tissues, including those of the kidney and heart, so that they can continuously perform their life-giving functions. It reinforces the immunity and provides clarity to the mind.

The three vital substances of Ayurveda are the three subtle nourishers of the mind and body and are also heavily emphasized in Yoga, the spiritual counterpart of Taoist internal martial arts practices like tai chi and qigong. In Yoga, one is first purifying the body, then the mind. The mind is stilled so more expansive, subtler states of awareness can be attained. For this to occur, prana/qi/energy, tejas/shen/spirit, and ojas/jing/essence must be in healthy quantity, quality, stability, and flow. In both Taoist and Yoga practice, the higher spiritual disciplines require these three to be in sufficient supply to assist the adept in achieving their esoteric goals. If not, advanced practices may be detrimental to the mind and body.

6

Consciousness

Consciousness is a fascinating topic. No one can completely say what it is, how it operates, or from where it arises. In fact, its origins are unknowable with our current awareness and technology, and its definitions are a hot topic in contemporary philosophy and science. Whether one is speaking from a background in neuroscience, philosophy, psychiatry, religion, or some other spiritual belief system, it seems that everyone has their own professional, as well as personal, take on what consciousness is, how it arises, where it is located, and if it follows us after death. Some believe it stays with us, others that it is us. Everyone has their own personal language for talking about what consciousness is.

In terms of describing the unseen, consciousness is even more difficult to write about than qi, or prana. Consciousness is subjective, intimate. Qi, or prana, is more objective and in many ways a tool at our disposal. Vital energy has distinct, definite pathways and behaviors that we can manipulate to some degree. We have a personal stake in the nature of consciousness, and that attachment is strongly rooted in our beliefs about the nature of life and existence and whether there is an afterlife and what that may be. What we think we know—or hope we are right about in our personal beliefs about consciousness—is tied to our morality, our rituals, our religious leanings, and whether or not we believe in God and what that means. It's also wired to our dharma, our dogma, and what we believe about karma.

Picking apart consciousness when we aren't fully, omnipotently, and objectively aware is quite a conundrum. People have an innate tendency to associate what consciousness is with their spiritual and religious personal truth. Because this is such a messy, emotionally charged topic, it might be helpful to identify the terminology we will use to describe it here in English, from a Western perspective, before going into what it means in Eastern medicine. It's helpful to do this with a little rooting in Western thought. A common ground for discussing the ground of existence, if you will.

In her book *Consciousness: An Introduction,* writer Susan Blackmore tells the reader that a serious study of consciousness has the power to cause big change. She further claims that this may be uncomfortable because deep personal, existential beliefs come into question.[1] One of the faculty in the Consciousness Studies department at Goddard College once told me that even as a lifelong student of Yoga and Sanatana Dharma, she herself did not dare delve into the philosophical or scientific studies of consciousness. This was because she didn't want to question her beliefs, she wanted to keep her mental, emotional, and spiritual toolkit intact because it worked for her and was strongly connected to her sense of well-being at a heart level.

When asking what consciousness is, the answer will vary based upon who is asked and in what context. In this book, we will cover many contexts. The first is universal consciousness, or "nonlocal" consciousness that connects all that is. This level of consciousness was perceptible to very ancient peoples and refers to the ground of being. It is the organizing principle of creation. It is the blueprint for the organization of universes and bodies and the driving force behind it. Nonlocal consciousness is what some Buddhists call "pure mind" and some "the void." Others have more personalized visions of a supreme being, God. Atheists may even have a view of a nonlocal consciousness—called "nature"—as a backbone for their existential belief system.

Dr. Stuart Hameroff, cofounder (with David Chalmers) and director of the University of Arizona Center for Consciousness Studies believes it is connected to fundamental space/time geometry at the most basic level of the universe. His theory holds that because of this, everything in existence is connected, and his work with Sir Roger Penrose provides a scientific argument for the concepts of nonlocal consciousness and spirituality.[2] The belief exists in some scientific circles that consciousness is a part of the original fabric of the universe, and that it is involved with everything in existence being connected.

NONLOCAL CONSCIOUSNESS

Nonlocal consciousness, to which we are all entangled or connected, is that which makes healing and communication at a distance possible. Reiki practitioners are trained in sending healing energy to persons and events at a distance, be that across the room, around the world, into the past, or into the future. They are utilizing their personal connection to nonlocal consciousness to connect to people, places, and things through time and space. Nonlocal consciousness is that which allows us to have an awareness of dreams that manifest in real life or to know who is on the phone before we answer it. Nonlocal consciousness also allows us to feel that those on the other side are still with us.

Unconsciousness is a state of complete immersion in nonlocal consciousness while in the body. It occurs during the deepest sleep, in deep meditative states, and sometimes under anesthesia. Some yogis are reported to have died while in trance because they completely disconnected their consciousness from their body. There are said to be various connectors between the two and severing the primary cord that binds them will result in bodily death. Just as the state between waking and sleeping is at the edge of conscious awareness falling into subconsciousness, transcendent awareness is local conscious awareness tipping into nonlocal consciousness. We may call this nonlocal consciousness a form of awareness because we become aware of it by experiencing it. Paradoxically, the thought that it is being experienced causes the experience to end. Nonlocal consciousness cannot be experienced fully at the same time that the mind is thinking.

Philosopher David Chalmers notes that not only is science lacking in specific theory concerning cognition, but that we have no good working theory for the science of consciousness. He notes that some people believe consciousness is an illusion. Chalmers suggests there needs to be a philosophical framework from which consciousness can be studied and understood, particularly the question of why sensory processing and thought is accompanied by a subjective inner experience.[3] This subjective perception of consciousness would arguably be what we are calling "local consciousness."

There is much detail and explanation of consciousness in Yoga and the related mental discipline of Buddhist mind training. In his book *Marma Points of Ayurveda,* Dr. Vasant Lad, director of the Ayurveda Institute in Albuquerque, New Mexico, describes the various aspects of consciousness; specifically, local consciousness and how we process information in great detail. He calls it "the flow of awareness."[4] The journey from perception to pure awareness happens in multiple steps, seemingly simultaneously. At first an object is perceived by the prana through one of the sense organs. It generates an automatic reaction in us or a feeling in the manas, or mind. We then can assess, label, and file away what we perceive. None of this is possible without reflection from the light of the soul, or pure awareness.

LOCAL CONSCIOUSNESS

Local consciousness is involved with the sensation, perception, and processing of our inner and outer worlds. The inner world is our own five or six senses, intuition, instinct, thought, past experience, and emotion. It is who we feel and believe we are. The outer world is that which we perceive, or the objects of our five or six senses. Some call local consciousness "mind," some equate it to the soul. Some say the mind and soul are not part of consciousness and vice versa.

Shinto, an ancient religion in Japan, involves an awareness that all objects, even inanimate ones, have a spirit or a consciousness that can exact cause and effect. Usually, this consciousness is imbued with natural forces and important concepts and beings, including the dead. Similarly, local consciousness is embedded in a defined object, entity, body, or being.

It is the local consciousness that Eastern medicine focuses on the most in diagnosis and treatment, but nonlocal consciousness is not overlooked as an important aspect of life. Our local consciousness includes the consciousness related to the mind and the consciousness related to the body. Consciousness related to the mind is broken into three states of awareness: conscious awareness, subconscious awareness, and unconsciousness. These are represented in the popular OM symbol (see fig. 6.1), which is a Sanskrit glyph whose shape represents the states of consciousness. The dot at the top is transcendent awareness. The curve it rests upon represents maya, or the illusory nature of existence that veils us from the higher self. The top of the 3 shape symbolizes deep sleep or the unconscious, and the bottom of it is the waking state. The curve to the right of the 3 represents the dream state and the subconscious.

Conscious awareness, or the waking state, is what you're using right now to read and process this text and, more specifically, the text's

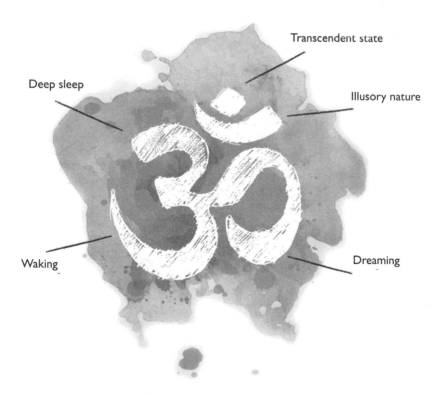

Fig. 6.1. The OM symbol

meaning. Subconscious awareness is the language stored under the radar of our conscious awareness. It can best be accessed by doing self-directed dream analysis. The idea behind this is that we all have an individual language stored deep within our minds. It speaks to us symbolically when we dream, processing the events of the day and communicating our own fears and hopes to us as we sleep. It uses objects, animals, natural forces, events, people, places, and emotions as its alphabet and words. It is the language that is encoded in the body.

In order to decipher what your personal symbolic subconscious dictionary is, write down your dreams. Pick out one theme or something in particular that jumps out at you from a particular dream or series of dreams and contemplate it. What does it feel like? What does it make *you* feel like? Does it remind you of something or someone? If so, what? If you could associate this impression with something in your life what would it be? When is the first time you remember experiencing this thing? How can this information help you understand yourself or someone/something else better or help you resolve a situation you are facing in your life?

Subconsciousness is very powerful. It's your inner child speaking to you. It's your own self speaking to you. It tells you regularly what is really going on with you emotionally and finds many clever ways to try and get you to listen. At first it may whisper. If ignored, this whisper gets louder and may manifest in physical patterns of holding, movement, or illness. This is not a form of punishment but a natural consequence of stifling energy flow and inner communication.

Conscious awareness of the subconscious mind begins to happen as you fall asleep. If you've ever had the experience of not being quite awake or not quite asleep, you understand what this is. Craniosacral therapists call this the "still point." Very simply put, it is a state they encourage the body to induce so that the craniosacral rhythm can reset, and it is healing. This is also the state of *yoga nidra,* or the yoga of sleep. It is in this state of awareness, on the precipice of the subconscious, that one can allow festering or random images to emerge and fade or release or process. This leads to a more integrated state of awareness and a sense of being light, more whole, and healed.

The local state of subconsciousness includes the physical body. In fact, all states include the physical body. Subconscious awareness manifests its imprint very clearly in the body, and it can be directly worked with through the musculoskeletal system. Indian yogis teach that any tension or areas of limited mobility in the body have their roots in the mind. Yoga is about becoming consciously aware of this connection between the mind and body and its implications for our well-being. This includes our ability to access an awareness of or establish a conscious connection to nonlocal consciousness. A yoga asana, or pose, is not just a way to feel good physically; it is a method of using the body to access and heal the mind, which in turn may heal the body.

According to Yogavisharada B. N. S. Iyengar of Mysore, India, there needs to be a vehicle that the local consciousness travels in or upon in order to allow awareness of nonlocal consciousness to happen. This, he says, is prana. Prana is the vehicle, it is the plane that you fly in to get to a state of blissful universal consciousness, or what is also called God consciousness. It is different from a state of self-awareness; it is transcendent awareness, beyond the self.

The terms soul, spirit, and mind are often used interchangeably, but they are not the same thing. Soul is the transcendental aspect of who you are. It is more aligned with nonlocal consciousness, or nonlocal consciousness projecting itself into an individual being. Spirit is your personal power. It is your energy and the personal spin you put on your energy, your vibe, but it is also beyond that. It is what we are animated by, and it is tinged with our natural inclinations. Mind is thinking, awareness, and the mental/emotional life.

CONSCIOUSNESS IN CHINESE MEDICINE: WU SHEN

In Chinese medicine, we talk about the *wu shen*, or the five spirits. In this sense, the word *spirit* is used to mean a force, or a vital part of being. It is also closely associated with the mind and how we come across to each other on the mental plane. Each spirit is related to an aspect of consciousness, emotional life, or mental activity and is housed in and influenced by bodily tissues and organs. The five spirits are interdependent. Inevitably, a long-term imbalance in one spirit will affect the others. Spirit disorders are closely linked to the health of the body. This is because spirit is a yang force and relies upon the yin material of the body to stay rooted and function optimally.

The five spirits are: *shen* (spirit), *po* (bodily soul), *yi* (intellect and conscience), *hun* (intangible soul), and *zhi* (will). The word *shen* is translated as "spirit" and refers both to the five spirits in general and to one spirit specifically. This is similar to there being a prana that refers to vital energy but also a particular prana that serves as one of the five subtypes of vata.

Shen

Shen refers to the clarity of mind. When we say someone has "good shen," we mean that when you look into his eyes you can see that he is fully present with his heart untroubled and his mind calm, happy, and clear. A shen disturbance means that the person is troubled or imbalanced mentally, emotionally, or both.

Shen is like the commander in chief of the other shen or spirits in the body. Just as the heart is top dog in the organ hierarchy of importance, the shen spirit is seen as the central spirit in the human body, and it is rooted in the physical heart. It is responsible for thoughts and emotions, clarity of mind, inner peace, and connection and communication with self and others. If the shen is disturbed it can lead to insomnia, agitation, paranoia, hallucinations, and generalized mental disturbance. Shen can become disturbed by conditions such as trauma, grief, unresolved emotions, other qi or vital forces harassing the heart, internal heat, and lack of fluids, to name a few.

Po

Po is the corporeal, or bodily, soul. In this context, the word *soul* is used to connote a specific entity that is attached to and guides the formation and growth of the body. It is not some generalized force or energy that dissipates upon the death of the body, but the entity that stays with the body at death. This may account for the abnormal preservation of some sages and saints for some time after death; the po in such individuals was probably very strong. The po is individualized. There is only one per body, and it doesn't float off somewhere once the consciousness leaves the body. Sometimes referred to as our animal spirit, po is the aspect of being that is the organizing principle behind the initial construction of the embryo and the aspect of DNA that tells which cells to differentiate into which tissues and which direction they should go in so the body can come into form.

The seat of the po is in the lungs, and the lungs are governed by the po. And because skin is part of the lung system in Chinese medicine, it is also related to po. Po is responsible for sensation and emotion. When the shen is disturbed, and a person isn't feeling well and maybe not sleeping or is fighting something off, she tends to be much more sensitive to the needles. This is because the po will be circulating more closely to the surface of the skin. It tends to lift up and outward in the presence of a perceived threat, invasion, or acute emotional disturbance, and like the lung's qi and yin, it is disturbed by grief.

Yi

Yi is translated as "intellect" and is responsible for reasoning. It is the self-reflective capacity of mind and is therefore linked to conscience. Overactive conscience, questioning your behavior or actions in a given situation again and again, rumination, and self-shaming are all symptoms of disturbed yi. Yi is easily imbalanced in our cerebral lives and results in overthinking and worry. Having its root in the spleen, yi imbalance adversely affects digestive functioning. This can be evidenced by the spleen qi deficiency often seen in the tongues of chronic severe worriers. A tongue with scalloped edges from teeth marks is indicative of digestive insufficiency. This usually occurs in the middle burner, in the realm of the spleen, stomach, liver, gallbladder, pancreas, and small intestine. In one of his classes, Dr. Lad suggested that these teeth marks at the edges of the tongue could indicate decreased enzymatic activity in the small intestine, which may cause malabsorption of nutrients.

Hun

The hun is most comparable to our Western notion of an intangible or noncorporeal soul. It has its root in the liver; specifically, the liver blood. When the liver qi is stagnated, or the liver blood is not at optimal sufficiency, the hun may become unsettled and cause poor or dream-disturbed sleep. This is because the hun is supposed to ground itself in the yin of the undisturbed liver blood at night. When this is not possible, it rises and follows its natural inclination to move. This disrupts the mind and causes dream-disturbed sleep. The liver time of day is 1 a.m. to 3 a.m., and people often wake up around these times when the hun is unsettled.

The hun is the aspect of shen that leaves the body at death and travels to the next place, taking with it aspects of who we were in this life. It is called soul as opposed to mind because it is individualized and more connected to nonlocal consciousness. This is a paradox in consciousness studies! For although the hun is individualized, it is all about connection and doesn't settle well in the body if the person feels disconnected from themselves, others, or the environment for any reason.

Zhi

Zhi is translated as "will." It is not just the will like the willpower we often speak of in our culture; it also includes the choices we make. It is not the decision-making process so much as the actual direction in which we end up going, or the track we put ourselves on. It is an amalgamation of our likes and dislikes, attachments and aversions. Zhi is housed in the kidneys. The kidneys are injured by fear, and chronic fear may negatively influence our decisions and therefore our life path. Have you ever had an impulse to do something fun or spectacular or life enhancing but then talked yourself out of it because of fear? This happens all the time. Fear can also affect our decision-making process by causing us to be stubborn about something that we might better reexamine or by causing us to procrastinate when it would be better to jump in and do what we need to do in a timely manner. Of course, it also has to do with our decision to not stick to integrating healthy habits into our lives.

CONSCIOUSNESS ACROSS TRADITIONS

In some respects it is a stretch to try to directly associate the five Chinese spirits with the five Indian bodily sheaths, but there are some strong similarities. We already discussed the Indian *triguna,* or the three states of mind in Indian philosophical thought known as sattva, rajas, and tamas. Sattva is the state that arises when there is mental clarity, peace, gratitude, compassion, and contentment. This is what we call "good shen" in the Chinese system. Rajas is the condition that occurs when a person is agitated, and the mind is overactive. It is closely related to disturbed shen, unsettled hun, and overactive yi. Tamas is the state that develops when the mind is dulled. It most closely relates to unsettled po, to an overall shen disturbance, and to any situation where our perception is not clear, where we aren't seeing things in their true nature, but clouded by misaligned judgments and misguided perceptions.

In Ayurveda, the states of mind also correlate to the streams of energy moving through the primordial psychic channels, or the ida, pingala, and sushumna nadis. The ida and pingala nadis relate more to local consciousness, and the sushumna channel relates to experiencing nonlocal consciousness. This is the channel craniosacral therapists try to free up. In addition to the energetic flow along the psychic channels, there is an aspect of esoteric anatomy in the Indian tradition that is somewhat congruent with the concept of shen, or spirit, in Chinese medicine and is called the kosha theory.

CONSCIOUSNESS IN AYURVEDA 101: KOSHAS

Kosha is translated as "sheath." Imagine that the physical body is the sheath that the other bodies fit sequentially into, like multiple daggers fitting into an actual sheath. Or you can think of it like a babushka, or nesting, doll where the outer doll is the physical body, and the smaller dolls inside are the subtler bodies. In kosha or sheath theory, we have an energy body that connects to each cell and connects each cell to the next. This energetic form within us, just under and within the skin, is what is accessed and manipulated by acupuncture. We have an overall energetic form that extends outward from the body into the surrounding space a few inches away from the skin's surface, but this is the auric field and is not what we're referring to specifically when we speak of koshas.

There are five koshas in the Indian system of energetic anatomy, and they are categorized from most gross to most subtle. They are: the *annamaya kosha,* or food sheath (physical body); the *pranamaya kosha,* or life force energy sheath; the *manomaya kosha,* or mental sheath; the *vijnanamaya kosha,* or intellect sheath; and the *anandamaya kosha,* or bliss sheath. These sheaths are the subtle physical counterparts that the various aspects of our being function in and travel through.

The annamaya kosha is the food sheath and the primary receptacle for the other sheaths; it is also the physical body. *Annam* means "food" in Sanskrit. The physical form is nourished by food, requires food, and essentially is food at its grossest level. Therefore, it was named the food sheath by the ancients.

The pranamaya kosha is the next sheath. It is the energy body, or pranic sheath. This means that it is the energetic body that holds and connects the physical form and is nourished by food, as is the physical body. It is part of the physical body, and it is in the physical body. The pranamaya kosha is associated with meridians, prana flow, brain-hemisphere balance, and chakras. In the sense that the pranamaya kosha is related to the balancing of the brain and the functioning of the chakras, it is also related to the heart spirit, or shen, in Chinese medicine. This is because the shen controls and is reflective of the emotions, which are related to the chakras, as well as sensory perception, which is transmitted from the body to the mind and brain where it is processed by the prana or qi. Prana also stimulates the beating of the heart and directs thoughts, which affect the state of mind or spirit of the person. This is another way in which the pranamaya kosha is associated with the shen spirit.

The annamaya kosha and more specifically, the grosser density of the pranamaya kosha, would be considered similar to the concept of the po in Chinese medicine. Although not all of the prana stays with the body at death like the po, a portion of it does. This portion is in plentiful supply in some spiritual aspirants, such as yogis and internal martial artists, at death. This is why their bodies do not decompose at the rate the rest of ours do. In fact, for years after the death of a spiritually advanced being, worshippers are said to be able to feel a potency around their graves and will sometimes meditate at their deceased mentor's grave sites.

The next subtle layer is the manomaya kosha, or the mental sheath, which fits within the physical and energy bodies. The mental sheath governs thinking and the emotions attached to thoughts. It pertains to rational thought, fantasy, memory, perception, and cognition. It is most similar to the Chinese medicine aspects of yi (intellect) or the shen spirit associated with thinking processes. More specifically, it is akin to the aspects of yi that are responsible for the way the mind works and those that are related to habitual patterns of thinking, overthinking, worrying, and replaying events as well as shyness, shame, and self-consciousness. The mental sheath is also connected to the heart, or shen spirit, in the Chinese system, as the spirit of the heart is related to the emotions.

The next subtle sheath is the vijnanamaya kosha, or the aspect of mind involved with the intellect and the knowledge of the truth. It is beyond the emotional mind in the sense that it is not affected by attachments or aversions but is concerned with truth. It can sometimes be difficult to differentiate between the manomaya kosha, or the mind sheath, and the vijnanamaya kosha, or the intellect, since we often use mind and intellect interchangeably in our culture. The manomaya kosha—and most of the function of the yi spirit for that matter—is not associated with wisdom but with the presence and processing of thoughts and emotions, which may or may not be rooted in truth or wisdom. The vijnanamaya kosha, on the other hand, deals only with wisdom and truth, without any emotional input.

When perception is accurate and untainted by ignorance or false belief, the action that follows is virtuous. This virtuous action is inspired by a healthy vijnanamaya kosha and is the epitome of a healthy zhi, or will, in Chinese medicine. When our lives are full of purposeful, right actions, we are most influenced by the vijnanamaya kosha, or our wisdom mind. And when we make decisions based on wisdom rather than emotion or false perception, then it is said our consciousness is operating primarily from the higher chakras—the ones associated with the wisdom mind sheath and the rational mind aspect of the manomaya kosha. Healthfully directed action indicates a healthy will and a strong mind, or vijnanamaya kosha, and making positive, sometimes difficult choices based in truth, for the betterment of ourselves and others, and without attachment or aversion, is akin to having a healthy zhi spirit or will.

The subtlest, most internal layer of being is the anandamaya kosha, or bliss sheath. This kosha is our connection to transcendental awareness, to cosmic consciousness, to existence without ego or attachment or defined boundaries. As Dr. Wayne Dyer would say, it is our connection to source. It is who we are at our most unattached, fundamental level. The anandamaya kosha can be most closely compared to the hun in Chinese theory. The hun is the transcendent spirit that survives the body after death and travels to other realms. It is the aspect of being that separates from the physical sheath of some yogis who have reached the highest states of meditative absorption, never to return. It is also what wakes you up at 3 a.m. when you are in a stressful time of life because it is not sufficiently rooted in a balanced, healthy annamaya kosha, or physical form, specifically, that of the liver.

In summary, the five bodily sheaths, or koshas, are associated with the energetic anatomy in the Yoga system and are related to the physical body, vital energy, the mind, consciousness, and the soul. In Ayurveda, we are addressing the first, second, and third sheaths directly and the other sheaths more indirectly by making them more accessible through the physical, with medicinal substances, lifestyle modification, and bodywork. Yogic inner cultivation practices are intentional practices that allow us to consciously access the innermost sheaths.

In Chinese medicine, we address the annamaya, pranamaya, and manomaya koshas physically and directly with herbs, acupuncture, and bodywork and support all of the five spirits, or wu shen. We do this in part by directly and physically helping to balance and heal the substrates—the organs, meridians, blood, fluids, yin, yang, qi, and jing essence—upon which they depend to ground in the body and operate optimally. When these are harmonized, not too cold or too hot, all flowing in good time, at the right pace, and in the right place, then the shen spirits can settle and shine, unencumbered and without shadow.

PART II

Heal Thyself
and Others

7

Understanding Imbalance and Treatment Modalities

According to both the Chinese and Indian medical traditions, diseases originate from a variety of sources and circumstances ranging from the supernatural to the common cold virus. Both Chinese medicine and Ayurveda have complete frameworks for how they perceive pathogens, pathogenesis, diagnosis, and treatment.

EIGHT PRINCIPLES

In Chinese medicine we look at an imbalance through a basic set of guidelines called the "eight principles." When looking at signs, symptoms, and causative factors we ask ourselves if the ailment is interior or exterior, hot or cold in nature, presenting as an excess or deficiency condition, and whether it is yin or yang. An internal cause means that the disease is a result of internal processes. These can be habitual negative thinking and unresolved, built-up emotional energy that disorders the qi. Oftentimes internal causes are the result of poor habits in daily living like not getting enough sleep, working too hard, not practicing good stress management, and eating a less-than-nutritious diet. They are also genetic in origin. We now know that our internal mental and emotional reactions to life can be profound enough to switch genes on and off. Lifestyle decisions encourage the health or well-being of the internal microbiome, which also turns genes on or off, and influences the health of the immune system. External causes start out as pathogens that invade the body or as physical and psychological traumas, such as car accidents, abuse, or falls for example.

Every ailment by nature is either hot or cold. For instance, if you hurt your knee playing basketball, does it feel hot or cold to the touch? Is arthritis discomfort relieved by heat or ice? Does an injury feel as though it is radiating heat? If we contract an external pathogen, do we display signs and symptoms of a cold or heat pathogen? These would include fever or chills (or both), a sore throat, sweating, a telltale mucus color, and so on.

Excess or deficiency is sometimes referred to as full or empty. When there is a deficiency we supplement, tonify, and nourish either with lifestyle changes, herbs, or bodywork. When there is an excess we disperse it by the same therapeutic modalities but use different substances and approaches. If something is in excess or full, it *feels* full. If you eat a meal and feel like it still hasn't left your belly hours later, this is a sensation of fullness. If a joint is swollen or puffy, this is excess or fullness. If an area feels more painful or tender when pressed or even lightly touched, it indicates an excess condition or fullness.

On the other hand, if an ache or a pain feels slightly relieved upon pressure this indicates that the pain is based on a deficiency of the body. Some people will even report feeling a vacuity or an emptiness in their chest or abdomen. This is also considered a deficiency symptom. Deficiency is usually the result of the body's resources being taxed. It may be a current cause that's taxing the body or the result of years of poor lifestyle choices. It can also be attributed to a previous ailment or injury that weakened a part of the body that now is more susceptible to invasion or imbalance.

Lastly, we ask if an imbalance is yin or yang. Remember the principles of yin. It is heavy, cool, wet, dense, potentially sluggish, stuck or still, and material in nature. Yang, as mentioned earlier, is light, hot, dry, quick, transient, moving, etheric, and, like heat in a room—especially presenting with an absence of yin—it rises. If something is more yin it tends to be more damp in nature. Dampness is like a stagnant pond. The extreme end of dampness is the actual formation of phlegm and beyond that a phlegm nodule. Sometimes people report that their limbs feel heavy. This is due to dampness, an excess of a pathogenic yin-like substance. Please know that yin is not a pathogen and in and of itself is not pathogenic. True yin is pure essence, which is a very good thing. The substance of your physical body is yin. It is when healthy secretions build up and become a hazard that yin-like qualities are said to be in excess.

When something is yang in nature it tends to be hot and dry, although heat and dampness can mix and cause a more complicated imbalance that can take some time to resolve. Oftentimes people experiencing damp heat conditions of an external origin end up taking antibiotics to resolve the infection. A urinary tract infection is a good example of this. Yeast infections are also a mix of dampness and heat. True yang, like yin, is a good thing. Yang is your spirit. It moves things and warms the body. An excess of yang usually presents as a hot bacterial or viral infection, a hot-blooded person with high blood pressure issues, or someone with chronic anger issues. Red, hot, swollen joints are more yang than yin.

A yin deficiency condition also presents with an element of heat. This is because there isn't a sufficient amount of yin in place to hold the yang. This happens in menopause. The hormone decline is akin to a yin deficiency, which means that the body doesn't have enough yin to remain symptom free. A yin deficiency can result in hot flashes, night sweats, palpitations, and troubled sleep. A yang deficiency usually results in feeling chronically tired or fatigued, susceptible to colds and flu, and sometimes depressed. Low thyroid or hypothyroidism presents as a yang deficient condition. If there is excess yin in the body, people tend toward weight gain, excessive sleeping, and sluggishness in the peristalsis of the bowels.

By understanding the nature of the pathogenic influence or imbalance we can understand how to treat the individual to restore harmony. The eight principles can apply to external pathogens invading the body or to internal patterns of disharmony. They help us to narrow our focus, simplify the often complex patterns that people present with, and move forward with treatment and future prevention. In terms of external pathogens in Chinese medicine theory, there are other models that serve to help us define an invader, determine where in the body it is located, and decide how to treat it. These are discussed below.

EXTERNAL PATHOGENS AND INTERNAL IMBALANCE

The actual cause of disease when considering external pathogenic factors differs slightly between Chinese medicine and Ayurveda. In addition to qi flow issues and mental/emotional imbalance being primary causative factors of internal imbalance, the Chinese also recognize what are called the "six pernicious influences" (see page 166) as the agents of external pathogenic invasion. Chinese medicine focuses on these external pathogens themselves in great depth, and this flow of thought is more clearly aligned with the Western model of thinking. This is not to say that Chinese practitioners do not recognize patterns of internal disharmony as underlying causes of disease. In fact, they do, and they differentiate between treating the root (cause) or the branch (symptom).

While Ayurveda recognizes the existence of external pathogens that invade the body, and have a pharmacopeia filled with antimicrobial substances to use in such cases, it comes more from the position that without the presence of internal disharmony, no pathogen could take root in the body. Because of this, the Ayurvedic practitioner's primary treatment protocol is to rebalance the doshas.

The idea behind this internal imbalance being the cause of a cold or a flu is that agni becomes damaged somewhere in the system. This can happen in the digestive tract, organs, or muscles for example. Agni transforms one thing to another. When it is damaged, ama, or toxin, can result. In China, the concept of toxin is attributed to severe heat somewhere in the body. In India, a toxin is any unresolved, untransformed residue that sticks somewhere and hampers agni even further, resulting in greater toxicity, or ama. This would probably coincide most closely with the idea of dampness in Chinese medicine, and with its more severe form, phlegm. The toxin can also combine with heat, making it very tricky to eradicate.

This idea of an inner weakness or disharmony leading the body to accept a pathogen has great merit. If you think about it, or if you ever took microbiology, you know there are many bacteria—staph, for example—on our skin and in our bodies that are harmful but to which we are rarely susceptible. We live with them all the time. When the agni weakens, ama accumulates and can migrate to a weak place in the body and become lodged there. This ama accumulation is the perfect breeding ground for bacteria. This is why some people may get more sinus symptoms, and others have more chest issues or GI problems when they catch a cold.

In both systems, one is trained to recognize patterns of imbalance long before symptoms arise. A pathogen can only thrive in an area of weak immunity. Once it does so, from an Ayurvedic perspective, it imbalances the doshas, and this is when we start to recognize signs and symptoms. We then treat the pattern of imbalance, the dosha imbalance. It is easier to address an imbalance before more than one dosha becomes affected.

SIX PERNICIOUS INFLUENCES

The six pernicious influences of Chinese medicine are: wind, cold, damp, heat, summer heat, and dryness. These concepts are not metaphors for what happens in the body but the reality of what is present. If a practitioner says there is cold someplace in the body, then there is a pocket of cold there, and that area of the body may contain one of these pernicious influences. Sometimes the practitioner can feel cold, for example, in an area when they palpate. This feeling is similar to when you walk into a lake and feel areas of water that are colder (or warmer) than the surrounding area. Practitioners may feel the cold in the pulse or in the belly during an abdominal examination. The patient may state that they feel cold somewhere, the hands and feet or a joint, perhaps. Sometimes people are always cold. We, as practitioners, take it very seriously when any one of the pernicious influences is described subjectively or palpated.

Wind

When wind enters the body from the outside it usually causes an occipital headache and a stiff neck/upper back. It can also cause sneezing, a runny nose, and an aversion to cold and chills. Wind is oftentimes the vehicle that carries the other pathogenic factors into the body. Sometimes wind sticks around and moves internally or is generated in other ways. This internal wind manifests as dizziness, blurry vision, vertigo, involuntary movements such as tics, tremors, and spasms, any kind of excessive movement, or, in a more severe form, a lack of movement. It also plays a role in Parkinson's-like disorders, stroke, and post-stroke damage. Internal wind usually manifests at a more subtle level as a facial twitch of some kind. This is usually due to a weakness and

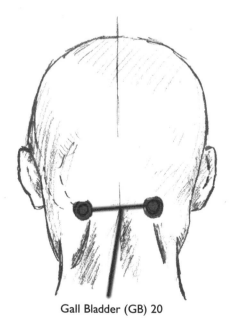

Gall Bladder (GB) 20

Fig. 7.1. GB 20, the feng chi acupoints

vata imbalance caused by stress. The best remedies are acupressure in the area, relaxation, and rest. You can also drink some warm, comforting tea or broth and do some yoga nidra or meditation. Internal wind manifests in the tongue as a quiver.

The best offense for external wind is defense. Always wear a scarf when it's windy and when it's cold. Make sure you cover the occipital points called the *feng chi,* or "wind gate" (see fig. 7.1 on page 167). They are just inside the hairline along the ridge of the back of the skull. If you must leave the house with your hair wet when it's windy or cold please cover it and your neck up well.

Cold

The pernicious influence of cold may bind with and ride into the body with the wind. When this happens there may be fever and chills, clear copious phlegm, sneezing, body aches, and possibly excessive sweating. Cold may also damage the spleen and stomach. This can cause all manner of digestive symptoms, including nausea, vomiting, loose or watery stools, diarrhea, abdominal pain, bloating, and loss of appetite. Internal cold is congealing and contracting. It can often cause pain because it obstructs the flow of yang qi through the system and therefore the warming, softening circulation of fluids that are propelled by yang.

External wind and cold can be hastened from the body through the use of warming substances. A great remedy for wind and cold invasion is a broth you can make to help push the pathogen out through the pores and warm the interior to extinguish the cold. Boil then cover and simmer together fresh ginger, cayenne pepper, scallion, black pepper, and radish. You can also use bouillon and add rice. Wrap yourself up in a warm, heavy blanket and sip the concoction until you start to feel quite warm and eventually get hot enough to lightly sweat. Continue to consume the mixture throughout the day without inducing the sweat, and maybe the next day as well if you feel so inclined. The warming, exterior-releasing effects of the broth should help you feel much better in a day or so.

When you feel internal cold, it is good to apply exterior heat—

usually moist heat—to the body in that area. This can be a heating pad on the moist heat setting or a microwavable pack. Warming teas like masala chai are good to drink. Use a pinch each of black pepper, ginger, cinnamon, cardamom, and nutmeg steeped in hot water. If you feel cold internally in your belly, drink this or just some ginger tea twenty minutes before meals to stimulate agni, improve digestion, and warm the middle of the body. Sometimes pathogens as well as patterns of internal disharmony present themselves through the tongue. Cold in the tongue usually appears as a pale purplish color to the tongue body, the part underneath the coating.

Dampness

Dampness is usually slow to manifest but can linger indefinitely if not treated consistently and diligently. It often accompanies wind when entering the body as an external pathogen. It can manifest in such symptoms as generalized body aches and heaviness, copious phlegm, mucusy bowel movements, nausea, and vomiting. Dampness mixed with heat can present as vaginitis, urinary tract infections, yeast infections, or acute hepatitis. Internal dampness can obstruct channels and result in heaviness, fatigue, mental fogginess, pain, and malabsorption. Dampness can only form in the presence of low agni. Therefore, using spices to enkindle agni is important, especially in the early stages. A tea made from a combination of cumin, coriander, fennel, and ginger is good for this.

Dampness is represented on the tongue by a thick tongue coating. This can be thicker in one area, indicating where in the body the dampness is, or it can extend to the edges of the tongue indicating a more systemic dampness issue. A normal tongue coating is very thin, covers only the back and front of the tongue but not sides, and you can see the color of the tongue body through it. When dampness is mixed with heat, the tongue coating is thicker with a yellow or gray tinge.

Heat/Summer Heat

Heat needs to be managed properly as it can quickly damage the body's yin and fluids. When it enters the body with wind it often causes more fever than chills, sore throat, yellow or green mucus, thirst, and redness.

Summer heat is a more severe heat reaction causing restlessness, fever, scanty urine, constipation, headache, and profuse sweating. Summer heat is an external cold pathogen that the person was exposed to in the winter or spring that hangs out and transforms internally later, manifesting as heat in the spring or summer.

Internally generated heat is associated with chronic inflammatory conditions and autoimmune disorders. The nature of heat is transformation. Heat cooks things, like the body's fluids. Heat also transforms substances from one thing to another as in chemical reactions. The presence of heat in the body may manifest as redness to the tongue body or in a colored coating.

Dryness

Dryness mixed with heat often creates dry cough, thirst, headache, fever, dry mouth, and dry nasal passages. Heat can also cause dryness if it cooks the fluids. Think about high cholesterol or plaque in the arteries. Heat (inflammation) cooks dampness, which adheres to the arterial walls, ultimately narrowing the passages and obstructing the blood flow. Externally contracted cold dryness causes a sensitivity to cold and stuffiness in the head. Internal cold and dryness can lead to bone deterioration and pain. Dryness can manifest as a dry tongue overall.

INTERNAL DISHARMONY AND DOSHA IMBALANCE

There are common patterns of internal disharmony outlined by Chinese medicine that correspond well to patterns of doshic imbalance in Ayurveda. If you go to an acupuncturist, you can ask them what your diagnosis is and then perhaps be able to make more sense of this section. See if you can't figure out your own predominant pattern here, though. The most common ones we see in the Chinese medicine clinic are spleen qi deficiency, liver qi stagnation, various bi (meridian obstruction pain) syndromes, blood deficiency, dampness, yang deficiency, and yin deficiency with heat signs.

Spleen Qi Deficiency

The spleen in Chinese medicine is considered the primary organ associated with what is considered the initial stages of digestion in Western biomedicine. It is an organ system that covers the functions we today associate with the stomach, small intestine, pancreas, and to some degree the liver. Spleen qi deficiency can mean that digestion isn't functioning optimally or that there is excessive menstrual blood loss, bleeding somewhere there shouldn't be, or easy bruising. This is because the spleen is associated with holding. In regard to blood, it's responsible for holding the blood in the vessels. What we usually see in the clinic on a daily basis is spleen qi deficiency associated with poor digestion. Spleen qi in this sense is responsible for the transformation of food and fluids and for balanced stomach acid, enzymatic activity, and metabolic functioning.

When spleen qi is deficient, we may suffer from lots of bloating, distention, and gas. There is probably a list of foods we have trouble digesting, and food may feel as though it passes through the system either too quickly or too slowly. The strength of the enzymes may be lacking or the enzymatic activity lagging for some reason in the small intestine. Stools may be loose, digestion sluggish, and energy low, and there may be an awareness of the abdomen. People who have spleen qi deficiency often report feeling better if they don't eat, or eat only little meals. They may also feel very tired after eating and crave sugar as a pick-me-up.

In Ayurveda, the above list of problems is attributed to damaged or depleted agni. Agni is the name of the Vedic fire deity associated with offering sacrifices to the gods. Interesting that the digestive or metabolic fire is named after this deity, or vice versa. Everything is considered sacred in Ayurveda, even something we Westerners would consider mundane, such as metabolism. It isn't mundane when it works well, though. When agni is good, everything feels good. We feel light, quick-witted, energetic, motivated, and inspired. Healthy agni means balanced stomach acidity, adequately functioning digestive enzymes, an absence of ama, a glow and good luster to the skin and eyes, a healthy strong physique, and a good quality and quantity of prana, tejas, and ojas. Thoughts are productive or imaginative without being heavy and cyclical, and emotions are processed instead of lingering or being suppressed. Colds and flus are few and far between.

Very generally speaking, spleen qi deficiency is synonymous with damaged agni. Again, signs and symptoms of spleen qi deficiency and damaged agni are loose stools, bloating, gas, distention, lack of appetite, fatigue, and worry. The person's tongue often will have edges scalloped by teeth marks. This is an indication of malabsorption in the intestines. Spleen qi and agni are responsible for the transformation of food and fluids in the digestive tract, and in their more refined aspects, of transforming thoughts and emotions.

Agni is responsible for the digestion, absorption, assimilation, and transformation of food into energy. In Ayurveda, digestive patterns are categorized according to four manifestations: irregular, hyper, slow, and balanced. When it manifests as irregular metabolism, or *vishama agni*, it is due to aggravation of the vata dosha. The person has difficulty digesting protein, and there is chronic gas, bloating, and even constipation. Hypermetabolism, or *tikshna agni,* is due to pitta being out of balance. These people have more difficulty digesting fats and oils. They are oftentimes hungry, irritable if they don't eat, and have a large appetite but not the digestive capacity to deal with the amount they are eating. They are prone to hyperacidity, gastritis, colitis, and loose bowel movements or diarrhea, especially if they have consumed fried, greasy foods. Slow metabolism is due to the kapha dosha and is called *manda agni*. These folks have the most difficulty digesting carbs and dairy, and usually crave both. If one feels phlegmy after eating dairy, or starts coughing or feels congested, this is an indication of manda agni. The slow metabolism, of course, makes one prone to gaining weight and can lead to metabolic disorders like diabetes. *Sama agni* is balanced agni. It is tridoshic and leads to proper absorption and assimilation and good elimination. One feels unencumbered by the digestive process, energized, light, grounded, and clearheaded. Keep in mind that agni can be dual doshic, meaning more than one pattern is happening. It can also vary according to age, season, or other changes.

Dampness, Phlegm, and Ama

As mentioned earlier, once agni is damaged or the spleen qi is deficient, toxins (ama in Ayurveda and heat/dampness in Chinese medicine) can be produced and become stuck in the system. Dampness often accompanies a spleen qi deficiency diagnosis in Chinese medicine. We call this "spleen qi deficiency with damp." Sometimes the dampness has progressed to phlegm accumulation as well. Dampness is considered thin and pervasive. Phlegm is thicker and in a more defined locale, unless it is accompanied or cooked by heat, which may cause it to turn to a mist that clouds the upper orifices. This may result in any manner of mental/emotional disorders or sensory perception issues. It can also affect equilibrium.

When phlegm congeals it can create a mass, like a ganglion or fatty cyst. In Ayurveda we might say this is vata pushing kapha into a place and form where it does not belong. Damp and phlegm are ama in Ayurveda. We would say the person has "damaged agni with ama accumulation." Ama can be greasy and sticky and can affect the absorption of nutrients by coating the intestinal wall. It can also veil the senses and cognitive functioning, leading to foggy-headedness.

Treat external wind damp similarly to external wind cold. For internal damp, the course of action varies depending upon where the dampness is and if it's mixed with heat. This can be local or dhatu agni, say, in a muscle, or agni in general, including but not limited to the digestive tract. On the whole, treat dampness from the root, damaged spleen qi agni. The best guideline for this would be to follow an Ayurvedic diet for your type. This is explained in more detail in chapter nine. Basically, not overeating, eating at regular mealtimes, and avoiding mucus-producing foods are recommended. If you eat something and then feel stuffy or mucusy, this is an indication that what you ate isn't best for you at this time.

Drink room temperature or warm water, and sip, don't gulp down cups at a time. Have a little ginger tea twenty minutes before meals. Drinking a tea made with cumin, coriander, and fennel throughout the day is also a good idea. For this recipe, see chapter 8, pages 205–6. If you tend toward anxiety or are experiencing stress, add tulsi to this. Make sure you are breathing well. Check in with your breath throughout the day. If you feel you can't take a deep breath, don't force one. Remain calm and pay attention to how you are breathing for a few minutes; your breath will naturally deepen and slow down. It is quite beneficial to do this before mealtimes. Make sure you are getting some exercise or movement in throughout the day. Do some brisk walking, jump up and down for a few minutes, or jog in place. Bouncing helps move the lymph. Remember that if you exercise regularly, it is only advisable in Chinese medicine to break a slight sweat and not to go much further. Otherwise, the qi and blood may become depleted.

Bi Syndromes

Like external dampness, internal damp, or ama, can create a feeling of heaviness and lethargy in the body. If it lodges in the joints it can cause swelling and pain. In Chinese medicine, any kind of chronic joint pain falls into the category of a bi syndrome. *Bi* refers to a painful obstruction along the meridians, usually with manifestations in the muscles, tendons, and joints. Wind, cold, damp, and heat can obstruct the channels causing pain, numbness, swelling, and heaviness. If ama and pitta mix it will create hot, swollen joints that are worse in humidity. This would be considered heat bi, maybe even heat bi with damp. If ama mixes with vata then joint symptoms will be activated by cold and/or wind. This is wind or cold bi or wind/cold bi. Oftentimes, since the nature of ama is damp and heavy, rainy, dark, cloudy days will make joints feel worse. This, of course, is considered damp bi. Oftentimes practitioners will prescribe herbal formulas that drain and transform dampness. As a home remedy, applying aromatic massage oils or castor oil packs to the affected joints once or twice daily can be helpful.

Liver Qi Stagnation

Liver qi stagnation is roughly imbalanced pitta and disrupted flow of prana vata. It presents as an inability to go with the flow. This pattern is usually habitual and oftentimes doesn't get acknowledged or addressed until the person is so angry, anxious, tired, or stressed that they can't stand it anymore, or they are manifesting physical symptoms. Liver qi stagnation can look like a like a type A personality. Perfectionism, over-work, and having to be in control are possible aspects of liver qi stagnation. The sides of the tongue are the liver areas. While liver issues may cause the entire tongue to be redder than usual, it is predominantly the sides or edges that will be reddened or redder. Sometimes they'll even be orange.

When liver qi stagnates, it can lead to a variety of signs and symptoms and may be the cause of more serious ailments long term. One of the liver system's responsibilities is to ensure the smooth flow of qi and blood throughout the body. When this flow is slowed, disrupted, or hastened, it can build up in the midsection of the body and cause aggravation, irritability, unreasonable expectations, and overly judgmental thinking, both toward oneself and others. Physically, this buildup needs someplace to go. Oftentimes it will travel across the body and impinge upon the proper functioning of the spleen and stomach. This can lead to overthinking, worry, and digestive complaints like excessive gas and bloating, belching, sluggish appetite, increased appetite (to dull the emotional discomfort of the stagnation), reflux, nausea, and loose stools. If liver qi rises upward and harasses the lungs, it can lead to shortness of breath, repressed grief, anxiety, cough, and fatigue.

The emotional/mental and digestive symptoms of liver qi stagnation are all associated with damaged pitta and agni and vata imbalance in Ayurveda. In fact, any qi stagnation is a vata imbalance because if something is stagnant, its movement is affected. However, if prana/qi flow is *obstructed*, that is different than saying that qi is stagnant. In the case of obstructions, there is an actual blockage impeding the flow. This blockage can be one of the six pernicious influences or a mass. Qi stagnation/prana flow issues can mean the energy is flowing in the wrong direction, in an unhealthy pattern, too slowly, too quickly, or there is not enough. Then, when qi or prana stagnates, there is a friction and/or a buildup that can create heat. This is how an internal heat condition or pitta imbalance can manifest. With liver qi stagnation, there is oftentimes an element of heat present, even if the person feels cold or has cold hands and feet. Sometimes the stagnation of energy creates an internal energy movement and holding that prevents the qi and blood from effectively circulating to the extremities.

When we are overly critical, easily frustrated or angered, aggravated, and impatient the pitta is considered to be out of balance. Damaged pitta and agni can cause acidity, nausea, and loose stools. Vata disorders can lead to worry, overthinking, gas and bloating, belching, irregular appetite and digestion, anxiety, and breathing issues. When liver qi stagnation intensifies, particularly in a person with a naturally pitta-predominant constitution, it can turn to liver yang rising. As we know from fire in the external environment, smoke and heat rise. Yang qi is warm. When liver yang rises, it causes extreme anger, sweating, shouting, angry outbursts, a red face, and an accelerated heart rate. As a repeated physiological and behavioral pattern this can be dangerous and in its most extreme form is called liver fire. It can lead to high blood pressure and certain kinds of stroke.

Liver wind issues cause paralysis, Bell's palsy, tics, tremors, muscle twitches, spasms, and any other involuntary movements. Liver wind, as wind implies, has to do with movement or the lack of it. Any movement is associated with air or vata in Ayurveda, and therefore is treated at its root as a vata imbalance. We try to calm the wind, or calm and regulate the vata. In Tibetan and Greek medicines, vata is called wind. This is because the most influential characteristic of vata is movement. The secondary aspects of vata include dryness, cold, and roughness.

Start treating liver qi stagnation before it progresses to something more serious like liver yang rising, liver fire, or liver wind, or is so chronic you are basically unhappy. Exercise is helpful for moving the qi and blood, as is deep abdominal breathing. When you breathe deeply, the diaphragm presses down and massages the liver. If the breath is shallow, the Chinese say the qi hits the liver and exits. They go on to say that when this happens that a zang, or yin, organ is depleted, namely the kidney. This means the in-breath isn't deep enough to nourish the kidneys. The kidney is the mother of the liver. If the mother is deficient how can the child thrive? The diaphragm is called the dynamic heat exchanger between the upper and lower aspects of the torso. If it isn't moving properly, heat is being trapped. Essentially, this is the heat caused by stagnation that has festered and triggered an imbalance. It then creates a catch-22 that encourages a lack of movement. Therefore, pay attention every so often throughout your day to your breathing. Your liver will thank you. Avoid greasy, fried, fatty foods, high-sugar foods, caffeine, and alcohol.

Blood Deficiency

In Chinese medicine we say the liver stores the blood, and sometimes the blood is depleted or consumed. Blood depletion can occur as a result of overactivity, trauma, intense prolonged stress, long illness, heat conditions, or excessive sweating. This can cause dryness or an increase in the vata dosha. A severe blood deficiency may be considered anemia in Western biomedicine. This also may be true in Chinese medicine at the more extreme end of blood deficiency's spectrum of manifestation, and we can often catch it before it progresses to anemia.

Someone with blood deficiency may be tired, forgetful, a light sleeper, a heavy dreamer, have difficulty concentrating or vision issues, have a pale complexion and tongue, a thin pulse, heart palpitations, and cold hands and feet, feel cold more easily than someone without blood deficiency, and experience dry skin, hair, and nails. Issues with the blood in Ayurveda usually fall into the category of pitta disorders. However, the lack of nourishment due to blood deficiency can cause not only deficiency heat but dryness. Dryness is a primary guna of vata. Since like increases like, the increase in dryness increases vata and its associated signs and symptoms. Blood deficiency is also a type of yin deficiency. This is because all the fluids of the body are yin.

Yin Deficiency

Although some would argue this point, menopause with its related symptoms is generally diagnosed as yin deficiency. Many of the symptoms of menopause present as insufficient yin. Yin, like kapha, is about body fluids and lubrication, and it also has to do with the hormones that are responsible for regulating the menstrual cycle and keeping the structure of the body strong and supple. Yin is a heavy, cool, dense, moist substrate. When it is not in sufficient supply in the body, the body becomes drier, warmer, and lighter or less dense. The bones become more porous, and the soft, plump, roundness and moistness associated with youth all wane. When this cooling, nourishing aspect of being diminishes, we may experience mucosal dryness in the eyes, mouth, and vagina. The skin, hair, and nails can become more dry, thin, and brittle. The joints become weaker and less supported, and heat can rise creating hot flashes, mood swings, irritability, palpitations, and insomnia. Yin deficiency looks like damaged pitta with vata imbalance.

Yin deficiency usually presents with a red tongue that has little to no coating or a mapped coating. The body typically needs to be nourished and cooled. Regular self-massage with a nourishing, constitutional-appropriate or tridoshic massage oil is best (see chapter eight), provided there is not ama present in the deeper tissues. Restful, adequate sleep is necessary, so focus on sleep hygiene. Do your best to take care of yourself and not overwork. Take baths and walk in nature, preferably around water. Shatavari and dang gui are good herbs for yin deficiency but always check with a practitioner before taking anything.

Yang Deficiency

Yang deficiency, like yin deficiency, can manifest at any age, but it usually gets worse as we get older. It is characterized by fatigue and coldness. Yang is light, dry, and hot in nature. When yang is deficient it can affect the circulation, resulting in channel obstruction, poor appetite, loose stools, excessive sleep without feeling rested, heaviness, lassitude, lack of motivation, sadness, depression, mental sluggishness, cold extremities, and a potential for fluid accumulation. Yang is associated with the kidney energy at its root, and the kidneys govern the low back, hips, legs, knees, ankles, and feet. Yang deficiency can commonly cause low back, hip, and knee pain, especially after exercise and at night. Yang deficiency can also be behind edema or lymphatic congestion, which can occur because fluids are yin, cool, and heavy and need the light, moving, warming nature of yang to move and transform. A yang-deficient tongue may be pale and puffy and wet or any combination of these. Yang deficiency is usually associated with a kapha imbalance, weak agni, and a possible ama accumulation.

Ashwagandha and ginseng are the most popular herbal products for yang-deficiency symptoms. Light exercise, energizing pranayama techniques, breath awareness, and keeping warm are helpful. Spicy teas that warm the interior and enkindle agni are also beneficial. A sprinkle of trikatu in a shot of warm water before meals can help with digestion. Bone broth is also good as it tonifies yin and blood and nourishes the body deeply, giving it a chance to restore itself. It is easy to digest and prebiotic. Getting out of the house and socializing with uplifting, kindred spirits is essential. Taking time for oneself is also important. Self-massage with warm sesame oil gets the circulation and lymph flowing and warms the body. Yoga nidra and mindfulness meditation are helpful as well. In fact, mindfulness meditation is recommended for preventing any pattern from manifesting or for catching them in their early stages so they can be reversed.

In Western medicine we wait until symptoms are already present before seeking treatment. In Chinese medicine this is often the case as well. For students of Chinese medicine, training is quite clinical and heavily geared toward treating both acute and chronic conditions. Cultivation practices may be introduced and encouraged, but it is largely up to the student, and later the practitioner, to explore what wellness is for himself or herself. In Ayurveda as it is taught in the West, the situation is reversed. We begin with exploring wellness, just scratching the surface of the clinical. In Chinese medicine there is some dietary and lifestyle guidance training in the West, but there is far more in an Ayurveda course. The Chinese system encourages a clinical experience for an acupuncture session, and insurances don't cover prevention. In many European countries you must be a licensed medical doctor in order to legally perform acupuncture. This causes people to think of the acupuncturist only for pain relief or symptom management as opposed to looking to a Chinese medical practitioner as a resource for better living. Looking at our health in terms of constitutional tendencies and personal patterns of thinking, feeling, and behavior is a paradigm shift in our beliefs about wellness, the mind, and the body.

An important thing to remember in both Chinese and Ayurvedic medicine theory and practice is that there is rarely an uncomplicated, simple pattern. Seldom do we see just qi stagnation, just a vata imbalance, just heat, just cold, or just damp. Oftentimes these pernicious influences and doshic patterns are complicated, occurring in tandem and mixing with each other. Damp and heat often mix, as do wind and damp, cold and heat, and excess and deficiency. It takes a well-trained, intuitive, experienced practitioner to regularly be able to correctly assess which layer to treat first and how to treat it.

8

Prevention and Maintenance

We've all heard the saying, "the best offense is a good defense," and this is certainly the case where health and wellness are concerned. It is always better not to get sick or too far out of balance in the first place. Once the balance is off severely enough or long enough, it is difficult or even impossible to reverse. Asian medicines recognize that there are diseases that are easily treated, those that take time and management to resolve, and those that are irreversible.

If you haven't already, now may be a good time to take the constitution quiz in chapter 4 and reread the sections on the elements and the doshas. By having that information fresh and keeping yourself in mind, you can read through the rest of this section, particularly the parts about daily routine and diet, and be able to more easily use the information for your own well-being.

Sometimes people think alternative medicine can offer miracle cures. This may on rare occasions be the case, as it can be in Western medicine, but it is important to note that Ayurveda and Chinese medicine are still medical systems that operate within the realm of nature just like allopathic biomedicine. This is why it is so important for us to understand our natural tendencies and how to manage them best to stay well. Another thing to consider is if you feel you suffer from any of the six pernicious influences. If so, know that like increases like, and that any change in weather, climate, or season will positively or adversely affect you based upon which influence(s) is the strongest. For example, if you regularly suffer from dryness and live someplace with forced-air heat, then you know winter will be aggravating to you, so you should get a good humidifier. Another example would be if you suffer from dampness and you live in a wet climate like Seattle. You will then be more susceptible to the effects of the damp weather there and will need to take steps to keep yourself warm and dry.

There are so many little adjustments we can make to improve our quality of life and well-being. Many are outlined in this chapter. Some take a little knowledge, like that provided in the morning and evening routine sections; others take getting yourself to a practitioner. Whatever you resonate with most is a great place to start. I recommend effecting change at a doable pace. Recently, many wonderful studies on habits have come to light. It turns out that if you start by changing one tiny thing, the rest of your life will start to shift and change for the better will naturally happen in other areas. So take it easy. If you try to do too much at once, it may not stick. As the salesman told me when I left the showroom with my new Vespa, "Slow and steady wins the race." I recommend that you choose an area that resonates with you and shift one thing. My personal favorite is to be mindful of the breath.

BREATHWORK

The number one thing we can do to improve our quality of life right now is to breathe well. This simple act restores an optimal flow of energy through our meridians, increases positivity and calm, and fully oxygenates and detoxifies our tissues. Seventy percent of bodily toxins are released through the breath. The way we breathe affects how we feel not just physically but emotionally. Breathing well can induce a sense of peace and calm and reduce stress. It can also help with circulation, digestion, immunity, and sleep.

Yoga master T. K. V. Krishnamacharya used to diagnose his clients' health issues by watching them breathe. This is because he could see and sense how people were breathing and how their breath was imbalanced. He could intuit how breathing patterns are connected to disease. He knew that emotional energy influences the flow of vitality through the body. Discomfort or trauma can adversely affect the body by creating a pattern of flow, or lack thereof, that lodges in the tissues and affects our posture and the way we move. This all affects the quality of the breath. When the breath is blocked or the body cannot breathe effortlessly, there is a subsequent imbalance in the flow of vitality. This can result in unconscious holding patterns in the body and negative thinking loops that affect our overall health.

Once these patterns are set they become reinforced over time, like a habit that becomes what we do moment to moment. These unconscious reactions to life are barely noticeable and can build up or get layered, one on top of another. When this happens we get further from the truth of ourselves. Through the breath, we can get back to a state of wholeness and well-being. This can be done by sitting quietly for just five or ten minutes a day and observing the breath. Although there is information included here on what an optimal breath looks like, it may not be what you experience while you are watching yours, and that's okay.

There is a process for using the breath to heal. The first step in this process is awareness. Self-awareness is the key to using the breath for healing, paradoxically, without trying to shift or change it. Allowing is the second step. Allowing leads to accepting the breath as it is. When a person is aware of the breath as it is without trying to change what it is doing, something magical happens: the body automatically begins to relax and breathing becomes more comfortable. When they begin observing the breath, people often notice that they start thinking it should be different from how it is. This makes them feel like something is wrong, and they are uncomfortable with their own breath. Although this may be a common reaction, it is not something to act upon. Simply notice the thoughts that are arising as you become the compassionate witness to your own breathing and the feelings that accompany those thoughts.

Allow feelings and thoughts buried beneath conscious awareness to surface for processing. Acceptance of what those thoughts and beliefs are, without judgment, is huge. And if you can do it with your breath, it may just start seeping into how you perceive the world at large. We formulate judgments about things to differentiate self from other and other from other. This is a developmental process that is important to the intake and assimilation of information. The problem arises when we use this skill against ourselves and others. Instead, just sit and watch the breath without attachment or aversion to it, simply be aware of it as an observer and allow it to breathe you. In this way, the conscious mind is letting the subconscious know that it is safe to breathe. By doing this practice, repeated patterns of unhealthy breathing that may be the holding pattern for suppression or misdirection of vital energy may begin to be corrected.

An optimal breath originates from the diaphragm. This means it is important to have the belly in a relaxed state. Tell that to a young gal trying to suck it in to look good, or someone suffering from chronic anxiety whose body is naturally holding their belly in due to the fight-or-flight reaction being chronically activated. The belly should be supple much of the time. On an in-breath, the abdomen protrudes, the rib cage opens, and air fills the space from the pelvic floor to the upper back and chest. On the out-breath the thorax deflates like a balloon, and air leaves the whole abdomen and chest, rushing most quickly from the lower portion of the thorax, then the middle, then the upper. It's that simple. Breaths flow in and out through the nose, shoulders are relaxed, inhales and exhales are about even, and there is no straining or holding of any kind. The entire breath cycle—the inhale, transition from inhale to exhale, the exhale, and the pause after the exhale—is effortless and free.

It is healthy to breathe, on average, about twelve times per minute. This of course will change with physical exertion, meditation, or illness. We also breathe faster and more shallowly under stress and if we are upset or angry. Anything above sixteen times per minute at rest indicates breathing trouble.

It is recommended to sit in a comfortable position and to observe the breath coming in and out through the nostrils. Is it cool or warm? Does it move equally through both sides?

Now notice how you are breathing further down in your body. What moves when you breathe? Your shoulders? Your back? Your belly? What doesn't move when you breathe? Ideally, over time, on a subtle level, your whole body will feel like it moves. Organs rock with the rhythm of the breath, and a subtle buzz hums through every cell and pore. But for now, you are observing and not trying to make anything happen.

Notice if you feel most comfortable with the inhale or the exhale. How is the transition? How is the pause? Which part of your breath cycle do you like the best? Which part do you like the least? You may find this will change over time. Please don't try to breathe over any areas of discomfort like you're trying to power through them or minimize their presence. This does not allow the life force to unearth deep unhealthy breathing patterns at the root. It only reinforces any misdirected flow or blockage that already exists. In fact, it may further cover it up. Just let it flow. Believe that with disciplined practice and the intention to heal, things will shift.

The breath cycle begins with the in-breath (see fig. 3.1 on page 59). After we inhale, there is a pause that happens between the inhalation and exhalation. This is where the spleen qi does its work in the lungs. There are enzymes in the alveoli, the little air pockets in the lungs. The Chinese classics state that between the inhale and the exhale "the spleen receives grains and flavors." This means that those little enzymes are digesting what is passing through the capillaries in the alveoli in that moment. Amazing, isn't it? After the pause, there is the exhale. At the bottom of the exhale there is another, longer pause. This is the place where yogis suspend the breath as they enter a state of transcendental awareness, samadhi, or enlightenment.

Breathwork can be very powerful, delightful, and sometimes even a little scary. Having a consistent intention to breathe well and establishing a practice sets the wheel in motion toward better well-being. Once you have established a practice, the body will start to breathe better when you aren't even thinking about it. Emotions you aren't expecting can surface at any time, whether it's convenient or not, and whether it makes sense or not. This can occur even when you aren't sitting and quietly witnessing. To know this may happen can help you feel safe if it does. Just breathe into it and through it and allow it to pass. When establishing a practice, start with short sessions, maybe two to three minutes at first, and let them lengthen gradually over time. Breathwork is not something to rush into or approach like you're training for the Olympics. If you try to pay attention to your breathing all day, you can actually create an imbalance. Breathing is largely meant to be an involuntary practice so give your observations a rest for most of the time and just let it be. Be patient. Sometimes big stuff can emerge, and if it does, it isn't always the best idea to try to manage it alone. If you find you are having trouble witnessing the breath, pick a different aspect of your life to shift and seek out a trained professional to assist you with anything your breathwork may have brought up.

MINDFULNESS

Mindfulness is such an amazing therapeutic tool. It is wonderful for calming anxiety and stress, and current research is finding that it's also linked to reducing systemic inflammation. More and more we are finding inflammation plays a key role in disease etiology. Reducing it in a way that is not only beneficial to us physically but also mentally and emotionally is such a gift. Mindfulness can be applied to any situation. *Any* situation. It can be utilized to deal with impatience when you're in line at the store, with pain, with uncomfortable emotional responses, and with typically uncomfortable situations ranging from dental procedures to childbirth.

To practice mindfulness you don't need special equipment or fancy clothes. It can be practiced when you are just lying in bed before you fall asleep. It can also be done as a meditation practice. If you are lying down in bed, simply make yourself comfortable. If you're comfortable being on your back, this is the best position. You can also do this seated if you're doing a meditative practice. Let your legs and arms relax and do a body scan by placing your awareness on each body part one at a time in a natural order as described below.

Start by following the breath in and out of your body. Once you are feeling settled, take your attention to the head. What does your head feel like? Is it achy? Heavy? How does it feel resting on whatever surface you are lying on? What does the temperature of your head feel like? Is there anything that feels uncomfortable in your head or face? If so, stay with this for a couple of moments and allow yourself to experience whatever this sensation is while continuing to breathe. Notice if there are any thoughts associated with the discomfort or any feelings associated with the discomfort or with the thoughts you are having about it. Do not try to change how you're feeling; just breathe and be aware of it.

Move on to the neck, shoulders, and upper back. Do the same awareness exercise in each area. Check in with your arms, elbows, wrists, hands, and fingers. Move to your chest, mid back, and ribs. Notice your belly, above and below the navel. Feel your sides, waist, and low back. Pay attention to your hips, pelvis, and pelvic floor. Go to your groin and legs, the upper then lower. Bring awareness to your knees, ankles, feet, and toes. Do this slowly. Take your time. After you've done a complete body scan go back through and see how things have shifted, if at all.

This exercise may take around twenty minutes and can be done seated as part of a meditation practice. If seated, sit with your legs crossed or in a chair with your feet on the floor and your spine lifted and long, but relaxed. You can check in with specific muscles or organs on the way. If you are in a hurry, just bring your awareness to what you notice the most in your body at the moment. Anchoring awareness in the body helps us to know ourselves better and allows the body to relax into what is. When it can do this, it is easier for it to heal. It also helps us to be with what is without trying to fight or change it. It can help us take our energy back from fearful thoughts and emotions because over time, awareness that we are more than what we think and feel somatically becomes more powerful than the discomfort.

There comes a time when most of us begin to contemplate our bodily mortality. Making our experience of our mortality part of our daily practice serves to open us to a greater truth, a deeper sense of connection, and daily gratitude. It better prepares us for life's constant change, of which we are all observers and experiencers in the grand scheme of things. Letting go and manifesting is such a balance. At some point though, we must release our grasp. Whether it is in letting go of the small ways in which we engage on a daily basis that cause us to be controlling or fearful and not able to fully enjoy our lives, or it is in the more existential way, it is the same muscle we are using. This surrender to the flow is what mindfulness helps us to achieve so that we may better enjoy our existence. It assists the body in healing, the mind in becoming more clear, the emotions in being more balanced, and our spirit in feeling free within the material confines of this body, in this life, in this place at this time.

When I was in India studying at Pattabhi Jois's yoga shala, he would host weekly question-and-answer sessions. At one of these sessions, a student asked how long one should remain in the pose called savasana. Savasana, pronounced sha-VA-sa-na, translates as "corpse pose." Savasana is usually done for about twenty minutes at the end of a yoga pose, or asana, practice. Mr. Jois went into a moment of deep thought. He then expounded a beautiful explanation of what savasana actually is. His reply was that it takes lifetimes to perfect savasana because it is practice for recognizing consciously and deeply to our core that we are not the body. This recognition assists us in leaving the body at the time of death through the proper energy channel and going on to the best place energetically in the afterlife without being overly attached to it or anything else in life. This is also why it is called the posture of the corpse—it is how the body is ultimately viewed in the later stages of yoga practice. Although the chap who asked the question was dissatisfied with the answer, as he was looking for a specific number of minutes, I was quite happy with it.

ESTABLISHING A DAILY ROUTINE

Ayurveda and Chinese medicine both have a system in place for organizing one's daily routine. On a grand scale, there are seasonal patterns, mostly having to do with the Sun cycle, and on a daily scale there are bodily patterns, also affected by the sun, that influence the energetic flow through the meridians and organs and indicate the most active doshas at any given time throughout the day. The body clocks are great guidelines for when to do or not do certain things in order to maintain the greatest sense of harmony. They are also diagnostics for understanding why things happen when they do at certain times of day. These bodily patterns fall into two four-hour time slots, around the clock. Ayurveda recognizes these four-hour periods as times when certain doshas are more active. Chinese medicine looks at the body clock in terms of meridian and organ activity changing every two hours.

In Ayurveda, the organ clock (see fig. 8.1) is ordered as follows:

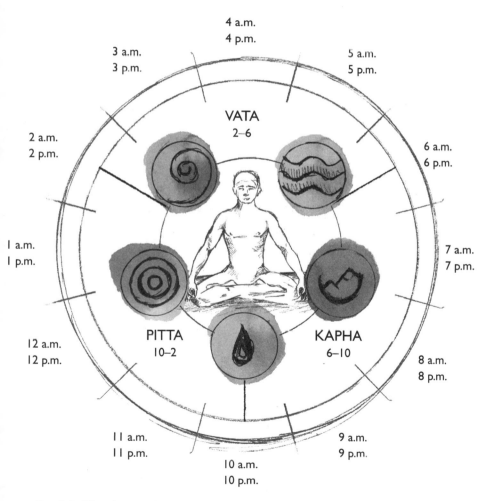

Fig. 8.1. The Ayurveda dosha clock that shows when the doshas are most active during the day and night

6 a.m.–10 a.m.: Kapha predominates. It is best to wake up by 6 a.m. since the heaviness of kapha encourages us to hit the snooze button. Since kapha is the energetic of sustainability and strength, it is best to exercise between 6 a.m. and 10 a.m.

10 a.m.–2 p.m.: Pitta is strongest. The transformative function of digestion is at its peak now, so it's better to eat your largest meal of the day for lunch.

2 p.m.–6 p.m.: Vata is dominant. When vata is more active, it's a good time to work, as thinking and creativity are at their peak.

6 p.m.–10 p.m.: Kapha increases again. And the heaviness of it causes the body and mind to settle for bedtime.

10 p.m.–2 a.m.: Pitta is dominant. Time to rest and digest!

2 a.m.–6 a.m.: Vata is stirring. It is gently waking the body and mind. In Yoga, it is advised to wake before sunrise, at around 4 a.m., to practice meditation.

The Chinese medicine body clock (see fig. 8.2) is organized according to meridian qi flow and organ qi activity. It is divided into two twelve-hour parts. The first twelve hours, beginning at 3 a.m., involve elimination and digestion. The second twelve hours involve filtering and cleansing. There is a path through the meridians that the qi takes, and it starts at the lung meridian.

3 a.m.–5 a.m.: Lung. Activity is dominant in the Lung meridian. It is a good time for elimination of gaseous waste from the blood through the lungs. Remember, 70 percent of bodily toxins are released through breathing. Usually the body begins to come close to waking in this phase. Traditionally and in the internal sciences of tai chi, qigong, and yoga, practitioners wake at this time and do breathing exercises, utilizing, cleansing, and charging the lungs. The lungs also govern the skin, throat, and sinuses. People with sinus or lung issues may wake at this time because of those problems. We may wake with a scratchy throat around this time when we're starting to come down with a cold.

5 a.m.–7 a.m.: Large intestine. The Large Intestine meridian and organ are most active now. This is a good time to evacuate the bowels, to let go of the previous day's metabolic waste.

7 a.m.–9 a.m.: Stomach. Eat a good, yet gentle breakfast. The stomach is tender first thing in the morning, so make it something only lightly spiced and flavored, that's warm and easy to digest. The largest meals of the day should be now and at lunch. This allows the food to be in the small intestine by the time the enzymatic activity is at its highest for the day.

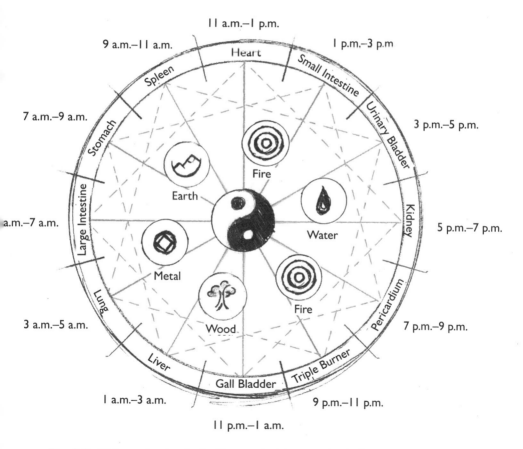

Fig. 8.2. Chinese body clock. Day and night are divided into two-hour segments, each representing the heightened activity of the corresponding meridian/organ system. The two-hour period directly opposite the clock from the meridian/organ that is at its peak is the time when the meridian/organ is at its lowest vitality level.

9 a.m.–11 a.m.: Spleen. Transformation is greatest at this time. Worry and self-esteem issues may be predominant now.

11 a.m.–1 p.m.: Heart. This is the time of day when the majority of biomedical heart-related issues occur. It is also when nutrients are best transported through the system by the heart for absorption by the tissues and other organs.

1 p.m.–3 p.m.: Small intestine. Foods from the earlier hours are completing their breakdown into nutrients.

3 p.m.–5 p.m.: Bladder. The bladder prepares the blood for filtration in the kidneys, works with the lungs to separate the clear from the turbid, and takes the turbid for release.

5 p.m.–7 p.m.: Kidney. The kidneys filter the blood, and because they are also related to the adrenals, this is a time when fear may begin to manifest.

7 p.m.–9 p.m.: Pericardium. The pericardium time is responsible for emotional stability and is traditionally recognized as the best time to engage in sexual activities. Perhaps this is because of the way the hormones shift in the next two-hour cycle.

9 p.m.–11 p.m.: Triple burner. Endocrine activity kicks in. The triple burner is responsible for hormonal balance.

11 p.m.–1 a.m.: Gallbladder. At gallbladder time cholesterol is processed, and the body is readied for sleep and regeneration. The yang qi dives inward to do its work of warming the interior and transforming toxins during the night for release in the morning.

1 a.m.–3 a.m.: Liver. The liver now filters toxins from the blood, and the hun settles in the liver blood for a good night's sleep.

There is a great deal of overlap between the two body clocks, particularly in terms of which element is predominant at any given time throughout the day. Something important to note is that the energetics may mix toward the end of one time and the beginning of the next as vital energy shifts its responsibilities. This is particularly true if there is an imbalance or an excess in one area; it may encroach upon the following time slot more than normal. One can see how the Ayurveda body clock integrates this overlap; its guidelines are more generalized. The Chinese body clock is more detailed and specific.

A good way to utilize these clocks is to look to the Ayurveda clock for generalized guidance on what to do when throughout the day in order to stay more in sync with natural rhythms. The vata/pitta/kapha times of day are not just guidelines for the body but for what is happening in the environment at that time as well. By going with the biorhythmic flow of life, we encourage balance in our own lives. For example, knowing that the kapha time of day is 6 a.m.–10 a.m., and taking into consideration the gunas or qualities of kapha, we know that if we are still asleep when this time comes that it will be more difficult to wake. It is actually advisable to awaken before 6 a.m., during vata time, because vata is light and mobile. We also know that kapha is great for routine. Establishing a healthy morning routine is easier to do between these hours than after them. This is evident if you've ever had the experience of oversleeping. The rest of the world is already on the go and more likely to interfere with our morning routine than if we get into it before the day is in full swing. We can use the qualities of the times of day to our benefit.

The Chinese medicine body clock is best used to understand what's happening to us when, particularly if there are any imbalances. If you always notice that you wake up at 3 a.m., perhaps your liver isn't happy. This is moving into lung time. Why is there activity going on that wakes you up as you transition from liver into lung time? Is the liver overtaxed and not able to let go of the energy? Or is its energy excessive and encroaching on the lungs? Are you also having issues with your lungs, such as grief or shortness of breath?

When looking at the Chinese body clock, note that when one organ is at its peak of activity, the organ directly across from it on the opposite side of the clock has the least amount of energy. For example, 5 a.m.–7 a.m. is large intestine time. It is the best time of day to clear out the debris from the previous day and set the body up for a new daily cycle. It will be difficult to wake, however, if the kidney yang energy is deficient and this is the time of day the kidneys are naturally at their lowest energetically. Since the kidney energy propels us and supports the overall well-being of the body, it makes sense that when their energy is low, the body will be tired. This also coincides with kapha time. If the kidneys are deficient, then the heaviness of kapha makes it even more difficult for the body to awaken.

The primary guna of sleep is tamas. It has to be because we need to dull the conscious thinking mind in order to fall asleep. Early morning is considered the sattva guna time of day. Therefore, it is advisable according to Ayurveda for all doshic types to awaken before sunrise, early in the morning. Vata types require the most sleep and are advised to wake around 5:30 a.m. Pitta types require a moderate amount of sleep, and it is suggested that they awaken around 5 a.m. Kapha types require the least amount of sleep, although they like it the most, and should try to awaken around 4 a.m.

Morning Routine

Generally speaking, what each type does at any given time of day is pretty much the same. The differences are in the foods they eat and products they use and how intensely they exercise. When you first wake up, give yourself a moment before getting out of bed. Check in with how you are feeling, maybe write down any dreams you had, then connect with your breath, and stretch out. Flex your feet and gently stretch your calves before stepping onto the floor. If your floor is ice cold, have socks on or slippers by your bed, so you can slip your feet into them. If you have the urge, evacuate your bladder and bowels. Wash your hands and rinse your face. Rinsing the face helps to clear tamasic energy from the night. Then, scrape your tongue.

Tongue Scraping

Tongue scraping should be done before brushing your teeth, as it eliminates the bacteria that accumulate during sleep. It's okay to brush your tongue, but that doesn't take the place of tongue scraping. Tongue scraping stimulates the internal organs. The tongue is a microcosm for the body. Every organ system opens to the tongue (see fig. 8.3). There are practitioners in China who *only* acupuncture the tongue. By stimulating the taste buds with the tongue scraper you are asking the body gently to wake up and let go of anything that's been stored from the previous day. In addition, you can see the sludge or slime that may come off. This is a good gauge of the strength of your agni and how much ama you accumulated overnight.

When your tongue coating is thicker than usual, it means you have eaten something your body did not assimilate well. It can also indicate that you are coming down with a respiratory or digestive ailment or are sick. If the goo is yellow it indicates that heat is present. This is not something you want to swallow first thing in the morning if you don't have to. The stomach is more delicate when we first wake up so why introduce unfriendly goo to it? Most health food stores carry

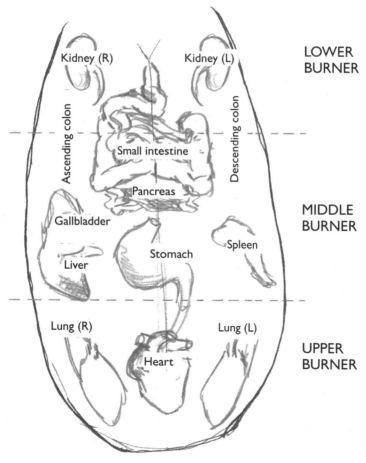

Fig. 8.3. Locations on the tongue that correspond to the internal organs

tongue scrapers. I recommend stainless steel as it is easy to keep clean. Just insert the *U* shape all the way to the back of the tongue. Drag it forward and off the tongue over the sink, then rinse it. Repeat until it is pretty clear. You shouldn't press too hard or try to scrape your entire coating off, as a light coating is normal. Just scrape lightly until you no longer see gunk on the scraper, only some normal moisture. Tongue scraping can make you gag a little sometimes. This is a positive thing, especially if you suffered from postnasal drip overnight, as it will help you to also clear mucus from your throat.

Oil Pulling

Oil pulling is recommended after scraping the tongue. This is an age-old mouth wash technique that is credited with reducing cavity- and odor-causing bacteria in the mouth. Basically, you swish your mouth with a teaspoon to a tablespoon—depending on the size of your mouth—of sesame oil for twenty minutes. As you swish, the oil will change consistency. It binds with fat soluble toxins in the oral cavity walls and pulls them out while eliminating potentially harmful bacteria. It is also used for breaking up plaque, which is why it needs to be done for twenty minutes. Oil pulling has been credited with soothing dry mouth and throat, reducing inflammation, strengthening and whitening teeth, preventing tooth decay, eliminating halitosis, and strengthening the gums. There is also evidence to suggest that sesame oil has antineoplastic (cancer inhibiting) properties, and is reportedly antiviral, antibacterial, and antifungal.

Speaking of oil pulling, the Charaka Samhita states:

In case of gum, teeth, and mouth diseases the same is prescribed for cure. The beneficial effects are given as: "It is beneficial for strength of jaws, depth of voice, flabbiness of face, improving gustatory sensation, and good taste for food. One used to this practice never gets dryness of throat, nor do his lips ever get cracked; his teeth will never be carious and will be deep rooted; he will not have any toothache nor will his teeth set on edge by sour intake; his teeth can chew even the hardest eatables."[1]

I generally recommend people start small with this and work up to a comfortable amount. Begin with one or two teaspoons of organic sesame oil (not toasted) and swish for up to five minutes. You can spit this out in the garbage to avoid too much oil getting in the pipes over time. If you don't notice anything uncomfortable about your gums or mouth, you may stick with the oil pulling. Over the course of a couple of weeks, work up to using one tablespoon of the oil for twenty minutes. If you notice your mouth feels hot or inflamed, oil pulling may not be right for you. While you're doing the oil pulling you can do *garshana* (dry brushing), *abhyanga* (self–oil massage), or little chores. After oil pulling, rinse the mouth with warm water and then brush your teeth.

Garshana

Garshana, or dry brushing, can be done before showering every day. In Ayurveda, it is recommended to have a set of garshana gloves to do this. They are basically nubby silk gloves that can be used to massage the skin. You can also use a natural loofah or shower brush for the body but use a special, gentle, natural sponge for the face. Garshana gloves are good for all surfaces, as you can change the pressure applied so as not to harm delicate skin. Basically, before performing a self-oil massage (see "Abhyanga" below) or showering, dry brushing is done by rubbing one of the above tools over the skin toward the heart. Dry brush from the toes toward the groin, do the buttocks and belly, and then do from the hands to the armpits and over the shoulders. All dry brushing should be done in comfortable strokes that move toward the heart. This is the direction in which lymph flows, and stroking in this manner helps to improve that flow. It also sloughs off dead skin, allowing the pores to breathe, and increases circulation.

Abhyanga

Abhyanga is self-oil massage. It is done to settle the nervous system, cleanse the body of fat-soluble toxins, keep the skin, muscles, and joints soft, flexible and supple, increase lymphatic drainage, improve circulation, and nourish the skin and hair. If you are a pitta type or have red, irritated, inflamed skin, use coconut oil. If you are a vata type, use sesame oil.

Kaphas can use sesame or safflower oil. Warm the oil by placing the bottle of it in some hot water. Apply the oil to your skin, all over your body. Use long strokes toward the heart. On the limbs you stroke toward the major lymph node areas of the armpits and groin. From the feet massage the oil toward the groin. Do circles on the abdomen and soak the belly button. Gently dredge with your fingertips between the ribs toward the armpits both above and below the nipples. Get your sides and your back as best as you can. Douse your head, face, and ears. Go from your fingers toward the armpits. Do circles on the joints. You should use enough oil that it soaks into your skin and then some. The oil should be left on the skin for up to twenty minutes so by the time you've massaged and waited to let the oil sink in, you should be done oil pulling as well.

Next, take a nice warm shower and wash the oil out of your hair. You can use soap in crucial areas, but no need to use it all over. Simply wipe the excess oil off with your hands. The oil will fill your pores instead of water, so there will most likely be no need for moisturizer when you're done. Abhyanga is like a little hug for every nerve ending that opens to the skin. It's very centering and relaxing. The oil binds to fat soluble toxins in the skin and the hot shower water opens your pores and rinses them off. People who do abhyanga on a regular basis have glowing skin that's supple and soft and their hair shines. Yoga practitioners report that with regular abhyanga their practice improves by leaps and bounds. They are more flexible and feel more solid in poses.

There are cautions when performing abhyanga. Many are common sense: don't put oil on broken skin and don't do abhyanga if you have swollen or red areas anywhere on your body. Avoid abhyanga if you are pregnant unless you get specific instructions from a qualified health care practitioner and refrain from it if you are menstruating or have an acute ailment like a cold, flu, injury, or infection. People with a great deal of ama or any illness are also encouraged to avoid abhyanga without the guidance of a qualified practitioner.

Food and Drink

The first thing that goes in the stomach in the morning should be a small cup of clean, pure, warm water. I say a small cup because there is a tendency for people to think giant mega-gulp-sized cups are considered a cup. They aren't. A cup in this case is four to six ounces. This is also true for coffee. Coffee is acidic, dehydrating, and can leach minerals namely, calcium, from your system. Coffee, like anything else, is medicinal for certain constitutions, under certain circumstances, in moderation. Big gulp-sized lattes are not, though. Usually, four to six ounces of coffee is recommended for medicinal purposes. Anything more than that, and on a regular basis, can increase vata and pitta and create dependency. There are coffee alternatives that have a similar earthy, emotionally satisfying vibe to them. They are usually roasted barley or chicory based instant coffee-substitute drinks.

First thing in the morning, drink that cup of warm water with a slice or a squeeze of lemon or lime. The warm water helps to stimulate the peristaltic action of the intestines, while the lemon or lime helps the body deal with ama. Although lemons are citrus fruits, their acidity should not adversely affect the body as they are alkalizing to the system. Some people with stomach acid imbalances may need to avoid them anyway. If you haven't already eliminated, you may now. Now is also a good time to do light exercise, yoga asana for well-being, pranayama (breathing exercises), and meditation. These should be done before eating and will further enkindle the agni, stimulating digestive function.

After all of this, it's time to eat! While eating, pay attention to the food. Eat nourishing, warm, unprocessed whole foods as often as possible. Do not overeat or overdrink at mealtimes. The stomach should roughly contain one-third air, one-third food, and one-third fluid. This fluid should include that which comes from your food, for instance if you have soup or congee or oatmeal that is not too thick. Eating larger meals and heavier foods earlier in the day is better for your body and mind than having them later in the day or at night. This is because your body is in the mode of digestion earlier in the day and can process things better. In the evening, it is more in the mode of winding down and uses its energy for things other than breaking down food at the front end of the digestive tract.

Chinese medicine advocates eating the largest meal of the day in the morning, and Ayurveda says to eat it between 11 a.m. and 2 p.m. This is because, according to the Chinese organ clock, the Stomach meridian and organ are most active during the breakfast hours. Ayurveda is looking at the strength of agni overall and follows the "as above so below" principle. The Sun is at its peak at noon—its light and heat are the strongest at this time. Since our bodies are in resonance with the atmosphere and environment, especially where the celestial bodies of the Moon and Sun are concerned, the digestive fire is influenced by the Sun's radiation and strongest when the Sun is at its most powerful.

Both times, breakfast and lunch, are good times to eat a hearty meal. If the agni is not strong, though, be careful not to overeat. Snack as you need to but always make sure you're giving your stomach time to empty before you add more food to it. It is not advisable to add fresh food to partially digested food as it overwhelms the stomach, dampens agni, and causes ama to form. Be sure to drink plenty of water each day, but refrain from having it all at once. It is best to sip on it throughout the day instead of overwhelming the body with a huge amount of fluid. Staying hydrated is good for all of your internal organs, for the smooth flow of qi and blood, for cognition, and for the skin, eyes, and even the discs in the back. Those discs typically contain a large amount of fluid and if there isn't enough, it can exacerbate things like arthritis, degenerative disc disease, herniations, and sciatica. It is also possible for a lack of hydration to cause pain in the soles of the feet when standing.

The general rule of thumb is to drink half of one's body weight in ounces of water per day.[2] The amount needed can fluctuate based upon humidity, or lack thereof, as well as how rigorously one exercises or sweats. Water should be either warm or at room temperature. Warmer water is for those afflicted by vata imbalance or a lot of constitutional vata. These are typically people who don't have a lot of insulation on their bodies and tend to run cold.

Sugar cravings can strike at any time but usually occur in that midday slump some people experience after eating a heavy lunch. A great way to satiate the sugar craving is to drink a tea made up of cumin, coriander, and fennel seeds. These can be purchased in bulk from a health food store. Basically, just put a pinch of each type of seed in a cup and pour boiling water over the mix. You can use a tea ball or allow the seeds to float freely through the water. If any get in your mouth, they're safe to chew and are wonderful digestive aids.

Evening Routine

In the evening, after work and dinner, drink some relaxing tea. Good choices are tulsi, lavender, or chamomile. It is best to avoid the news or anything overly engaging or disturbing. The mind is winding down and stimulating it can aggravate pitta before bed and provide a second wind that adversely affects sleep. Refrain from overdrinking water before bed. It is best to pace oneself so as to not have to keep getting up during the night to urinate. An oil, such as brahmi or bhringraj in a sesame base, may be massaged into the feet and scalp. Brahmi clears the mind and calms the nervous system, and bhringraj is good for the skin and hair. In fact, bhringraj is used in Ayurveda for premature graying, hair loss, and blood support. In Chinese medicine it is also used for supporting the liver and kidney yin.

What we eat can affect the quality of our sleep. This is largely because foods can have a calming or energizing effect on the mind. We all know caffeine and sugar are good to avoid before bedtime, but what about garlic and onions? People practicing rigorous yoga and meditation refrain from eating raw onions and garlic because they have a rajasic effect on the mind. This means they increase mental activity and make it difficult to attain higher states of realization. I don't advocate avoiding these foods for the average person, as they have many health-promoting benefits. However, refraining from eating them for dinner can help you to get more restful sleep. This is especially true if you are someone who suffers from insomnia. Alcohol can also disturb the mind. It may initially make the mind rajasic, then tamasic, or dull, so it's easier to fall asleep, but its heating, sour qualities aggravate the liver and cause the mind to become rajasic in the middle of the night, leading to restlessness, difficulty staying asleep, and disturbed sleep.

Technology can also stimulate the mind. Try reading a real, paper book with a night-light, or if you must have a screen, engage the blue-light block in the evening or dim the light. Also, keep the phone away from the body at night. Some people sleep with their phone under their pillow. Why be exposed to excess radiation? Best to leave the phone in another room entirely, if possible, or to shut it off.

These guidelines for daily living were established long before we had technology and night shifts. Of course follow these guidelines in a reasonable way and to the best of your ability, within the framework of your life and without stressing about whether you've done enough or not. If abhyanga and oil pulling aren't in the cards every morning, maybe you can fit in a little self-oil massage when there is time, like on a day off, for example. Just know that this daily morning routine, part of what Ayurveda calls "dinacharya," is a recommended ideal. Tweak it however you must, and if you have questions, consult an Ayurvedic practitioner to help you understand how you can work some of these principles seamlessly into your life.

Peppered throughout the daily hubbub there should be windows of opportunity to take better care of yourself, even if it only means taking a breath or having a cup of tea. If the breath is shallow, create regular moments to take a deeper breath, allow the space to do this within yourself and your day or evening. It doesn't have to be the deepest breath ever, this won't happen on the heels of hours of restricted, choppy, or shallow breathing. But the mindfulness to give your breath attention for a moment will help establish a regular habit of better, deeper, more healthy breaths that can positively affect the body and the mind.

ESSENTIAL OIL AND HERBAL THERAPIES

Essential oils and herbal medicine are very powerful tools used for healing. "Natural" medicines, like foods, have an effect on the subtle energetic and gross physical aspects of ones being. Please keep this in mind and remember to follow the guidelines outlined below, as well as any other information you come across, with caution and awareness. In recent years there's been a surge in essential oil usage, and some of the information being circulated may actually cause harm. In terms of herbal medicine, I always recommend that people see a well-educated herbal practitioner.

Aromatherapy

Aromatherapy has become increasingly popular over the past decade. It is a part of both Chinese medicine and Ayurveda in the sense that aroma affects us, but not traditionally, as in the way essential oils are used today. There are massive multilevel marketing companies and probably hundreds of small businesses distributing essential oils and educating people about how to use them. I mention it here because it has become such a huge business that traditional medicine practitioners have had to start categorizing the oils according to elements and doshas. There are even lines of essential oils created specifically for Chinese and Ayurvedic medicine practitioners.

If you are seeking guidance about essential oils, my recommendation is to seek out a practitioner with credentials from a reputable school. The National Association for Holistic Aromatherapy (NAHA) has a list on their website.[3] There is an enormous amount of information widely available and accepted as true about how to use essential oils. Some of this information, although popular, is actually causing harm to people. Even licensed health care professionals are being misinformed about how to safely use essential oils. Please use discretion, and as a general rule of thumb, do not ingest oils or place them undiluted on your skin. Unless directed to do so by a licensed health care professional with proper training, do not use oils on small children or pets.

Some oils, like lavender for example, are considered safe in general to diffuse and even to wear. It is, however, contraindicated for people who have suffered from a certain kind of breast cancer. Many of the citrus oils create sensitivity to sunlight when placed on the skin and can result in burns. Even the gentlest of oils can cause contact dermatitis. Playing with oils all the time can irritate the respiratory tract, and overuse of oils in general can aggravate all the doshas, starting with vata. As a traditionally trained aromatherapist and registered nurse once told me, we don't know how the body processes oils. We don't know if it processes oils. They may sit in a glob on the liver or burn through mucosal membranes. If you are offered a glass of water with essential oil in it, pleasantly pass.

It boils down to this: essential oils are not oils like cooking or massage oils. Olive oil, for example, is created in such a way as to make it easily bioavailable to the human digestive system. Essential oils are very highly concentrated chemicals. They are chemicals meant to work on the olfactory system primarily. Yes, they are natural, but so is poison ivy, so are peanuts. As David Crow, founder of Floracopeia, once said in a class I attended, essential oils are the concentrated immune system of the plant. As such, their presence is helpful for stimulating our own immunity through resonance. There is no need to eat harsh oils to effect this stimulation; we need only diffuse them. All this being said, included below is a basic list of oils to diffuse, use for cleaning, or place in a carrier oil and apply to adult skin. Essential oils are beautiful healing tools; they just need to be utilized properly, so they do no harm.

Lavender oil is very popular. It's lovely for calming the nervous system, and lavender flowers are added to products like eye pillows and under-the-pillow sachets to encourage restful sleep. Tea tree oil has been found in vivo to kill MRSA, the bacteria that are resistant to methicillin and other related antibiotics. It is generally recognized as being antifungal, antiviral, and antimicrobial. It can be used to clean your floors with just a few drops in a bucket of water, or diffused to keep the air clear in a space. People also use it in a carrier oil (another type of oil like olive oil or coconut oil used to dilute essential oils) as an antifungal for the toes. Ravensara is also great to diffuse—in an office, for example—as it is widely recognized for its immune boosting properties. A drop of clove oil in a carrier oil can be rubbed on a sore gum to help ease a toothache. Lemon oil is great for cleaning. Rose oil is pricey, but it's worth it; it lasts a long time, and it doesn't take much to have an effect, so small quantities are fine. It sooths emotional distress and the heart chakra, and calms the pitta dosha, heat, or inflammatory conditions.

Essential oils powerfully affect the mind and emotions. We are so inundated with information and energy waves from so many sources that our bodies are bombarded in a way they never have been before. Because of this, it is easy to become less aware and just inundate ourselves with essential oils. However, if we strive to live more simply and with balance, our attention will naturally be more centered, and we will be able to focus on the ideal quantity and the quality of an oil without overdoing it.

Steam Inhalation to Clear the Orifices

A drop of eucalyptus oil in a steam inhalation is great for clearing the sinuses. To do this, boil water in a small pot, move the pot to a safe pot holder on a table, and add a few drops of eucalyptus oil to the water. Once it is safe to be near the steam, sit with the head several inches over the pot. Place a towel over the head to get the benefits of the rising steam. Breathe this in through the nose as much as possible. The steam will help the sinuses to drain and the little bit of oil will help to open the orifices and assist the body in ridding itself of pathogens. This is also a great practice for chest congestion.

Teas

There are many teas readily available for a home pharmacy. Some favorites are the Ayurvedic combination of cumin, coriander, and fennel, or CCF. These three seeds combine to create a tridoshic (balancing for all constitutional types) tea that not only helps improve digestion and provide mild detoxification but also reduces sugar cravings. This tea is highly beneficial during seasonal Ayurvedic cleansing, as it dulls these harmful cravings. To make it, simply purchase loose cumin, coriander, and fennel seeds. Place a pinch of each in a cup of hot water, or in a tea ball, steep in hot water for five to ten minutes, then drink. If you're not using a tea ball, chewing on some of the seeds that inevitably end up in the mouth is fine. Cumin is warming, it decreases vata and kapha while mildly stimulating pitta and enkindling agni. Coriander is cooling. It calms high pitta and is somewhat calming to the mind. Fennel is cooling and sweet, hence the assistance with ameliorating sugar cravings, and enkindles agni without aggravating the pitta dosha. It is balancing for vata and kapha and is touted for its ability to reduce gas and bloating, transform fat, and stimulate water metabolism. Please note, drinking a cup of tea is not a substitute for that glass of water.

Other herbs or spices may be added to CCF tea or consumed on their own to assist in absorption and assimilation or help calm the mind. Tulsi is one of them. It can be purchased loose leaf or in teabags. Tulsi is balancing to vata and kapha, but if pitta is already aggravated it may make it worse. It is heating and useful for easing respiratory ailments and digestive ailments like bloating and gas and for boosting immunity.

Ginger is another wonderful addition to either CCF tea or to have on its own. It is used in both systems of medicine as a digestive aid. It helps with absorption and reduces nausea. In Chinese medicine the skin of fresh ginger is used to move dampness and swelling from the surface fo the body. Fresh ginger is not considered as heating as the dried variety. In fact, dried ginger is classified as hot and only used in small quantities in formulations for very yang-deficient conditions. Sipping fresh ginger tea a half an hour before a meal is recommended. Slice up several quarter-sized pieces of fresh ginger root. If it is organic and clean, leave the skin right on it. Place it in a pot of water, bring it to a boil, then simmer it a few minutes with the lid on so that the volatile oils don't escape. Strain and enjoy!

Licorice tea is a wonderful aid to cool a hot liver or stomach. It is balancing to vata and pitta while increasing kapha. In this sense, it is nourishing and has been used for things like acid reflux or heartburn, gastrointestinal ulcerations, and calming an inflamed liver, especially after an infection like Epstein-Barr or mononucleosis. Licorice root is sweet and can help deter sugar cravings. It is used in small doses in Chinese medicinal formulas to harmonize the actions of the other ingredients.

Herbalism

Herbalism is a highly refined method of treatment in both Chinese and Ayurvedic medicine. Practitioners are very well-trained in administering herbs, minerals, and animal products and in their known potential side effects with pharmaceuticals. There is an entirely complex medical theory underlying Chinese medicine and Ayurvedic remedies. It is not like Western herbalism where a symptom is addressed by administering a tea or tincture. Instead, all of the aforementioned constitutional factors and imbalances are taken into consideration. Formulas made up of two to dozens of herbs are administered to help not only alleviate the symptoms but to do so by addressing the cause of the disease as well. In Chinese medicine this method is called "root and branch." It is important to treat the branch, or the symptom, in order to alleviate suffering and gain the patient's trust and faith that the medicine will work. However, the root, or cause, must also be treated in order to alleviate suffering in the long term and restore harmony. Ayurveda also says we must remove the cause of the disease. Sometimes this cause is not something that can be treated with a pill, but there are circumstances whereby using a pill or herbal decoction can help loosen or right the energy flow so that causative lifestyle factors can be identified and dealt with.

Each medicinal substance in the Chinese pharmacopeia has thermal properties, in that it is either heating, cooling, or neutral to the system. Each substance also has one or more tastes associated with it. Each taste increases or decreases various physiological processes. For example, the sourness of a lemon increases salivation, or the saltiness of something causes water retention. In addition to a temperature and a taste, Chinese herbs are classified according to the channels they enter and their primary modes of action. In constructing a formula, the practitioner takes all of this into account to create a balanced prescription with no side effects or interactions. Most Chinese herbalists use classic formulas, often thousands of years in the making, as base formulas for what they give their patients. Some practitioners stick only to the formulas in the classical texts. There is a growing group of practitioners that categorize medicinal substances and formulas into constitutional types and prescribe them accordingly.

Ayurvedic medicinal substances have classifications similar to those of the Chinese. They also have specific temperatures and tastes. Interestingly, the Indians found that there is an immediate effect from a medicinal substance, called *virya,* as well as a post-digestive effect, called *vipaka*. This post-digestive action on the body can cause either a sour, pungent, or sweet effect cascade in the system. Therefore, in taking into account the actions of herbs and other substances like minerals, metals, and animal products, practitioners are mindful of the post-digestive effect. So in Ayurveda, there is rasa, or taste, quality of a substance, a virya, or thermal potency, and vipaka, or post-digestive effect. All of these aspects are taken into consideration in terms of how they affect the doshas. Some Ayurveda practitioners construct their own formulations, usually with less than ten herbs or substances. Traditional formulas can include dozens of medicinals.

Chinese and Ayurvedic medicinals can be used topically or internally. In Chinese medicine, formulas are cooked into honey pills, prepared as decoctions, ground into powders and cooked with water, made into granules that are dissolvable in water, mixed with egg, cooked in congee, or administered topically for relief of physical traumas or open wounds. In Ayurveda, medicated oils are applied to the skin, hair, eyes, or ears. They can also be taken rectally. Modern formulations are usually encapsulated or made into pills for ingestion, as they are in Chinese medicine today. Traditionally, certain formulations in both systems were meant to be taken only as teas or powders. However, the demand for modern convenience and the aversion to the medicinal tastes has caused this practice to fall out of favor. This is not optimal, as tasting the medicinal has an immediate effect on balancing the system.

These days many single herbs and formulas are available for purchase over the counter like in drugstores, supplement outlets, in health food stores, and online. The quality of these products varies widely, and their construction is usually so specific that many should only be used for certain constitutions or under certain circumstances. Take Yin Qiao San, for example. This is a traditional Chinese medicine for the onset of an external pathogenic invasion. However, if it's taken after the initial tickle in the throat, it's pretty useless in treating the infection. If the average person doesn't know this and starts taking it three days into their cold, they will assume it doesn't work. It actually works magically taken at the right time, in the correct dosage. This is not information the average supplement shopper is privy to, however.

The intestinal regulating and mildly cleansing formula Triphala is very popular in the Ayurveda and yoga communities. It is a combination of three fruits that help to regulate the bowels and gently pull toxins to the large intestine for elimination. It is usually sold in capsule form. Triphala has a very distinctive taste that activates your body to start this process. If you are swallowing a pill, you skip this step. Triphala should be taken as a powder and washed down with a small amount of warm or hot water. Most people wouldn't take it if they knew this. Some people's bodies have so many toxins that Triphala can be too stimulating for them, and they should only take it when agni is at its highest so as to utilize the strength of the digestive fire to burn through the toxins or ama. Otherwise, they may end up suffering from dream-disturbed sleep while taking it. It is always advisable to seek the guidance of a qualified practitioner when considering starting any therapeutic regimen.

Castor Oil

Castor oil has been used for millennia in Egypt and India as a medicinal substance. It came back into vogue in the West with the teachings of modern-day prophet Edgar Cayce, who would go into a trance and speak of cures for various maladies to an assistant, who would write them all down. Taken internally, castor oil is used as a strong purgative, cleansing the small and large intestines. Some Ayurvedic practitioners use it in their seasonal cleanse routine. Many people are familiar with it as a dreaded childhood treatment for constipation. It can also be used to stimulate labor as it activates apana vayu so strongly.

Castor oil packs can be used on the joints to balance vata and reduce ama. When ama accumulates in the joints, pain increases with cold, damp, heat, or a combination of the three. Vata in the joints creates cracking, popping, pain with movement, and tenderness to the touch. According to Ayurveda, castor oil is cooling when used externally, but heating when used internally. Although it is externally cooling, it is successfully used for most disorders involving vata, pitta, or kapha. In addition to joint pain, castor oil packs can be used to improve digestion, relieve constipation, reduce gas and bloating, detoxify the liver, break up tumors, cysts, and scar tissue, improve lymphatic circulation, and alleviate sore, swollen, inflamed, or tight muscles. For digestion, place it over the area of concern.

Castor oil packs are wonderful for gently soothing, cleansing, and nourishing the liver and surrounding tissues. Unlike herbs, castor oil does this slowly over time by pulling the toxins toward the surface of the body for elimination. For a castor oil pack over the liver, place the pack over the side of the right lower rib and the front of the abdomen, just below the lower ribs. Wherever it is used, the castor oil penetrates through the skin and binds to fat soluble chemicals and toxins, pulling them out of the underlying tissue for elimination from the body. It is soothing, nourishing, ama clearing, and anti-inflammatory.

To do a castor oil pack requires castor oil, a piece of flannel that can be folded to a ¼-inch thickness, a piece of plastic, such as saran wrap or part of an old shopping bag, a hot water bottle or heating pad with a moist heat setting, time, and patience. Once the pack is on it's very relaxing; it's just getting it ready that can be a drag for some people. Please do not use a castor oil pack over an open wound, if you're suffering from a malignancy, while pregnant or menstruating, or without your doctor's approval in any situation where you are under a doctor's care. Be mindful if you feel cranky or uncomfortable from the heat and either turn it down or remove it.

Here are the steps to making and using a castor oil pack:

1. Place the bottle of oil in hot water in the sink to warm it up.
2. Once heated, drizzle the oil onto the flannel. It is quite viscous and spreads easily, so a little goes a long way.
3. Massage a bit of oil into your skin where you're going to place the pack.
4. Apply the pack to your skin, oil side down.
5. Put the plastic over the pack. This is so it doesn't leach out into your clothing or any surrounding fabric. Castor oil does stain, so keep this in mind when using it.
6. Place the heat source over the pack.
7. Cover yourself and the pack with a blanket and relax for thirty to sixty minutes.

The pack can be used daily for a week or so, or as needed. After each use, place the pack in a clean container in the refrigerator. Each time you use it, warm the oil and add more to the cloth. This cloth may be used a dozen or so times before it needs to be discarded. Do not wash it; throw it out. Otherwise the oil will get all over everything.

Sterile castor oil makes a wonderful eye drop as well! It's great for red, irritated, itchy, dry, or puffy eyes. Before bedtime, gently massage around the eyes, then place one or two drops in each eye. Massage again after the oil is in, but be sure to be gentle. Allow excess oil to flow onto the eyelids and around the eyes, especially if you have wrinkles, puffiness, or scanty eyelashes. You can also use the oil if you have glaucoma or cataracts, but if you're already using a prescription eye drop, please consult your eye doctor first. Some pharmaceutical eye drops are actually made from a constituent in castor oil! For chapped lips, apply the oil to the lips at bedtime. It's the best natural remedy for chapped lips I've seen.

MOVEMENT THERAPIES

It is imperative that we move. Movement helps to circulate the qi or prana, blood, and lymph. Movement maintains and increases mobility where needed, loosens tight muscles and tissues, increases circulation to those tissues, and serves to stabilize the mind and body when done in the correct intensity and proportion. Some people are so busy they feel as though they can't make time for movement, and other people move excessively or overexercise. This can actually tax the body and lead to high vata, damaged pitta, and believe it or not, qi stagnation. Incorporating a movement routine, and looking at it as more of a therapeutic time carved into the schedule not only serves to supplement good health, but may be preventive for a variety of ailments.

Qigong

Qigong (pronounced, chee gung) is a traditional Chinese internal martial art where the practitioner learns to circulate and store qi in his body. There is an aspect of this practice that is called medical qigong, which is similar to Reiki and tapping, but the practitioner is not only channeling energy from the environment, he is also using what is stored. In Reiki, the practitioner channels the energy and uses intuition to direct it. In tapping, there is no channeling, but there is a system in place for redirecting energy flow. Qigong uses a system for helping the energy to flow and some channeling, but the energy is channeled intentionally from the Sun, Moon, stars, and Earth. It is also radiated and projected. In fact, martial artists who describe accounts of a well-trained, experienced opponent barely touching them and sending them flying across the room are talking about this kind of skill and the power of qigong.

Like yoga, qigong practice utilizes the breath. This is the case for personal qigong and for medical qigong. Oftentimes, the practitioner will also use sounds to help move, break up, or store qi. It is a highly effective energy healing modality for self-care and for healing others. Well-trained qigong masters—those who come from a bona fide lineage and have been refining their practice for decades—have the capacity to greatly affect another person's physiology. They are like the Jedi in *Star Wars* to some extent and perhaps where George Lucas drew his inspiration for them. There are accounts of qigong masters turning light bulbs on and off, light bulbs that aren't attached to anything but the practitioner's hands. Some have been reported to have the ability to shrink tumors. Stan Lee had a show where a qigong practitioner demonstrated the ability of putting a bull to sleep with his hands.

Because qigong involves manipulating the circulation of energy, it is definitely advisable to find a reliable source for training. There are probably thousands of qigong forms. Generally speaking, most qigong exercises utilize movement, even if it's just visualizing it. Most of the time though, the body is moving to some extent, even if the practitioner is seated. The movements are repetitive, fairly slow, controlled, and easy to do, but they're difficult to describe and should be taught by a qualified practitioner.

Constitutional Yoga

Yoga practice is used as a form of *chikitsa,* or therapy, in India. It is highly effective at treating respiratory ailments, aches and pains, digestive issues, sleep problems, and a wide variety of other ailments.

B. N. S. Iyengar is a famous yogi from Puna who as a young man actually cured himself of tuberculosis using a yoga practice. His teacher, T. K. V. Krishnamacharya, could diagnose a person's ailment by watching their breathing and prescribe a daily practice accordingly. Yoga was traditionally practiced early in the morning. Nowadays, classes are scheduled at all times of the day. It is best to do yoga when you have plenty of time, preferably in the morning, and it should be done indoors in a space that is at a comfortable temperature and away from drafts and direct sunlight.

Yoga practice includes breathing exercises, visualizations, asanas, and mudras, which consciously redirect, seal, and store the energy flow in the body. Below is a sequence of suggested breathing practices and postures that arc useful for balancing each dosha. How one does a pose is as important as which pose one does. Of course it is always best to consult a professional before establishing a new routine, especially if health issues are present. Because pranayama and mudra techniques redirect the flow of vital energy, they should be learned and practiced initially under the supervision of a qualified teacher.

Vata Yoga

Vata yoga calms the nervous system. Most vata types love movement. They are usually drawn to fast-paced classes where poses are not held for long and savasanas are short. That is, unless their vata is so out of balance that they are exhausted and welcome the rest. Poses that encourage strength and stability are best for vata or vata-out-of-balance types (See fig. 8.4 on page 214). Forward bends and twists are helpful because they assist with moving energy in the lower jiao and alleviating bloating, gas, distention, and constipation. Postures that place pressure on bones and joints should be avoided, as should fast, rigorous sun salutations and *vinyasa* practices. In addition, there should be balance in the poses themselves, and they should be calming to the nervous system. They should also be held, but not for so long as to stimulate mental agitation or overstretching as is the case with some yin yoga classes. Focus should be on the breath and in the body.

Everyone's mind wanders regardless of one's constitution, but those with imbalanced vata can experience "monkey mind," or nervous, agitated thoughts and fearful imaginings of the future. Vata types need to focus more on their bodies, moving their attention out of the head, away from the nervous energy, and into the consistent ebb and flow of the breath and the stability and stillness of the earth element in the

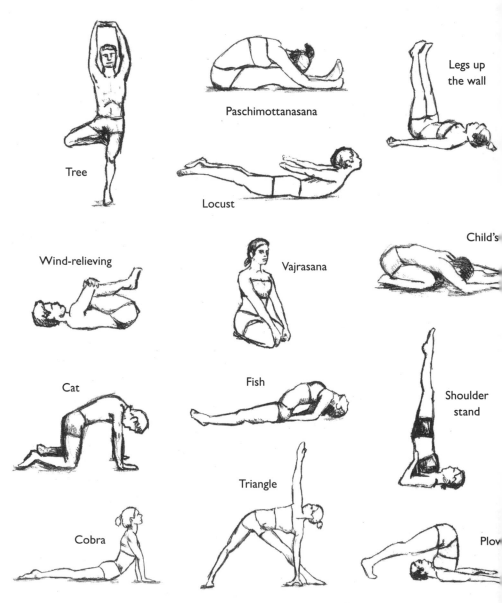

Fig. 8.4. Recommended poses for vata

body. In general, vata types need more stillness in their practice and to hold poses longer. Vatas tend to dissipate vital energy and may suffer from joint laxity, so strength-building poses are generally best. Focusing on the body parts that are touching the ground in practice is very helpful for vata types. Noticing whatever you can about how heavy you feel, how the ground feels—if it is warm, hard, or soft—and where the edges of a foot or arm or glute touches the ground can take the attention away from thoughts of fleeing the moment and direct it into the body for grounding and calming.

Poses that encourage stillness, spaciousness, kidney tonification and decrease gas, bloating, and constipation are particularly important. These include forward bends like *paschimottanasana* or intense western facing pose, gentle backbends like cobra and locust pose variations, cat/cow pose, *vajrasana* or thunderbolt pose, triangle pose, tree pose, wind-relieving pose, child's pose, legs-up-the-wall pose, and corpse pose. Poses should be held for ten breaths at least or ten on each side if alternating sides. Slow, deep breaths in general and alternate nostril breathing are recommended.

Pitta Yoga

Pitta yoga is good for balancing intensity, metabolism, and heat. Pitta types may also need to settle, not because they are scattered or nervous but because their more aggressive natures oftentimes need to be counteracted. They benefit from a more moderate practice than vata types with slightly more movement, additional cooling poses, and relaxation. Pitta types may also have monkey mind, but theirs is less nervous and more critical, even of themselves. For pittas, yoga can be a competition against themselves as well as everyone else in the room. They benefit from focusing on the breath and the body but with the intention of relaxing into what is, without judgment. In their practice, it may be helpful for pitta types to focus on compassion and acceptance and on their connection to all that is.

Pitta poses (see fig. 8.5 on page 216) focus on circulating excess energy and encouraging flow of liver qi. They help to alternate expansion and compression in areas of high pitta in the body. These

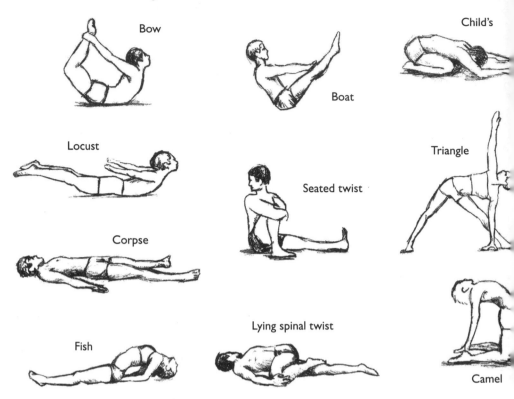

Fig. 8.5. Recommended poses for pitta

include triangle pose, revolving triangle pose, seated twists, backbends such as bow pose and bridge pose, boat pose or half boat pose, camel pose, fish pose, locust pose, child's pose with the knees apart, lying spinal twist, and corpse pose, along with gentle sun salutations, twelve total, as in pitta yoga we are being mindful of not overly increasing internal heat. Avoiding inversions, particularly the headstand, is recommended as these greatly increase pitta dosha. Easy, relaxed breathing and sitali pranayama are also recommended.

Kapha Yoga

Kapha yoga is done for support and stability and to energize sluggish physicality and mentality. Kaphas, in general, tend to be more ambivalent toward exercise but benefit greatly from the movement. Sun salutations, heat-building movement, and less stillness are recommended for them (see fig. 8.6). Although some kaphas may be thinking, "God, when can I do savasana?" they should focus on keeping the breath flowing and on how good it feels to move. In the Yoga Sutras of Patanjali it says *sthira sukham asanam* or, "posture is that which is steady and

Sun salutations in motion

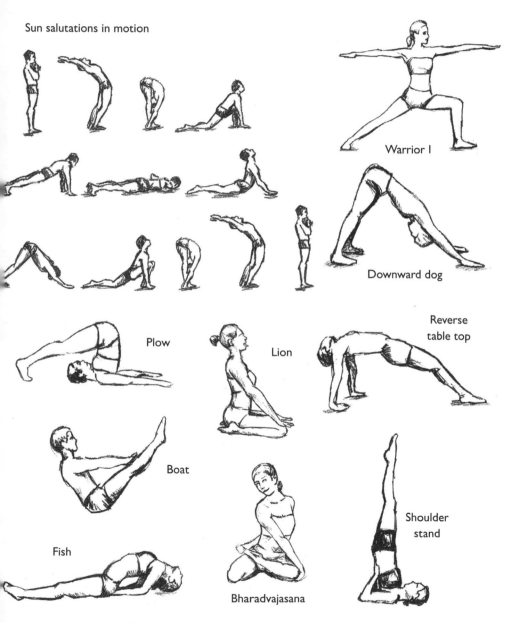

Warrior I

Downward dog

Plow

Lion

Reverse table top

Boat

Fish

Bharadvajasana

Shoulder stand

Fig. 8.6. Recommended poses for kapha

comfortable." Kaphas can also focus on this saying when their tendency to want to be still arises. Another good practice for these types is to mentally focus on the grounded energy within themselves during and between poses and movement. The poses, overall, should be stimulating and challenging and increase the heart rate.

A sample kapha routine would include sun salutations in which poses are not held but move fluidly, intentionally, and consistently. Hero pose and the warrior poses offer stimulation and challenge. Other effective poses include downward dog pose, boat pose, *purvottasana* or upward plank or reverse table top pose, Bharadvaja's twisting pose, lion pose, shoulder stand, plow pose, and fish pose. Breathing with visualization is recommended, e.g., imagine breathing in infinite space and allowing that space to expand throughout the room around you on the exhale. *Bhastrika* pranayama or bellow's breath is also recommended.

Yoga Nidra

Yoga nidra is good for all body and mind types. As mentioned earlier, it is the yoga of sleep, or the state of consciousness between waking and sleeping that addresses the subconscious mind. It is wonderfully relaxing and allows for a deep release from residual emotional energy and traumas held by connective and muscle tissue. Yoga nidra includes only a few postures, and they are done in a gentle, repetitive fashion to help the body settle into a comfortable supine position. A yoga nidra practice can be as short as twenty minutes or as long as an hour. More and more teachers are providing this style of class. It is also safe enough to do at home to a CD or DVD.

BODYWORK THERAPIES

Regardless of your ability to work the above lifestyle regime into your daily schedule, it is important to seek outside support in achieving optimal preventative self-care. There are many different types of practitioners available, and it is often difficult to know which modality to choose. While the best first step is to get a positive word-of-mouth referral, this is not always possible, and we oftentimes end up heading into a new experience blindly. The descriptions below should help clarify what each technique focuses on and what to expect in your first session. With any bodywork modality, it's often three steps forward and two steps back. Do not expect to go one time to one form of treatment and be healed. It usually doesn't work that way. It typically takes years to get off balance and you cannot expect to resolve it in an hour or two. Be patient, commit to a treatment schedule, and follow through with your practitioner.

Acupuncture

Acupuncture involves the insertion of thin, flexible needles into the body. These needles are FDA-approved, made of surgical stainless steel, and packaged to be used one time only. Every practitioner has their own personal style. Very generally speaking, Chinese style practitioners tend to be more aggressive needlers. This is not a bad thing at all. It just means that when they insert the needles, they are trying to get you to feel what is called a "qi response." This is usually an achy sensation at the needle insertion site that dissipates or dulls by the end of the session. This can be startling for some people, while others don't believe they've been treated if they don't feel it. Japanese-style acupuncturists may not even insert the needle. Sometimes they just set it on the skin inside the guide tube, pull the tube off, and connect with your qi through the needle barely touching the skin. Interestingly, this can be just as powerful as an insertion with a strong needling sensation.

When referring a client to an acupuncture practitioner, it's good to familiarize oneself with the different styles of the acupuncturists in the area. More-sensitive patients will most likely follow through with a treatment plan if they aren't anxious about feeling the needles as much, so send them to a gentler practitioner. This could be a Japanese-trained acupuncturist or a Chinese-trained practitioner who errs on the side of gentleness.

Trigger-point acupuncturists are also becoming more popular. They utilize Chinese acupuncture theory, but the needling style is quite aggressive. Trigger-point needling is similar to what some physical therapists are doing, but physical therapists are not as well-trained in this area as acupuncturists, and their treatments are recognized by the acupuncture community as carrying greater risk of a pneumothorax puncture, for example. This style of acupuncture involves inserting a longer needle, usually into a muscle belly, and trying to stimulate a neuromuscular reaction. Often the needle needs to be moved back and forth inside the skin until it hits the neuromuscular junction and the muscle twitches. This creates a release and is great for athletes with repetitive strain issues or people who are really locked up in an area. It can create more bruising and discomfort, but many people swear by it.

Moxibustion

Moxibustion, or moxa for short, is the burning of dried mugwort over points to effect healing. It is usually done in conjunction with acupuncture. It can be burned on the handles of inserted needles, smoldered in a moxa box over the belly, held over points, or burned in rice-sized bits directly on the skin. Moxa tonifies the yang qi, reduces inflammation and swelling, stimulates the immune system, and regulates intestinal activity. It is used over the Spleen (SP) 1 point to stop excessive uterine bleeding, and when used over the Urinary Bladder (UB) 67 point, it can turn a breeched baby. It is warming and comforting.

Gua Sha

Gua sha is basically skin rubbing or scraping. Medicated oil is applied, and the skin is rubbed with a smooth object like the edge of a Chinese soup spoon. It is usually done during a session of acupuncture and is useful for relieving muscle tension and respiratory ailments. The practitioner usually scrapes along areas of profound tension to help relieve congestion in the tissue. The marks left behind usually clear in a matter of days and are called the *sha*, meaning "sand." The idea is that this gunk is expelled from the tissue so the body can eliminate it. The darker it is, the more necessary it was for the person to have had the treatment. Some gua sha is so intense it should not be done more than once every six months.

Cupping

Cupping is also usually done in conjunction with acupuncture. Like gua sha, it is helpful for breaking up adhesions in the tissue, dredging and elimination of toxins, and increasing circulation of qi and blood. The power of cupping can reach up to four inches into the body, so it is quite useful for respiratory conditions like asthma, allergies, and cough. I've seen it cure exercise-induced asthma in a matter of weeks. Cupping is done by placing oil on the skin and then sealing bulbous cups to the skin via vacuum action. The cups are then slid across the skin.

Practitioners use various methods and many types of cups. Flash cupping involves taking cups on and off quickly over and over again. Stationary cupping is when cups are applied and left on for up to twenty minutes. They suck the skin up, which is quite the opposite of the pressing action of gua sha. While gua sha can be quite intense, cupping tends to grant a sense of relief and release to the client. Cups can be glass, plastic with pumps attached, silicone, or natural rubber. They can be used on many parts of the body. Silicone and rubber cups in the smaller sizes are becoming quite popular for facial rejuvenation treatments and useful on the jaw for people who clench, grind, or suffer from temporomandibular joint dysfunction, or TMJD. In these cases, they can be used at home but only if there are no active dental issues like an infection or abscess.

Acupressure/Shiatsu/Marma Therapy

Acupressure is the stimulation of points using the finger pads, thumbs, and sometimes the elbows following Chinese acupuncture theory. Japanese practitioners and those trained to treat young children will also use little tools with blunt or rounded edges to treat a point. Points may be tender, so this isn't necessarily completely relaxing while it's happening but should be afterward. Shiatsu is Japanese acupressure. Oftentimes a shiatsu practitioner will stimulate a point while moving a limb or stroking along the channel the point lies upon. Most Shiatsu practitioners in the United States are licensed massage therapists because there is an aspect of muscle manipulation involved. Marma therapy is Indian acupressure using the principles of Ayurveda and Yoga and oftentimes involves the application of poultices and herbal oils to the points.

Reflexology

Reflexology is a form of acupressure. The idea with reflexology is that the sole of the foot is a microcosm of the rest of the body. The practitioner can use sensitive areas of the foot diagnostically to better understand what is happening with a person's glands and organs and then use that information to treat the affected areas using pressure on the points. Reflexologists also massage up to the knees, and many will do a little hand, forearm, and sometimes a light head massage as well. Although they treat these other areas, the primary focus is on the feet. They are wonderful resources for people suffering from circulation issues and diabetic and post-chemotherapeutic neuropathy. Those with lymphatic pooling in the legs and ankles can also greatly benefit from reflexology.

Tapping

Tapping is becoming increasingly popular and is a great modality for those who want a simple practice they don't need specialized training for. It involves tapping meridians, points, and other areas of the body to effect a very specific healing response. Tapping has its origins in qigong practice and has recently been standardized in the West. It now includes specific mantras or affirmations that go along with prescribed patterns of tapping to alleviate everything from physical pain to addictions to negative patterns of thinking. The Emotional Freedom Technique (EFT), Thought Field Therapy (TFT), and Donna Eden's Energy Medicine are at the forefront of this form of therapy. EFT and TFT are nice because most practitioners will give the client specific exercises to do at home that can be used for the rest of one's life if needed.

Neuro-Linguistic Programming

Neuro-linguistic programming (NLP) is another increasingly popular form of therapy that involves imagination, guided imagery, Q&A, and intention. NLP helps the person who is seeking healing to reprogram their own mind using words and images. It can be highly effective for addictions, physical reactions, and phobias.

Craniosacral Therapy

Craniosacral therapy is gentle and can be profoundly relaxing. It is based on the principle that there is a specific rhythm to the circulation of the craniosacral fluid through the brain and spinal cord. This rhythm gets disrupted when lesions develop in connective tissue anywhere in the body. The idea is that the bodily fasciae, including connective tissue and the dura mater around the spine and brain, are like a giant stocking. If there is a snag in a stocking it pulls the rest of the stocking toward it and quickly progresses into a run that ruins the integrity of the stocking. In the body, this pulling can actually pull the micro-movable plates of the skull and other bodily structures out of place or cause them to be stuck or to move out of sync with the correct craniosacral rhythm.

Craniosacral therapists sensitize themselves to this rhythm, which is different from the respiratory rhythm or the heartbeat. They then work to correct the rhythm by placing their hands at various key fascial points on the body, including the back of the head, clavicular area, waist, and hips. Doing so helps the body to relax where it is snagged. While holding their hands at these key places, they feel for the rhythm and where it is out of balance. They then allow the body to reset itself. The rhythm basically stops for a moment—this is called the still point—then reestablishes itself to an optimal cadence. This treatment is wonderful for people with anxiety, head injuries, and post-concussion syndrome, and anyone who has experienced a trauma. It's rather noninvasive, the client remains clothed, and the touch is very light.

Craniosacral therapy is a wonderful choice for new mothers and their infants, provided the practitioner is trained in performing this specialized kind of work. It's a good opportunity to overcome any birth trauma for the mother or the child, and for mother and baby to bond and be in sync with one another. The still point aspect of craniosacral work can be quite a powerful, transformative experience. It can sometimes feel as though there is a transcendence of time and space. Craniosacral therapy teaches that the still point is where profound healing can occur. It is possible to experience still point in other treatment modalities, but it is the conscious intention of the craniosacral practitioner to get the client there.

In terms of experiencing the benefits of craniosacral therapy at home, there are ways to touch in on it. One is to practice yoga nidra. The other is to utilize a still point inducer. This is a foam apparatus that you lie down on with the apparatus placed under the base of your skull. It is best to do this on a stiff massage table or lying down on the floor. Always check with a qualified practitioner before doing this, particularly if you're troubled with neck or proprioceptive issues.

Massage

Massage therapy is an umbrella term that includes a number of techniques that manipulate the muscles to facilitate healing. It can be either relaxing or rigorous depending on the style of the practitioner. Usually, clients disrobe and climb under sheets and blankets on a massage table that is often heated. Therapists are conscious of differing levels of modesty and will always ask permission before touching a questionable area of the body, like the inner thighs, groin, or near the breasts. They also try to keep the areas of the body that aren't being massaged covered.

Pressure will vary based on the practitioner and style of massage. Deep-tissue massage is just that. They dig in and work toward loosening up tight muscles and fascial restrictions with their fingers, thumbs, forearms, elbows, and sometimes specialized massage tools. Some practitioners apply heat, and some slide hot stones on the body. Swedish massage is basic Western massage. If referring a client, be sure to send more sensitive vata types to someone who does more gentle work. Pittas often say they like deep work because of their competitive nature, but actually need moderate pressure because they need to relax. Kaphas usually do best with deeper work.

Nowadays, massage therapists are using more cupping and gua sha. While these are great, they're usually not as strong a stimulation as one would receive from a Chinese medicine practitioner. A massage is not recommended if you're feeling like you're coming down with something, or if you have the initial tingling of a current herpes outbreak. Massage is spreading by nature. It spreads you out. It also spreads pathogens out. Reschedule if you feel that cold or flu coming on. Massage can push it deeper. Instead, have acupuncture to release it, or practice optimum self-care with a day off from work, adequate rest and fluids, and a little extra vitamin C or antimicrobial immune-strengthening herbals.

Tui Na

Tui na is a form of massage from China that means "push pull." It involves fairly aggressive muscle manipulation that includes techniques such as dredging and plucking that are as "pleasant" as they sound. However, while uncomfortable in the moment, the aftereffects can be quite profound. Tui na is a great modality for athletes such as martial artists, who are often overtraining and getting injured. In China, bonesetters (what we would call chiropractors) and Chinese medicine doctors practice tui na.

Abhyanga

Abhyanga is Ayurvedic massage. It involves *a lot* of oil and oftentimes two practitioners, one on each side of the body. Traditional Ayurvedic massage is done on a wooden table that has a ditch around the edges for directing used oil off the table and into receptacles underneath it. Usually the client wears a pair of panties provided by the therapists, and women use a towel folded over the breasts. In India, this may not be the case. The therapists start with long strokes and deepen them as time goes on. The stroking is done in a synchronized pattern. This is much different from the average Swedish massage in that they don't just go right into a specific area. They are trying to move lymph, blood, prana, and toxins by gently sneaking their way in and generating heat. The oil is heated and helps to soften the skin, bind to and pull out toxins, and nourish the tissues and nervous system. It is extremely relaxing.

Thai Massage

Thai massage is gaining in popularity as the yoga crowd from India, largely already trained in some form of bodywork, travels to Thailand for a break, then learns Thai massage and brings it back home with them. It is like a combination of acupressure, massage, and yoga. Largely, it entails being stretched by the practitioner. While they are doing the stretching, they may focus on pressure points or do a little massage to loosen up blocked areas of energy.

Shirodhara

Shirodhara is a wonderful technique for alleviating vata disorders and relaxing the mind. It is done on the Ayurvedic massage table and involves hot medicated sesame oil being poured evenly over the third eye and forehead. The rhythm by which the shirodhara pot is moved, along with the oil's temperature, the rate at which it leaves the pot, and the distance it travels to the head are all very specific. Since it is directly affecting the mind, the practitioner should be well-trained in the technique and be highly attentive and intuitive during the session.

Dough Dam Basti

Dough dam *basti* is a therapy in which an Ayurvedic bodyworker creates a dough dam on or around the particular area that needs healing such as an afflicted joint, the belly in cases of digestive distress, or the head if mental/emotional or sensorial issues are concerned, and then fills the area with hot medicated oil. Practitioners use natural sponges or cloths to sop up the cooling oil and continually refill the dam until the treatment is finished. Basti is a specific treatment that can help regulate digestion, reduce joint swelling and pain, and provide clarity to the mind and five senses.

Chiropractic Therapy

Many people are leery of chiropractors, but there are a lot of great practitioners who are attentive to their client's concerns. The idea behind chiropractic therapy is that the bones can move slightly out of place. They can slightly twist, or subluxate. When this happens in the back, it can affect nerve impulses between the brain and the areas of the body that the nerve innervates. When this happens we can suffer not only localized pain but also digestive, urinary, and respiratory functioning issues, just to name a few. Ribs can shift out of place, as can toes and fingers. By stretching or massaging the client's body or using ultrasound or heat, the chiropractor relaxes the body enough to be able to adjust the bones without the muscles pulling them out of place again.

Oftentimes, bones are pulled out of place by tight muscles, so it's important to have a regular yoga practice or massage that can relax the muscles enough to prevent them from doing this. Nowadays there are chiropractors trained in more gentle forms of adjustment such as the use of activators, which are handheld devices that very specifically nudge a vertebra back into alignment. Many also use kinesiology, or muscle testing. This involves asking the body a question and observing its response, then treating accordingly. Chiropractors also employ various energy-healing modalities.

REIKI

Reiki is a hands-on energy-healing modality that originated in Japan and involves the pure intention of the practitioner to be a vessel for life force energy so they can send it through their hands and into the client. Sessions are usually about an hour and the client remains fully clothed. Reiki is a wonderfully gentle touch and nontouch technique that can create profound states of relaxation. Some people report having visions and remembering favorite childhood memories. Practitioners are often very interested in the unseen world of mystic experience as they regularly experience the unexplained while treating others and themselves. The wonderful thing about Reiki is that anyone can do it, young or old. It doesn't require a particular belief other than that prana/qi, or ki, exists.

The word *Reiki* means "universally guided life force energy." Practitioners center themselves, clear their minds, and set their intention for effecting healing on the recipient. They then tune in to the client's energy field and allow themselves to be a conduit for universal life force energy to pour through them and into the person or pet receiving the healing. They place their hands in the space occupied by the client's energy field and directly on the client's body. They may work directly on an affected area or on the body using a generalized, standardized hand-position protocol. At this time Reiki is not regulated, but that doesn't mean practitioners aren't sincere. Use your gut feeling and word of mouth when choosing a practitioner. Resources for self-governing bodies are through the International Center for Reiki Training, the Reiki Council, and the International Association of Reiki Professionals.

9

Taste and Nutrition

Diet is an enormous topic in Ayurveda and Chinese medicine. In fact, it is probably the number one feature that draws people to Ayurveda in the first place. Everyone is concerned about their diet these days. With genetically modified organisms (GMOs), environmental pollutants, hormone and antibiotic treatments, and factory farming in general, there is good reason for concern. The beef industry isn't just one of the primary causes of global warming, beef is also detrimental to our well-being if we consume too much of it. Proponents of family farming and vegetarian diets note not only the cancer risk associated with beef consumption, but also the energetics that go into the meat. Many believe there is an effect on our consciousness when we consume factory-farmed beef specifically, but also meat, poultry, or eggs, in general.

The idea is that the chemicals produced in the animal's brain flood its body and remain in the meat we consume. In factory farming, animals are crushed together and live in utter filth. Sometimes they attack each other out of frustration and crazed mental imbalances. They are fed junk and pumped with hormones and antibiotics. Not only do these substances get into the meat and milk, they get excreted and end up in the ground and the water table. Some scientists warn this is contributing to the rise in antibiotic-resistant bacteria.

Living under such horrific circumstances and being fed pharmaceuticals affects the prana, or lack thereof, in what humans end up consuming. For an experienced meditator, this consumption will lead to a marked recognition of a tamasic or rajasic alteration in consciousness. I was told that in India, even though 80 percent of the population is Hindu, and many of them vegetarian, the police and military are encouraged to eat meat because it makes them more aggressive, and this is deemed a necessary quality in those professions. If this is true, imagine how it may be affecting a modern-day, overstimulated, prepubescent male. Hormones already agitate one's mind, and defiance is aggressive. For these reasons, it is advisable to limit meat intake and to gravitate toward family-farmed, organically raised meats and to drink milk that has not been produced with artificial growth hormones or antibiotics.

I was recently informed that in India, the milk of cows is gathered at specific times of the year based upon whether the farmer wants it to taste sweet or not and upon the fat content they want in their product.[1] Milk from cows at certain times changes in composition and medicinal quality. This is also true of food and herbal remedies. Certain herbs are only considered medicinally potent if they are harvested at certain times. Some herbs are harvested early in their growing season to create a different medicinal effect than those gathered when they are fully grown.

What changes in these gifts from the earth are their chemical properties that cause them to act in certain ways within the body. These properties are reflected in the tastes we perceive when we ingest them and the influence they have over our doshas and our minds. Inherently, food is either anabolic or catabolic. It either builds tissue or assists the body in breaking things down. We know when we eat something whether it has an anabolic or catabolic effect based upon its primary taste.

TASTES IN AYURVEDA AND CHINESE MEDICINE

In Ayurveda, there are six tastes—sweet, salty, sour, pungent, bitter, and astringent. Chinese medicine recognizes sweet, sour, salty, acrid, and bitter. In the West we typically identify sweet, salty, sour, bitter, and spicy. Ayurveda and Chinese medicine classify foods and medicinals according to taste, and ultimately the taste reflects the dominant elements present in the item. To achieve a taste sensation, one or more of the five elements must be present. In both systems, each taste has an affinity for a specific organ or organs and can increase the functioning of the organ it is associated with. It is interesting to note that scientists recently found taste receptors for bitter on human heart tissue. In Chinese medicine, bitter is the taste associated with the heart system, and in Ayurveda, it aids in circulation, the purview of the heart. It is so exciting when modern science confirms ancient wisdom. The tissue-building tastes are sweet, sour, and salty. Flavors that move, circulate, and clear are bitter and pungent (acrid or spicy). Astringent does a little of both. Let's look at the elements associated with each flavor.

Sweet

Sweetness is considered tonifying in Chinese medicine, and its associated organ is the spleen. When we eat something sweet, the Nei Jing says the sweet taste goes to the spleen first. Children whose spleens are still developing strength, and people who are spleen-qi deficient crave sweetness because it (in moderation, of course) tonifies the spleen qi. It also promotes tissue growth, which is another reason that infants and young children crave it.

By breaking down the elemental influence of sweetness, we can better understand what it is and how it works. Sweetness comprises the earth and water elements in Ayurvedic terms. The attributes of earth, remember, are heavy, solid, dense, stable, dull, and slow. Water's qualities are liquid, moist, cold, slow, soft, smooth. The primary attributes that end up qualifying sweetness are cool and heavy. Because of the cooling effect, sweetness helps to relieve thirst, burning sensations, agitation, and irritation. It also nourishes, sustains, and moistens and provides stability. Energy is contained in food and drink having a sweet taste. The solid, dense aspects of earth, then, are also included in sweetness in the sense that structure, which holds energy, is present here. Carbohydrates and proteins fall into this category.

Like increases like, so if the qualities of a particular element or dosha are ingested, that element or dosha increases. The opposite is also true: if one refrains from ingesting the qualities of a specific element or dosha, the dosha may stop accumulation or become less aggravated. This is why sweetness increases kapha but decreases vata and pitta. Sweetness prevents vata from going into excess mode because it is heavy and moist, while vata is light and dry. Yes, pitta is fire *and* water, but it is more fire, less water. Sweetness is used to balance pitta because it has the effect of cooling the fire.

Fats often accompany and take on a sweet taste. Good examples are meats and nuts. Simple sugars are highly addictive and difficult to cut from the diet. They are also the favorite food of bacteria and parasites. When sweetness is in excess, it can increase kapha beyond balance. This will result in any combination of the following symptoms: colds and coughs, mucusy excretions, weight gain (obesity), heaviness, fatigue, lymphatic congestion, and sluggishness. With regard to cravings, which are usually for sweet or salty foods, if the person is in balance they will crave the taste(s) that decreases the dosha that is currently going out of balance. Oftentimes, we ignore this or overindulge in something and whatever is out of balance is beyond a simple fix with a medicinal craving. In this case, a craving is due to the severely imbalanced dosha(s).

Sweetness should not and cannot be eliminated from the diet, as the majority of foodstuffs that nourish the brain and body have some sweetness to them. However, it is advisable to really limit the intake of simple sugars—refined white sugar, for example. Behavioral and emotional kapha qualities that may arise from an overabundance of sweetness are attachment and grasping. Sweetness, when functioning to support the system, results in sensations of satiation and satisfaction. It can also contribute to feelings of contentment, joy, happiness, connection, love, and compassion.

Sour

Sourness in Chinese medicine has an affinity for the liver. The liver energy system is the first place it goes during the process of digestion. Sourness softens and moistens. For this reason we use it to "soften" the liver. This means that sourness can calm aggression or other aspects of liver qi stagnation, as well as soften and smooth tense tendons and ligaments. In addition, sourness has a holding quality—sort of like a gentle hug. It helps to hold fluids. The Chinese did not add a sixth taste, astringent, as the Indians did; foods and drinks that have the power to astringe fluids are included in the sour taste in Chinese medicine. In the Chinese system, any fluid, including sweat, urine, semen, blood, and vaginal secretions, can be astringed with the sour taste.

This holding quality is due to the earth element's influence on a sour taste's action in the body, which is to increase water. In excess sourness can pull the fluid from the membranes into the deeper tissues, which can lead to dry membranes. Because earth is present, sourness is increasing for kapha and balancing for vata, and because it also contains the fire element (hot, intense, subtle, dry, and clear), it is heating and increasing for pitta.

Sourness stimulates the mind, enhancing discrimination. If too much of it makes its way into the diet it can increase feelings of envy. Overall, sourness is warming and heavy. It can enkindle agni (i.e., stimulate metabolism), activate salivation and gastric secretions, and increase the appetite. Examples of sour foodstuffs are yogurt, cheese, fermented foods, rose hips, and hawthorn berries.

Salty

Saltiness goes to the kidneys. Chinese medicine states that an excess of salt in the diet can injure the kidneys, but salty medicinals can actually tonify them. Certain salty substances are useful for nourishing and holding the jing, or essence. Salt is also used to bring forth other tastes in foods. Good examples of salty foods are sea vegetables and rock salt. Functionally, salty-tasting medicinals are used to soften hardness and dissolve masses and phlegm. In small amounts, they can increase good digestive functioning and moisten tissue. In excess, they can dry and lead to tissue degeneration.

Saltiness is a combination of water and fire, so it is heavy and heating. It can be used as a laxative and antiflatulent and can help ease spasms and maintain electrolyte balance. It also brings confidence and enthusiasm. When ingested out of balance, it can thicken the blood, mess with the blood pressure, and cause water retention, heat sensations, hair loss, and vomiting.

> *I once made the mistake of attempting a saltwater cleanse. It was a perfect example of not listening to the body when it screams, "No, don't do it!" It was a bad combination of ignoring my own better judgment, deferring to other people's beliefs, and not possessing enough knowledge to rationally understand why it might be wrong for me. It was spring, and I was in a pattern of getting a stuck sensation in my diaphragm at that time every year. A yogi was staying with me at the time, and the yoga studio I was affiliated with was leading the cleanse. I knew I didn't want to do it in public, so I decided to try it at home. It is something that's becoming more popular in the yoga community, and the yogi staying at my house promised to guide me through it.*
>
> *Basically, it calls for drinking a gallon of salt water. I do not recommend this to anyone, by the way. As I began drinking, I became fuller and fuller. The water wasn't going through me, and the stuck feeling just got worse. Finally, the water made me throw up. It's supposed to go through and clean out the whole gastrointestinal (GI) tract. Nope, not in my case. I basically did* virechana *(vomiting therapy) without proper preparation. Long story short, I can attest to the fact that too much salt causes vomiting, and that one of the other side effects of excess salt consumption is irritability—believe me, I was irritable!*

Saltiness increases pitta (fire) and kapha (water), so in addition to irritability (pitta out of balance), it also causes greed, possessiveness, and attachment issues (kapha out of balance). Saltiness brings a zest for life that, in excess, can be seen as hedonism. On the other hand, an insufficiency of salt can contribute to depressed feelings or dullness. It can also lead to fatigue. There needs to be fire in the system, and the jing, or essence, needs to be held. This is why both systems of medicine recommend that we have each of the tastes in our diet every day. It is just that some need to be eaten in greater quantities than others, depending on one's dosha and imbalances. In fact, it is ideal to have each of the five or six tastes present in every meal, in a healthy form.

Sweet, sour, and salty are all anabolic, or tissue supporting, building, and nourishing. They all contain either earth or water, or both. Earth and water are heavy and downward moving. Now we will move into the more subtle tastes that are mostly influenced by the elements of fire, air, and ether. These have a lighter quality and an upward and outward movement. They are more catabolic, meaning that they help to break down, transform, and move substances, toxins, or doshas out of the body.

Pungent/Acrid/Spicy

Pungency is useful for releasing the surface level. This means that it activates the lung qi (pungency is associated with the lungs in Chinese medicine) and wei qi to disperse incoming pathogenic influences. Pungency also helps to clear the upper orifices and sinuses, also the domain of the lungs, as many pungent medicinals contain volatile oils. Certain medicinals that are pungent in nature actually help the lung qi descend, thereby stopping coughs. Pepper, if inhaled, causes sneezing, a lung qi activity that clears the upper part of the body. Pungency activates the circulation of qi, especially superficially, and disperses damp accumulation.

Pungency is composed of air and fire. It is balancing to the kapha dosha, as the dispersion of damp accumulation would indicate, but can increase pitta and vata. Pungency is used to stoke the fire of digestion. Many pungent ingredients are useful in this way. This is because they are light and hot and need only be taken in small quantities. Foods that are pungent are penetrating, light, dry, and sharp. Some examples are peppers, chilies, mustard seed, ginger, cardamom, onions, radishes, and garlic. Taken in balancing moderation, these substances can bring vigor and clarity and improve the metabolism and the absorption, circulation, and elimination of mucus and wastes. In excess, pungent foods and substances can create gastrointestinal pitta disorders like heartburn, nausea, and loose bowel movements. Too much pungency can disrupt sleep, and lead to inflammation, thirst, and burning sensations. Ultimately, pungency can damage the jing, which may bring harm to sperm and eggs. Pungent foods create a sense of excitement and passion. In excess they bring anger.

Bitter

Bitterness goes first to the heart. Excess heat, or what we may recognize as inflammation, is very damaging to the heart and to the circulatory and nervous systems that the Chinese associate with it. In Western biomedicine, inflammation is recognized as a root cause of circulatory system issues such as high cholesterol. Inflammation is also damaging to mental balance, the domain of the heart shen, or spirit. The active constituents in bitter-tasting medicinals are now known to help decrease inflammation in the body. Bitters also tend to be antimicrobial, have a cleansing action, remove heat and toxins, and dry dampness.

Bitter substances are very cold. They are primarily composed of the air and space elements and therefore are aggravating to vata. Ever drink too much coffee and feel fidgety with a racing mind? This is a good example. Bitterness, in moderation, is like a cool breeze that clears away the damp, hot gunk in the body and mind, and it is purifying to the liver and blood. Its qualities are cool, light, and dry. Bitterness decreases pitta (inflammation) and kapha (dampness or mucusy excretions). Bitterness creates a desire for change (again, vata), and in excess, it does this by causing one to become acutely aware of one's dissatisfaction with life. It is, in this sense, the opposite of sweetness.

Bitterness is the most cooling taste of them all. In excess, it leads to resentment, cynicism, separation, and, potentially, isolation. It can be depleting and cause dizziness, decreased libido, and dryness. Think air and ether. We would describe most medicinals and formulas as tasting bitter. Good examples of substances that are bitter are goldenseal, echinacea, turmeric, dandelion, and coffee.

Astringent

In Chinese medicine, astringency is in the sour taste spectrum in terms of flavor and action in the body. In Ayurveda, astringency is very interesting. It is the combination of the most intangible element, space, and the most dense, earth. This makes it cooling, but also lifting. Perhaps this is why the Indians recognize it as a sixth taste. While sourness is heavy and heating, astringency is light. It increases vata but decreases pitta and kapha. It is tonifying and drying, and it squeezes the tissues, almost puckering them.

Astringency improves absorption, helps combat or prevent inflammation, and has decongestant properties. It can help to bind loose stools, dry excretions, and stop bleeding. Good examples of astringency are pomegranate, uva ursi, alfalfa sprouts, and unripe bananas. Foods that have a hint of astringent taste or action are chickpeas, green beans, yellow split peas, and okra. Turmeric is also slightly astringent. It helps one to mentally feel grounded, yet open, and organized. Astringency directs the mind inward. In excess, it can cause muscle spasms, mouth dryness, constipation, increased coagulation, and introversion. It can cause vata to become imbalanced, leading one to feel scattered and disorganized while exaggerating the earthlike holding quality of attachment.

Post-Digestive Effects

In addition to the elements having lifting or sinking qualities, the energy of everything lies on a spectrum of cold to hot. This is called thermal potency, or virya. Substances that are heating (not hot) are dilating. They open channels and vessels, increase circulation, and stimulate agni, improving digestive capability. Things that have a cooling effect on the body decrease agni and constrict the channels. And as in any rule-based system, there are always exceptions. These exceptions are said in Ayurveda to have special qualities, or *prabhav*. This means that in spite of what we know of its qualities, a substance has a specific action that doesn't make sense, but happens anyway.

Sometimes, we don't experience taste with our taste buds; it is only after agni has worked on a substance that its taste is released into the system. In addition, most substances have more than one taste, although one or two are usually dominant to our tongue. In Ayurveda, taste that happens after digestion is completed is called vipaka. There are three vipakas: sweet, sour, and pungent. Ayurveda teaches that there is a pre- and a post-digestive effect. The Ayurvedic physician must know what these are in order to best prescribe the appropriate formulas. The post-digestive effects of sweetness and saltiness include sweet excreta and a laxative action. Sourness has a sour vipaka and an acidic bowel movement. Pungency/acridness/spiciness, bitterness, and astringency all turn pungent and may create burning sensations on the way out. Knowing vipaka or post-digestive effect can be very helpful for practitioners in ascertaining the cause of imbalance, for prevention, and for treatment. For the layperson, I recommend that people look at the things they eat and drink and their primary tastes and actions. It's best to choose those that the ancients have suggested as benefitting their constitutional tendencies.

RASA

In order to fully understand taste from the perspective of Ayurveda and Chinese medicine, it's important to know it from more than the perspective of the taste buds. Taste is called rasa in Ayurvedic medicine. In traditional medicine, when we talk about taste, we are talking also about nutrition and the nourishment of the entire being. Taste is pivotal because of its effects on the body and the mind. The word *rasa* means many different things in Sanskrit. It means "taste" and it means "juice." It also means "essence," "comprehension," "melody," and "nourishment." Rasa is also the first tissue that becomes nourished in Ayurveda, and it transports nourishment to the other tissues. A lack of any one of the tastes creates a natural craving for it. Unhealthy cravings are usually due to ama that is confusing the system.

Triguna, Rasa, and the Mind

Beyond food and drink, what we bring in through our other sensory organs also has an effect on our consciousness and therefore our physiology through the pharmacy in the brain. Ideally, we want to encourage the sattva guna, clarity. Clarity of mind leads to sensations that make life feel more pleasant, safe, and comfortable and help us to accept things about life that are contrary to what we want. Ask yourself if what you're doing creates mental clarity, inner peace regardless of circumstances, and a truthful perception of reality. Look at the books or materials you read, the kinds of conversations you engage in, and the movies and TV shows you watch.

Anything that unsettles the mind, makes it restless, anxious, worried, or angry is encouraging a predominance of the rajas guna. This is the aggravated quality of mind. Things that foster complacency, dullness, or zoning out are tamasic in nature. Try moving away from these things. Loud noises and overexposure to light can be stimulating. Itchy clothes or cold air can be stimulating as well. All of the senses are processing information that is either calming and vitality promoting or stimulating and draining. Certain smells can also be pacifying or stimulating or even create severe adverse reactions. Anything we soak up or react to is rasa. Rasa is literally taste, but it also refers to how and what we feed the senses. It is sweetness in life, and being drawn to beauty.

What we feed the body and spirit affects the mind. Everything can be categorized as primarily one of the three mental/emotional gunas. In terms of diet, each food has qualities that either stimulate, dull, or bring clarity to the mind. Foodstuffs can be classified not only according to taste but also to which of the mental states they encourage. Sattva is mental clarity and equanimity, rajas is stimulation and at its extreme, aggression, and tamas is inertia and dullness.

Of course, it is best to eat a diet that leans toward being sattvic. This is calming and clarifying to the physical and emotional bodies. It provides mental clarity and more even energy throughout the day. This does not mean that it is bad to eat foods that enhance the other gunas. Sometimes a little rajasic boost is good—before a competition or a game, for example. Or maybe if you're feeling overstimulated, something tamasic may be grounding and helpful, particularly at dinner. These are just guidelines and to be taken with the proverbial grain of salt. They are useful at times when you find yourself feeling a certain way and can trace it back to what you ate. Ayurveda is about knowing the self and what the best choices for you are so that you can live more harmoniously.

Eating sattvically partially means eating a balanced quantity. The stomach, according to Ayurveda, should be one third solid food, one third fluid, and one third air in order for proper combustion to occur. Sattvic foods enhance clarity and the light qualities of vata, the heating and sharp qualities of pitta, and the liquid and oily qualities of kapha. The quality and types of foods that are sattvic include organic, fresh fruits and vegetables, whole grains, seeds, nuts, seed and nut milks, legumes, sprouted seeds, leafy greens, honey, raw milk (specifically acquired and prepared and best when fresh and warm), and ghee. Specific examples of fruits and vegetables are: pomegranates, figs, dates, coconuts, mangos, sweet potatoes, sprouts, leafy greens, squash, and asparagus. Preferred grains are whole grains like rice and barley. Powdered proteins and processed, canned, frozen, and leftover foods are not sattvic.

Rajasic foods tend to increase mental activity in a way that may cause one to overthink and become more competitive and aggressive. Other aspects of a rajasic mental and emotional state are fear, anxiety, anger, and jealousy. Rajasic foods tend to increase the mobile aspect of vata, be unbalancing to pitta, and increase the cloudy and slimy aspects of kapha. Fleshy foods that are particularly rajas promoting are fish, shrimp, chicken, and eggs. In terms of dairy, sour cream, cream, and ice cream are rajasic. Specific fruits and vegetables that are rajasic include apple, guava, and banana, white potatoes, broccoli, pickled foods, and pretty much all nightshades such as eggplant and tomatoes. Millet, buckwheat, and corn are also rajas promoting. In addition, eating all day long can be rajasic. Whenever we eat, the entire digestive tract becomes mildly inflamed. This is to increase absorption, but it's a lot of activity. It is better to have periods of rest from food.

Lastly, tamas is the dullest of the mental states. It's associated problems may include feeling lonely, attached, chronically tired, and depressed. Being stuck in any negative emotional pattern is also tamasic. Foods that are tamasic encourage vata to slow and kapha to be more heavy. The foul smell sometimes associated with pathological heat in the body is also an aspect of tamas. Tamas is increased by a diet high in meat, specifically beef, pork, and lamb. Milk and hard cheeses can also increase a dull mental attitude. Wheat and brown rice are considered tamasic, probably because they are heavy, but this does not mean they shouldn't be eaten, remember. Mushrooms are considered tamasic, as are garlic and onion, depending on the source. Some categorize them as being rajasic. Avocado, watermelons, plums, and apricots fall into the tamasic category.

Keep in mind these categorizations are generalities. The specifics often vary depending on which lineage the information came through. Teachers have different outlooks on these things, but in general, they encourage leaning toward being more sattvic physically in order to more easily achieve mental clarity and inner peace. So the categorizations are most important for experienced meditators, as they will most notice the effects of the foods on their experience during practice and their personal outlook.

I recommend eating according to what your body wants/needs. All of the above foods are medicinal, and depending upon the circumstances, some are recommended over others at any given time. These are basic guidelines, and really, apply the strongest to situations where any of the rajasic or tamasic foods are being eaten regularly. For example, if you eat beef twice a day and are feeling heavy and sluggish, it makes sense. If you're feeling a generalized anxiety for no good reason and have a diet high in sour foods, nightshades, and shrimp, then perhaps this rajasic eating is contributing to your worry. These categorizations are all good food for thought.

FOOD COMBINING

Food combining means creating combinations or pairs of foods that digest well together. It also means being aware of the ones that don't. Interestingly, foods we tend to combine are ones that confuse or spread the agni too thin. Good examples of this are fruit and yogurt or cheese and eggs. When we combine foods that don't go well together inside the body at the same time, it can lead to indigestion, flatulence, and mucus production. If we do it often and long enough, it will eventually lead to ama. Other foods that lead to ama accumulation include those that are powdered, processed, canned, jarred, frozen, and left over.

One basic rule of thumb is to eat fruits separately from other things. This brings up smoothies/juicing. Those of you who are tossing everything under the sun into the blender, especially if there's some sort of powder involved, usually come into the clinic with spleen qi deficiency. Let's look at why. Powders are processed, and processed anything can tax the digestion. Powder is dry and rough, which increases the vata dosha, or the air and ether qualities of the body. Powder is good for snuffing out a fire; it is like throwing dirt on a campfire. If you're having a smoothie because eating actual food causes you to feel too heavy, you have deficient agni. Usually, having a smoothie only compounds the problem.

The same with raw food diets. Cold puts out fire. Since the cavemen first threw meat on the fire, our bodies have been evolving to eat cooked foods. We are not wild animals anymore, especially in terms of digestive capacity. We are more refined. Eating largely dense, uncooked meals on a regular basis will eventually weaken agni, and the food will either bind you up or go right through you. If you've ever had a raw meal, you may have found yourself filled up without having eaten much at all. And it may have caused you to feel full for a long time. It may have also encouraged the sense of lightness and mobility associated with the vata dosha and not being tied down to eating all the time, but it is not good for the body long term. One reason is because it requires too much time, effort (and money) to eat a balanced raw diet. I have observed several people who have been on raw diets for a long time. They tend to be thin and wiry, have a grayish tint to their skin, and may actually look older than they are. The skin lacks a healthy glow as a result of the difficult-to-digest meals they eat regularly, which overtax their agni.

Smoothies, when mixed just shy of heating the ingredients to beyond being raw, which is what most good juicers/mixers do, are difficult to digest for most people. Protein is already complex to digest on its own and turning it into a concentrated powder doesn't help. Piling this into a machine with fruit is poor food combining. Add honey or some other sweetener, some form of milk, raw vegetables, flaxseeds, and whatever else is in the fridge or freezer, and it becomes a lot for the body to process. In addition, it's usually consumed year round on an empty stomach first thing in the morning, which is when

Chinese medicine considers the stomach is at its most delicate. Even if protein powder isn't used, the combination of anything with fruit is poor food combining. This is because the fruit is easy to break down and starts to ferment in the stomach pretty much right away. Think about something fermenting when everything else is barely digesting. Ideally the fruit should be able to pass from the stomach at this point, but it gets trapped in there with everything else. This is not an ideal situation for keeping agni strong and preventing ama accumulation.

The general rule of thumb is that fruit should be eaten one hour before or after other foods. This especially applies to melon. Melon forms a mucusy ball in the stomach, and this mucus can coat the other foods that may have been ingested, making it difficult to transform and absorb them. For this reason, melon should be eaten alone. Unbelievable, right? It's always in fruit salad! Most likely because it's an inexpensive filler.

Cheese and apples is another combination that isn't great for the agni/spleen qi. Sometimes the agni isn't damaged enough yet for poor food combinations to be an issue. And sometimes these foods may have been eaten regularly enough that the body has adjusted. Other times, though, undesirable food combinations are eaten regularly, and the agni is weak or the body hasn't adjusted, and they do end up causing indigestion, flatulence, bloating, constipation, brain fog, or any number of other symptoms. This is cause to examine regular patterns of eating, and if anything being consumed, even if it is categorized by society as healthy or normal, could be the culprit.

Overeating, eating leftovers, eating while upset or angry, before the previous meal is digested, or late at night, or not eating regularly can also weaken spleen qi and agni. Leftovers and processed foods have very dull prana. Food that lacks prana or qi is subtly identifiable by the wisdom of the body. We don't just need nourishment in the form of nutrients and minerals. In order to have strong, healthy, thriving minds, bodies, and spirits we need pranic nourishment. This comes from the ground, the air, the atmosphere, the energy of the Moon, stars, and Sun and through the food we eat and water we drink.

Processed foods and drinks, frozen and canned foods, and leftovers are deficient in prana. So are substances that shouldn't be consumed regularly by anyone like artificial flavorings and colors, most canola oils, and products with added sugar and salt. If you were to compare a lightly steamed stalk of broccoli to one that had been boiled for half an hour, you would clearly see that the overcooked one had less prana or qi than the one that is bright green and intact. If you were to drink water fresh from a spring and compare it to a purified water product, you'd observe an obvious difference there too.

Of course we need to weigh what is really good for us to eat against our busy lives. Sometimes leftovers are very necessary. Oftentimes stocks and sauces are prepared in bulk then frozen. This is just what we need to do to save time, and it makes sense. When shopping for ingredients for said stocks and sauces, find non-GMO, organic ones whenever possible, and eat fresh, local foods whenever you can. A carrot from 3,000 miles away has less prana than an organically grown local carrot that just came out of the ground a mile away. Something prepared at home is most likely going to be better for you than something at a restaurant. You never know the state of health or the thoughts and intentions of the food preparer when you eat out. The energy from their mental body can and does infuse the food at a subtle level. Just do the best you can. Find the best alternative for you and your family whenever fresh foods aren't available.

Remember, these are guidelines. Of course it is not possible for most of us to follow everything to the letter, but having the information that can best serve your greatest well-being is helpful for the times you follow it. I'm a big proponent of the middle path.

DIETARY GUIDANCE FOR THE VATA DOSHA

Vata types do well with easy-to-digest foods that are moist, warm, and oily. Remember, the primary qualities of vata are cold, rough, dry, and light, so anything having the opposites of those qualities will pacify vata, and anything containing those qualities will increase it. The tastes that decrease vata are sweet, salty, and sour, and the tastes that increase it are bitter, pungent, and astringent.

The following is not a complete list and, other than a few oils to avoid, only includes the foods to favor. I don't generally love food lists, but since everybody wants them, I'm providing them here. I ask, though, that you learn to hone and follow your body's guidance.

The foods that balance the vata dosha are as follows:

Fruits (all fresh, cooked, or soaked)

apples	dates	melons
apricots	figs	oranges
avocados	grapefruits	papayas
bananas	grapes	peaches
berries	kiwis	pineapples
cantaloupes	lemons	plums
cherries	limes	prunes
coconuts	mangos	raisins

Vegetables (all cooked)

asparagus	green chilies	rutabagas
beets	leeks	squash
black olives	mustard greens	sweet potatoes
carrots	okra	spinach
cucumbers	parsnips	watercress
fennel	peas	zucchini
green beans	pumpkins	

Grains

amaranth	quinoa	seitan
oats	rice	wheat

Legumes

miso	yellow mung dal	tofu
mung beans	red lentils	

Dairy

butter	cottage cheese	ghee
buttermilk	cow's milk*	goat's milk
cheese		

Meats

beef	dark meat chicken	sardines
buffalo	dark meat turkey	shrimp
eggs	salmon	tuna

Nuts and Seeds

almonds	pecans	flaxseeds
brazil nuts	pine nuts	pumpkin seeds
cashews	pistachio nuts	sesame seeds
macadamia nuts	walnuts	sunflower seeds
peanuts	chia seeds	

Oils (all but the following are good for vata)

canola	flax	soy
corn		

Spices

allspice	cinnamon	nutmeg
anise	clove	orange peel
asafetida (hing)	cumin	oregano
basil	curry	rosemary
black pepper (in moderation)	fennel	sage
caraway	ginger	salt
cardamom	licorice	tarragon
cilantro	marjoram	
coriander	mustard	

*Boil, then skim the skin off and store the rest in the fridge.

DIETARY GUIDANCE FOR THE PITTA DOSHA

Pitta types do well with foods that are cool, cooling, dense, grounding, and nourishing. Remember, the primary qualities of pitta are hot, sharp, intense, and light. Anything having the opposites of those qualities will pacify pitta, and anything containing those qualities will increase it. The tastes that decrease pitta are sweet, bitter, and astringent, and the tastes that increase it are pungent, sour, and salty.

The following is not a complete list and only includes the foods to favor. Note that even though pitta types are sensitive to hot, light, and sharp, there are some spices included here because they may actually be cooling. Also keep in mind that instead of relying on food lists, it is best that you learn to hone and follow your body's guidance.

The foods that balance the pitta dosha are as follows:

Fruits (These should be sweet and ripe. Sour fruits will aggravate pitta.)

apricots	melons	sweet apples
avocados	pears	sweet berries
coconuts	prunes	sweet cherries
dates	raisins	sweet plums
figs	ripe pineapples	watermelon

Vegetables (Favor sweet and bitter.)

asparagus	green beans	peas
broccoli	leafy greens	pumpkin
brussels sprouts	leeks (cooked)	sprouts
cabbage	lettuce	squash
cauliflower	mushrooms	sweet green peppers
celery	okra	sweet potatoes
cucumber (if agni is strong)	parsley	zucchini

Grains

barley	rice	wheat
oats		

Dairy

butter	ghee	milk
egg whites		

Legumes

adzuki beans	lentils	split peas
black beans	lima beans	tempeh
chickpeas	mung beans	tofu
kidney beans	soy	

Meats

chicken	turkey	venison

Nuts and Seeds

almonds (peeled)	pumpkin seeds
flaxseeds	sunflower seeds

Spices

cardamom	dill	spearmint
cilantro	fennel	turmeric
cinnamon	mint	
coriander	saffron	

Oils

coconut	soy	sunflower
olive		

DIETARY GUIDANCE FOR THE KAPHA DOSHA

Kapha types do well with easy-to-digest foods that are light, dry, and warming. Remember, the primary qualities of kapha are cool, heavy, and moist, so anything having the opposites of those qualities will pacify kapha, and anything containing those qualities will increase kapha. The tastes that decrease kapha are pungent, bitter, and some astringent, and the tastes that increase kapha are sweet, sour, and salty.

The following is by no means a complete list and only includes the foods to favor. It is always best to learn to follow your body's guidance.

The foods that balance the kapha dosha are as follows:

Fruits

apples	lemons	peaches
apricots	limes	pears
cranberries	cherries	prunes
figs	pomegranates	raspberries

Vegetables (Favor pungent and/or bitter.)

asparagus	celery	onions
beets	chilies	peppers
broccoli	corn (non-GMO)	radishes
brussels sprouts	garlic	spinach
cabbage	leafy greens	sprouts
carrots	leeks	turnips
cauliflower	lettuce	

Grains

amaranth	oat bran	spelt
barley	millet	wheat bran
buckwheat	quinoa	
corn (non-GMO)	rye	

Meats

chicken (white meat)	freshwater fish	venison
eggs	turkey (white meat)	

Legumes

adzuki beans	lentils	pinto beans
black beans	lima beans	tur dal
black-eyed peas	mung beans	
chickpeas	navy beans	

Nuts and Seeds

sunflower seeds	pumpkin seeds

Oils

almond	flax	safflower
corn	ghee	

Spices

Favor everything but salt.

Dairy

Favor ghee, but use it in moderation.

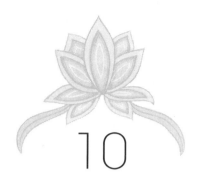

10

Cleansing
and the Seasons

One of the benefits of Ayurveda is that it has a well-thought-out, time-tested protocol for eliminating unwanted substances, or ama, from the body. Chinese medicine also includes a concept of toxins, but they are recorded in the classical texts as being heat or fire toxins, which would only cover severe heat that depletes the fluids, or pitta imbalances consuming kapha in Ayurveda, and are not the norm. In Chinese medicine the closest thing to ama, or insidious, chronic toxin accumulation, is dampness and phlegm. To treat chronic dampness and phlegm, Chinese practitioners recommend some foods to avoid and some to favor and ultimately herbal formulas to deal with the excess. They have a clinical approach to what the Indians call ama elimination, but the substances being targeted aren't perceived as toxins; they are seen as an unhealthy buildup of natural substances in the body, usually dampness that can often mix with heat, or as a fluid metabolism issue.

The modern Western mind recognizes toxicity on a spectrum. There is the subjective feeling of being toxic when one doesn't eliminate daily or goes on a junk food binge. Then there is an actual toxic exposure to pesticides, heavy metals, or radiation that may require more serious allopathic interventions. The vague subjective sensation of toxicity, or a mental impression or fear of it, causes people to attempt to cleanse, detox, or purge themselves in myriad ways. These ways are usually based on the current fad cleanse or therapy, and seldom do they take the age-old, time-tested concept of constitution into consideration. These self-cleansing efforts may lead to the person feeling better, but it is usually temporary, and they could also lead to greater imbalance and sometimes even cause immediate negative side effects.

Most people usually end up doing some kind of a juice cleanse or a fast. If their agni is damaged and they have ama, or toxins, and they don't have blood-sugar regulation issues, then they will probably feel great while they are doing it. They will have more energy, they'll poop a lot, and probably pee a lot too. They may feel lighter and like they need less sleep. On one hand they are giving their body a break from dealing with food and simple sugars. On the other hand, that break doesn't change the fact that their agni is damaged, and they have ama accumulation. It just gives them a break from noticing it. The burst of energy and sensation of lightness can actually be the beginning of what leads to a fasting addiction that causes a real vata imbalance.

Agni and ama are complete opposites. Agni must be protected and enkindled, not weighed down or dampened. Ama does just this to agni, which eventually cannot resist and in turn more ama is created. The qualities of agni are hot, sharp, light, dry, subtle, clear, stable, and fragrant. Those of ama are dull, heavy, viscous, wet, gross, sticky, slimy, spreading, stagnant, and foul. Ama is not easy to get rid of, and oftentimes it is really stuck. It can lead to inflammation, or heat. It then gets cooked by the heat and really caked on. This is why it's so important to have a well-thought-out process for loosening ama and moving it out of the body. Afterward, the body needs to be built back up with healthy fluids and tissues and transformative energy. Ayurveda does this by gently coaxing ama and disordered doshas out of their hiding places and into the digestive tract for elimination.

PANCHAKARMA

Panchakarma is the Sanskrit term for Ayurvedic detoxification or cleansing. It often is a done as a practice to support the branch of Ayurveda known as Rasayana, or rejuvenation and longevity. As mentioned in chapter 1, *pancha* means "five," and *karma* means "action." Deep detoxification in Ayurveda involves five actions to cleanse the body by balancing the doshas. These five actions are: *vamana,* or emesis (vomiting therapy), virechana, or purgation (intestinal purge), basti, or enema (colon cleanse), *nasya,* or nasal cleansing, and *rakta mokshana,* or bloodletting. Sounds intense, right? It is. True detoxification of the body is an involved process, requiring clinical aptitude and skilled practitioners. This is because it is not a one-size-fits-all process. Everyone needs something tailored to their individual needs. True panchakarma is, from my experience and research to date, rarely found outside of India. Many of its techniques are not something that falls under the scope of practice of a massage therapist or even a licensed acupuncturist.

The fact that panchakarma is actually inaccessible to most in the West doesn't make the concept of cleansing the body of ama useless or beyond grasp. There are steps we can take to begin anew, namely, short, safe, home cleansing, lifestyle changes, and long-term modifications to our diets that are rooted in Ayurveda. We can incorporate many of the techniques for detoxification and rejuvenation found in the classical texts in a safe, gentle, consistent manner. If one wants a more serious cleanse, there are Ayurvedic doctors from India with BAMS degrees, who may be able to guide an individual on a one-on-one basis in how to use the more intense or involved techniques in their own homes.

What has become popular in the West for Ayurvedic home cleansing is actually *purvakarma,* potentially with a hint of panchakarma practices like mild purgation, enemas, and or nasya treatments toward the end. *Purva* means "before." Therefore, purvakarma is what is done in India to prepare the body for panchakarma. It is a preparatory phase where a simple diet is eaten, only mild exercise is done, and lots of medicated oil is applied to the body, both internally and externally, in a process called "oleation."

Slight, monitored sweating from the neck down is also a part of purvakarma. This is called *swedana,* where the person is seated in a box with their head on the outside. In Ayurveda, it is not recommended to heat the head like one would do in a Western sauna; it is considered unhealthy. The mild sweating is done because the combination of it and oil massage gently encourages imbalanced doshas and ama to loosen from the tissues where they are lodged so that they can move back to the digestive tract for elimination. In terms of the oil treatment, warm, medicated oil is applied to the body, in various ways, often by two practitioners. This oil penetrates deep into the body and binds with fat soluble toxins in the deeper tissue. The combination of oleation and light therapeutic sweating helps to soften and open the channels for purification. The oil massage also calms the mind and relaxes and strengthens the body for the next stage in the process. A growing number of licensed massage therapists in the United States are trained in how to administer these oil treatments.

Purvakarma is an important part of the cleansing process. Ayurvedic doctors know that it is detrimental to throw the body into a detox without preparing it first. It's like trying to clean a grease-caked pot with cold water and no scrubber or soap. If the body is caked with ama, it needs the right amount of heat and lubricant to loosen it and the proper diet, herbs, and bodywork to help scrape it out. The fact that warm oil is relaxing to the nervous system is a bonus. Relaxation is important to balance the mind. It is also much easier to enter areas of the body if it is relaxed, as tension helps to hold the imbalanced doshas and toxins in place. When undergoing any cleansing process, the mind may become easily disturbed or agitated. One must work their way in gently, with trust and patience. Forcing the body to expel toxins may create many adverse mental effects like sleep difficulty, nervousness, and anxiety, to name a few. In essence, it can create vata imbalance and further injure the agni.

The doshas that are out of balance need to be culled out of dormancy from the places they don't belong and driven back to the digestive tract for elimination from the system. For example, there is no sense in doing vomiting therapy before kapha is in the stomach, or in purging if pitta has not moved into the opening of the small intestine. Thus, purvakarma is essential.

After purvakarma come the primary five actions of panchakarma—vamana, virechana, basti, nasya, and rakta mokshana as described above. This is the second of three stages in classical panchakarma. *Pradhana* means "main" or "most important." *Pradhana karma* therefore means the "most important actions" in panchakarma.

The third aspect of Ayurvedic cleansing involves paschatkarma, or rehabilitative measures post panchakarma. It is a time of rest and rejuvenation. After purvakarma and pradhana karma, the body is more like a clean slate. It is now slowly nourished to build the energy back up by administering easy-to-digest grain soups and tonifying herbs that build agni. By rebuilding or enkindling agni, the body can again transform properly and thereby prevent further ama accumulation. If one were to go to a good panchakarma center in India, especially for their first time, the entire process would take about thirty to forty days, depending upon the amount of ama and the strength of the agni. *Ayurveda* means "wisdom of life." It cannot be rushed. To paraphrase Lao-tzu in the Tao Te Ching, "Nature does not hurry, yet everything is accomplished." Humans hurry, but what of any substance is accomplished?

Obviously, the average person cannot take a month off to be massaged and purged halfway across the world. Perhaps this is why the ancient Chinese did not develop or adopt this branch of medicine. It was simply too much of a commitment, or they were more invested in practicality or too consumed with operating in survival mode to spend time exploring something that is today linked to privilege and disposable income. Or they may have been so desperate to maintain some semblance of health in the population that they may have foregone the idea entirely. The Chinese culture does, however, include the concept of longevity and practices that cultivate it that parallel the idea of rejuvenation in Ayurveda, or the building-up phase of paschatkarma.

Although most people will never experience complete Ayurvedic cleansing and rejuvenation in their lifetime, there is an alternative: we can gently cleanse a little at a time while cumulatively improving our environment and lifestyle, thereby minimizing harmful causative factors. Many people do regular seasonal cleanses, regular purvakarmas, along with a little panchakarma and paschatkarma. These can be done at any change of season if need be, but the early spring, ideally, and early fall are preferred. This is because the qualities of change in those two seasons greatly enhance the release of toxins from the body. The ancients were adept enough at perceiving the many facets of our interrelationship with the "outer world," regardless of subtlety. Drawing from this knowledge they deduced the optimal times to build the body up or to cleanse it throughout the yearly cycle.

RITUCHARYA: SEASONAL ROUTINE

Ritucharya is the term used for living in harmony with the seasons. *Ritu* means "seasons" and *charya* refers to a routine to be followed. Ritucharya is based upon the strength of the Sun upon Earth's atmosphere in its yearly orbit. Most of the time, it is interpreted as being more tied to weather patterns. Weather patterns predispose us to certain weaknesses. If we are pretty well-balanced, we will not be too affected by shifts in the weather and should still follow the principles of ritucharya in order to maintain wellness. However, when we have one or more doshas a fair degree out of balance, we will really notice shifts in the weather and seasons. One seasonal change may be worse than another depending upon the preexisting imbalance.

The seasonal factors that we may feel afflicted by are a result of the deeper, subtler effect of Earth's year-long voyage around the Sun and the moistening or drying effect the Sun has on our atmosphere. The angle of the Earth in relationship to the Sun is the backbone of ritucharya. The weather that accompanies a given season and its qualities of cold, hot, windy, or damp do affect us, but they are more branch issues, or symptoms, that may or may not have a major impact on our bodies and minds. The body naturally responds to the heat or cold in the air by cooling or heating internally to balance itself. An example of this would be agni strengthening internally in the fall as the balancing mechanism to the weather cooling externally. In addition, as pitta rises in the body, the Earth above the equator is still in Moon time, and moonlight is naturally soothing to pitta! This is an exquisite balancing mechanism.

Each time of year has certain qualities that increase or decrease one of the doshas. This equates to an increase or decrease in the five elements. The increase of qualities in nature can cause a dosha to accumulate, aggravate, then settle or calm. The body is designed to sense the change in sunlight or the dominance of moonlight, dryness, wetness, cold, and heat and adjust itself accordingly to maintain homeostasis. Only if there is an imbalance too great for the natural rhythm to calm will it continue throughout the year and be exacerbated by even slight barometric pressure changes, weather changes, or even the time of day.

It is important to explain why Ayurveda recommends cleansing at specific times of year and what those times are. Many people cleanse willy-nilly any time of year and may do cleansing practices that are potentially damaging to their specific constitution. An example of this might be a vata-aggravated individual doing a colon cleanse in the late summer or fall. This is naturally when the vata dosha is at its highest and moving into the time it should naturally be calm. Instead, this person flushes out the colon (vata's seat in the body) with plain water (not nourishing enough to balance vata), without preparing properly (purvakarma), or nourishing afterward (paschatkarma), during the most depleting half of the year, headed into the coldest time of year. So they are totally aggravating vata, leaving a gaping space (vata is space and air), and weakening the system.

Now, they head into winter (cold and dry) and the dry heat indoors with the qualities of vata heightened instead of calmed. As a result, vata is not calmed for the year and appears to be exacerbated that winter, all year long, and the following autumn. When it begins its accumulation phase after the spring, the person probably has a greater vata derangement than the previous year and feels so unsettled and exhausted from it they just think they are toxic from eating all winter and want to cleanse again in the summer, when vata naturally accumulates. This is a vicious cycle. Colon cleansing doesn't always necessarily cause a great imbalance; the scenario outlined above simply serves as a single example of the myriad ways in which we may unintentionally contribute to our own imbalance if the timing isn't right or the therapy isn't right for our particular constitution.

Let's take a closer look at how the year is broken down. It is divided into two parts. The first begins around the winter solstice and lasts until the summer solstice. It is the time of light, as there is more daylight over a larger portion of the globe at this time of year, at least in the northern hemisphere. Because of the increase in the Sun's rays, the Earth experiences the transformation of water: evaporation. There are also many storms bringing with them great winds. In addition, as we move toward summer it gets hotter outside. The increased temperatures heat the body, evaporating kapha (water) and increasing vata (air) dosha. Therefore, this time of year leads to increased internal dryness. It is the solar half of the year and is yang in nature because there is greater light, heat, radiation, and expansion. The dominant doshas at this time of year are kapha and vata initially and vata and pitta later on in the summer. This is felt in the body as lingering late-winter colds and flu, mucusy spring seasonal allergies, and summertime weakness, sleep disturbance, dehydration, and dryness.

During the other half of the year, the days are getting shorter. The portion of the Earth that is exposed to the Sun is smaller from just after the summer solstice in late June to around the winter solstice in late December. This is considered the wet time of year. There is not as much solar energy evaporating water. The days are shorter, the nights are longer, and storms are more prevalent. This time of year starts out warm but begins to cool as we head from late summer into early fall. This is the lunar or Moon-dominant time. The Moon is associated with water, the feminine, and yin energies. It is a time where bodily energy is decreasing, when vata, then pitta dominate, and where, clinically, practitioners see a lot of chronic inflammatory flare-ups and wind-related conditions. This time begins in July and lasts through mid-January.

In terms of doshic influence (see fig. 10.1), kapha begins accumulating late in winter, from about mid-January to mid-March. It aggravates in the spring, from mid-March through mid-May, and calms in early to midsummer, from May to July. In midsummer, vata begins to accumulate. It aggravates in the later summer, from July through the middle of September, and calms in the fall. In late summer, mid-July through mid-September, pitta begins accumulating in

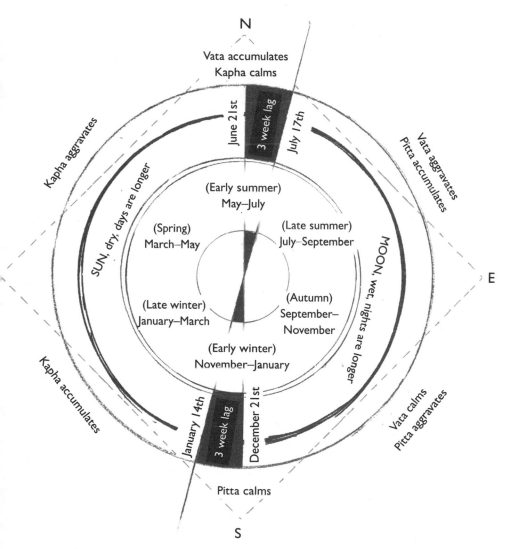

Fig. 10.1. The doshas accumulating, aggravating, and calming

the body. In autumn, from September through November, pitta aggravates and then calms back down in early to midwinter, from mid-November to mid-January.[1] Then the cycle repeats.

Remember that doshas or elements can go out of balance in a person at any time of the year. Another contributing factor to this phenomenon is that, sometimes, the energetic of the dominant underlying force at work actually takes some time to manifest externally. At first it may only be perceptible in the pulse. An example of this may be someone under stress, great pressure, emotional turmoil, or a major life change, who thinks, feels, and appears as though they are handling themselves and managing life well in spite of it. It is only after they've passed through this trying time that they begin to fall apart. This falling apart can manifest as any number of physical or mental patterns or illnesses.

In looking at seasonal effects on the body and mind, climates also need to be taken into account as subcycles under the umbrella of the Sun's yearly cycle. Is an area considered a desert or temperate climate? Is it at altitude or sea level? Global weather patterns like El Niño that change some years may also influence internal balance. So we have daily cycles, Moon cycles, Sun cycles, and lifetime cycles along with environment, lifestyle, and current vikruti, or constitutional imbalance, to take into account when assessing an individual or ourselves. These factors are also important in determining whether to cleanse and when. Before determining that, let's look at the seasons in more depth.

Spring

According to Ayurveda the best time to cleanse is at the change of seasons. Depending upon one's constitution and imbalance pattern, one seasonal change may be a more advantageous time for a cleanse than another. At the change of seasons, energy is moving and shifting, and this change is felt within the body. This makes it easier to withstand the change from the cleanse and to work with the energy of seasonal change to derive the best outcome. It's about moving with the seasonal energy and using it to our advantage. In general, spring, usually late March to mid-April, is my favorite time for a cleanse. This is because the energy of the liver is strong, and the kapha dosha dominates. Some may notice this manifesting as a kapha-type inflammation or spring allergies.

The body is coming from the strength-building dormancy of winter and strong agni into a time of decreasing agni and increasing kapha. The increase of kapha means that the bodily secretions are also increasing. It is like we are fertile ground for co-creating good health. If one is interested in cleansing, why not work with this energy to flush the toxins from the deeper tissues? Since the kapha-like secretions are already doing this, using that momentum saves bodily energy and works with the natural processes at that time of year. The kapha dosha is a combination of water and earth elements, and in the spring one can smell the dominance of the earth element in the air. The ground is loosening as new growth stirs within it, and the earth is nourished by snow and ice melt before moving into the dry summer season.

In Chinese medicine, there is also a correspondence between Earth's journey around the Sun and the effect it has on the body. The Chinese draw parallels between the seasons and the elements and their associated organs. In Chinese medicine, springtime is governed by the wood element and the liver. The Chinese were probably looking to the action of budding leaves on the trees and buds on flowering plants. The liver correlates to the wood element and to the act of stretching, as this is one of the qualities of wood. If not cared for properly, this stretching can become invasive. This means that its overactivity may harass the spleen and stomach, causing digestive issues, create heat in the diaphragm, or harass the lungs, creating heat conditions and making it difficult to take a deep breath. The Chinese recommend avoiding sour foods and increasing sweet foods in the spring. This is because sour is holding, which can lead to a disruption in liver energetic flow and congestion. This congestion can build in the liver (wood), move across the torso, and inhibit the action of the spleen/stomach (earth). So if one's digestion is upset in the spring, it's helpful to limit sour foods and have more sweet. A tiny bit of sweet is cooling for the liver, but not cold, and it enhances digestion. In fact, all those kids (and kids at heart) who want dessert before their meal don't have it wrong. It is naturally best for us to have some sweet taste early in the meal to stimulate digestive secretions.

When kapha is aggravated in the spring, instead of an increase of secretions, there is an inflammatory kapha response and a corresponding increase in excretions. Secretions are considered healthy, physiological fluids, while excretions are the result of imbalance. Excretions are excessive activity and may manifest as congestion. Kapha aggravation saps the energy, makes one sensitive to changes in the atmosphere and environment, and manifests as a myriad of allergic symptoms. It also can create an increased susceptibility to colds and the flu. Remember, kapha time is at its peak late January through May.

When the liver qi stretches in the spring, it may stretch sideways across the body and into the domain of the spleen and stomach (earth element organs). A useful visual for both the spring/wood/liver energy in Chinese medicine and the spring/akasha energy in Ayurveda is a sprout pushing up through the earth and moving it out of the way to get to the sunlight. The Chinese say this is yin moving to yang. That same energetic of pressing through the former winter dormancy from deep in the tissues toward the space of the digestive tract is the mode of action we are using in our favor in the spring to cleanse. It is an upward, outward, spreading movement. If the spleen/stomach/earth energy is weak, this spreading will naturally flow over to fill it.

The stomach comfortably holds and prepares, while the spleen transforms and transports food and fluids. The liver harassing the spleen and stomach may create reflux, upper abdominal pain, distension, malabsorption, and discomfort. It can weaken the spleen so that mucusy secretions or excretions go unchecked by the spleen yang, which is supposed to transform them. This can create increased congestion and all the problems that arise in response to it like imbalanced immune response, postnasal drip, watery eyes, and so on. Adding insult to injury, everything that was consumed during the winter in excess has been building in the body, and the ama, or toxins, from it can really be felt in the spring. They will either naturally rise up and out or be weighed down by kapha congestion. This is a catch-22 as it can in turn create more liver qi stagnation.

By doing a cleanse in the spring, the liver energy is used to help clear the body of toxins accumulated during the winter, which naturally begin to get pushed out of deep tissues. The liver has a lot of energy in the spring, which is why the Chinese caution one to mind it well with diet and exercise in fresh air. It is like leaving a child or a puppy with an abundance of energy that needs to get circulated in a small area or indoors. They get cranky, frustrated, angry, and eventually may get sick. This is what happens to all of us if liver qi congests, especially if it is chronic. By doing a cleanse when the liver energy is most active, its functions are being utilized to their potential instead of rambling out of control.

Given the right circumstances, the liver secretes something that causes the body to shift from building tissue mode (kapha) to cleanse and detoxify mode (pitta-agni). This happens when a proportionate-to-weight caloric intake occurs one or two days per week. There are guidelines for this and a diet out there on the market that uses this information to help people not only lose weight but bring down inflammatory markers and balance blood sugar. Perhaps Ayurveda recommends regular cleansing because these benefits are what they intuitively and experientially recognized thousands of years ago. In fact, it is part of Indian culture to fast one day per week to give the body a break from assimilating food, so it can work instead on purification.

We need space to breathe in the spring, and it is a good time to get some distance and reflect on what behavior, attitudes, mental/emotional patterns, and lifestyle choices are no longer beneficial, healthy, or desired. We spring clean our environment and our mind and body. Some people start this process in the winter months. Spring is a good time to do it because the kapha energy creates a stability from which one can more clearly view desired change. Chinese medicine recommends letting one's hair down a bit, both figuratively and literally, and getting out in the fresh air for regular walks in nature. This helps the liver qi to course and relaxes the nervous system. In fact, there are

Native American tribes that believe the hair is an extension of the nervous system that plays a role in our connection to the natural world and intuition. Clearing out closets, attics, and basements makes space. Airing out the home brings freshness and lightness.

Because of the Sun's naturally increased presence, we are affected by more light and it shines on those dark places within us. We are also increasing our exposure to the air, which is wonderful in that we are not cooped up, breathing recycled or hot-forced air, and we are not in air conditioning mode yet. It can be a bittersweet time, however, in that we feel better with more light and outdoor time but also rough because if we don't acknowledge and shift out of or transform what no longer serves our highest good, wood can stagnate, harass earth, and lead to issues related to the digestion of thoughts and emotions, as well as worry and pensiveness.

Things to do in the spring to stay balanced are as follows:

Clean out closets, drawers, and attics.
Get rid of excess stuff, just as the body is releasing accumulated toxins.
Go for walks in nature on nice days.
Let your hair down.
Relax.
Increase movement.
Eat light meals with spices.
Drink warm water with honey in the morning.
Breathe well.
Air out your living quarters.
Notice what feels oppressive to you and make shifts that allow for greater space within.

Summer

The nervous system is the domain of the vata dosha, which starts to perk up as kapha time wanes in early summer. This is not the best time for a cleanse, as vata is governed by air and space and is easily ungrounded. It is heightened by the dryness of longer, sunshiny days and many summertime lifestyle changes. It can be increased by all the travel that happens in summer, fluctuating weather patterns, sharp forceful winds, a late-to-bed-late-to-rise schedule, cold or iced foods and drinks, not enough sleep, increased alcohol intake, decreased food consumption, and generally erratic living and eating. Inconsistency in schedule and diet is a major contributing factor to vata imbalances and heightened nervous system activity.

In the summer, Ayurveda focuses on the dry, light aspects of vata and how its increase can be weakening to the body, and the Chinese see it as the fire time of year related most closely to the heart organ. This is not surprising because many characteristics of fire in Chinese medicine match qualities of vata in Ayurveda. Fire is drying, subtle, and moving, and it contains air and space. The common ground here is that the king of organs, the heart, is a fire organ. It helps circulate qi and blood and is driven to beat by prana vayu, a subtype of vata. The stimulation of the atrioventricular node that causes the heart to beat regularly and steadily is vata in nature. It comes from prana vata communicating from the brain to the heart. The heart houses the shen spirit and is in charge of the other spirits, and the spirit is moved, or not, by vata.

Many fire qualities are vata in nature. Fire dries, has movement, requires air to exist, and contributes to vata-type disturbances common in the summer like irregularity in schedule and diet, restless sleep, digestive complaints, dryness, and insomnia. Small intestine heat resulting in loose bowel movements and diarrhea can also be the result of heart fire. The small intestine is the heart's paired yang organ. It is like a reservoir for excess heart heat, and the Small Intestine meridian is often treated for this. In addition, since the Small Intestine meridian forms a single pathway with the Bladder meridian, this heat can in turn affect the urinary bladder, causing bladder infections. This is not uncommon given the external heat of the summer months, pathological obsession with overheating in the sun, exercising in the sun, sunbathing, spicy barbecues, increased alcohol consumption, and oftentimes increased caffeine.

Summer naturally saps the energy, and it decreases agni. The days get shorter and, in addition to the natural weakness of agni, people are overindulging in damaging habits and foods. Look at animals in the summer. They naturally lie around. Elderly dogs are not as active in the summer months. This is a time for us to rest and take it easy. It is not natural to run in the sun and heat, lie on hot dry sand in the wind and bake, or do yoga at noon in the park. It may be the norm, but that doesn't make it good for us. It is a time of natural dehydration, and our society and culture are certainly going with that flow because dehydration, heat stroke, and sun poisoning are all prevalent in the summer. Additionally, sweat is the fluid of the heart, and the heart's vitality can be depleted by too much sweating. This is especially true for those who exercise in the heat, especially right in the sun, as they are provoking heart fire as they deplete the system of fluids.

The increased heat and solar power can be used to our advantage in the summer. Chinese medicine has a practice for treating future seasonal allergies. At the time the Sun is at its greatest light, before the Moon time begins to take over, dry moxa treatment is recommended. It involves the application of caustic paste to several yang points on the back, over the area of the lungs. This paste actually burns the skin. It's not comfortable or pretty, but it works. It charges the body's yang qi before heading into Moon time using the power of the heating, drying herbs and harnessing the energy of the Sun on the summer solstice. By charging the yang, one is enkindling the agni and strengthening the immune response, which is designed to balance the immune system in preparation for fall and spring allergies. This is repeated three times around the solstice, three years in a row for complete treatment.

People become more tired at this time of year and really need to push themselves physically to do things not only because of the naturally occurring diminished agni but also because of the popular, but poor, lifestyle choices they make that aren't in tandem with what is healthy for the summer. People tend to increase their intake of iced tea, iced coffee, and ice cream, freeze their water bottles, and drink ice water. In addition to increased caffeine, a diuretic, there is an increase in sweating and a potential decrease in overall water consumption as other drinks are often substituted for water. In an effort to decrease the urge to urinate because they're going out on a boat or to the pool or don't want to look bloated in their bikini, people drink less hydrating substances than they should. The excess of iced food and drink they consume leads to a further decrease in agni, which facilitates low energy and ama formation and sets the stage for fall pitta imbalance. This is much more difficult to treat than a straight-up pitta aggravation.

Believe it or not, we are vulnerable to wind, manmade or otherwise, in the summer months, which can be quite vata provoking. Wind is present outdoors, on scooters, motorcycles, and boats and indoors from air conditioners and fans. Since the pores are more open in the summer because of the heat, it is not advisable to be in drafts. They carry pestilential qi into the body. Unfortunately, it is not uncommon for people to sit in front of air conditioning units or fans and sleep with fans blowing on them. Summer colds are not nice, and Chinese medicine teaches that pathogens caught in the summer can linger in the body, then emerge in the fall or winter as full-blown problems. Ayurveda and Chinese medicine give similar advice about the seasons and how to stay healthy during each one.

Since vata dominates and easily aggravates by late summer, and agni is naturally low, summer is not a good time to cleanse. Instead, take the time to relax as much as possible and in proper fashion for the season. Hydrate well and nourish the body gently. Tone down physical activity and eat light, nutrient rich, seasonally appropriate, easily digestible food and drink with some spice. Also remember to back off on the ice. Chinese medicine actually recommends taking warm medicinals during the summer to allay potential stomach cold, which is due largely to the interplay of diminished agni and an inappropriate lifestyle at this time of year.

Spices, light foods, regular meal times, and smaller portions can all help to keep agni enkindled. Remember that vata is cold, and that cold can cause diarrhea just as heat can. Cold can actually cause heat to flare in some cases. Bitter tasting foods and drinks can drain heat from the body, so it is recommended to keep them in check in the summer. Pungent foods are more warming and are recommended for balance in the summer months. Garlic and onion are very popular in warm climates, as are chilies. The pungency comes out through the pores and may aid in repelling insects.

Pay attention to what your body craves in summer. Notice if the craving is emotional, nostalgic, or coming from a place within that enhances good health. If you pay attention, you can discern the difference. If it's an emotional craving, ask your body why it needs that particular food or drink. If it's nostalgic, eat or drink it in moderation. Healthy cravings feel different from cravings that occur due to an imbalance. They are more easily ignored. Pay attention, notice how you feel after you eat, and favor foods that don't weigh you down too much, cause indigestion, or make you want to take a nap. Moderation, as in all things, is key. It is not good for energy flow to be rigid about these guidelines to the point where not having certain foods becomes obsessive. Merely be aware of them and make the best choice. Keep in mind that Ayurveda says the greatest imbalance is to have knowledge of truth and go against it.

Things you can do to stay balanced in the summer are as follows:

Exercise early in the morning before the sun is strong if exercising outdoors.
Stay out of the sun and wind when practicing yoga.
Do only what you feel you have the energy for when exercising.
Limit iced food and drink.
Use alcohol and sugar in moderation.
Eat raw or cold foods for lunch.
Continue to eat soups, stews, and cooked foods regularly.
Try to stay on a regular schedule.

Autumn

After spring, autumn is the second best time of the year to cleanse. It runs from late September through November. Cleansing earlier in the season is best and only if pitta has been maintained well through the late summer months, July to September. Since pitta is naturally heightened right now, a cleanse at this time can work with this natural ebb and flow and help to purge it. Ama may have accumulated from poor summertime digestion and eating habits. In addition, aggravated vata has calmed by this time, and in that sense the body and mind are more grounded, and vata is less likely to be disharmonized by cleansing. In both Chinese and Indian thought, spring and fall are the most changeable, in-flux times of the year. That makes them the perfect times to make a change physiologically as well.

The atmospheric vibe of autumn is that of letting go. In terms of Chinese theory, it correlates to the metal element and to the lungs and large intestine organs. Autumn is lung time in Ayurveda too. The lung qi is responsible for processing grief. Unresolved grief often comes to the surface at this time. If the energy of the lungs becomes overactive, it can adversely affect the liver. Fall is a time when clinicians often see wind disturbances like skin issues and tremors, seizures, and tics. These are all related to the wood element, and in Chinese theory we call this metal (lung qi) overacting on wood (liver qi). It is important at this time to keep a good balance. Breathe well and eat regular meals of light, seasonal, good quality, and easily digestible foods.

When grief is unprocessed and arises in the fall, do your best to understand and work through it. It is possible to feel grief and still be happy. Find the bittersweet, so to speak, look toward beauty, recognize this energy as part of the natural ebb and flow of life, part of the yin and yang balance. Do your best to breathe well, meditate, and appreciate nature. The leaves fall from a tree because the tree's energy is drawing inward like our own in preparation for winter. It is a time of extreme change and remembrance. Allow the thoughts and emotions that come up to flow through you or fall away into space. Nothing is ever gone, merely transformed. It is our attachment to static objects and unmet expectations, like people and pets not living forever or happy times passing, that causes us to live with unprocessed emotional energy.

In Indian philosophy there is a concept called the *kleshas*. The kleshas are the five obstacles that keep us from realizing the true nature of the self, or the Tao. These are ignorance, egoism, attachment, aversion, and clinging to life. In fact this last obstacle, alternately translated as fear of death, is said to be the greatest one for even the most enlightened individuals. Really, all obstacles to inner peace, knowing, and contentment can be traced to our attachments and aversions. Whatever we are attached to causes us pain when it goes away. What we have aversion to causes pain and suffering as it comes closer to us. Our awareness of these things is heightened in the fall, as they all can cause grief in one form or another, and that grief needs to be processed by the lungs.

The lungs breathe. Without the breath there is no life. With the breath there is life, movement, transformation, and sustainability, however fleeting. Keeping the bigger picture in mind and allowing the discomfort to arise into consciousness will help us stay balanced in the autumn. We ordinarily have an aversion to grief and hence try to avoid it, but being with, witnessing, or allowing the grief actually helps us. In fact, scientists are finding that sadness, the kind that flows through you at times, not clinical depression, is beneficial to our growth as humans. In fall, we move from a time of decreasing fire (agni) and light (solar energy) toward a time of yin/darkness, to the inner world of the self. The energy that was distracted and dissipated over the summer is forced to draw inward, making it difficult to ignore.

In Chinese terms we call this the yang qi moving in deep to the core. It does this every night, but every winter it does it on a grander scale. If there is stuff inside we don't want to acknowledge it makes us very uncomfortable, and this discomfort is only exacerbated by the urge to suppress the things that unnerve us. It can be things about ourselves we don't like or the grief that haunts us when we have lost a loved one. This affects our breathing, our lungs, our minds, and our bodies systemically. A fall cleanse may help with the process of sensing these things and processing them before moving into winter. As the energy of the dark increases, transient sadness may escalate to chronic sadness or depression, as opposed to just a heightened time and awareness of our resistances, attachments, and grief.

Overall, autumn is a time when pitta aggravates, and vata may be provoked by increasing wind and dryness. It is a time to tend to the health of the lung qi and be mindful of how the liver qi is managing the change in season. The change from late winter into spring and late summer into autumn are the greatest times of change and fluctuation during the year. It is at these times we are the most internally stirred. It is important to remain centered at these times, and being present with what is going on inside of us is paramount to good health. The ancients prescribed these times to be the best for cleansing just for these reasons.

Things to do to stay balanced in autumn are as follows:

Wear a scarf.

Avoid iced foods and beverages.

Integrate self-oil massage if it fits with your current constitutional state.

Begin a breath awareness practice.

Exercise moderately, being mindful of avoiding excess wind.

Assimilate more herbs and spices into your cooking. Examples include turmeric, ginger, cardamon, nutmeg, coriander, pepper, and cinnamon.

Winter

Early winter is generally mid-November to mid-January. As we move from fall to winter, the cooler air and increased lunar energy cause heat to move inward, calming pitta and increasing agni. As the digestive fire increases, it helps our bodies cope with the heavier foods we are naturally drawn to at this time of year. Kapha is increasing, and this strengthened agni helps us maintain its balance. The increase in agni and kapha create greater strength in the winter, so it is a good time to increase the intensity of exercise. It is also important to keep the circulation flowing at this time, as it assists in lymph flow and in heart health.

According to Chinese medicine, the heart may be susceptible to imbalance in the winter time. This is interesting since we now recognize

February to be heart health month in the United States. In terms of Chinese theory, the yang qi has moved within. The Chinese caution against being too hot in the winter as it can damage the heart qi. Too much heat applied externally—taking saunas or sitting in front of hot fires or heaters—can imbalance the heart qi and cause restlessness. The transition from early winter to late winter, which is mid-January to mid-March, marks a shift from the wet, yin time of year to the drier time of late winter. Fire is dry, and the heart is a fire organ and therefore easily damaged by excess fire and its dry quality.

Chinese medicine practitioners also recognize winter as being a good time to conserve the kidney qi. The kidneys are naturally dominant in the winter, particularly kidney yang. It helps that the yang goes inward in winter, and the agni strengthens. If agni is strong and kidney yin and yang are strong and balanced, immunity should be high and the person should have good stamina. If, however, the kidneys are depleted for any reason, the person may be more susceptible to the cold, wind, and dryness and feel like they have a vata imbalance rather than increased strength. Winter is a good time to tonify the kidneys and conserve essence, or jing, and yin and yang.

Even if one is very healthy, it is best to avoid cold drafts, especially with the ears exposed. The kidneys open to the ears. This makes the ears a weak point and an entry point to the kidney system. If wind gets in the ear canal in the winter, it can be potentially harmful to the kidney qi, especially if it is already deficient. The low belly, low back, and feet should also be kept warm and dry in the winter. These areas are governed by the kidney qi and store the essence. The soles of the feet connect directly to the earth through the Kidney channel and when the ground is cold and dry it can tax the kidney yang. For this reason, it is best to keep the feet covered to avoid cold entering the Kidney channel and depleting the yang qi or contributing to issues with the low back, ankles, or knees.

The low belly and back are also susceptible to wind attack and cold, particularly in the winter months. Chinese medicine advises against wearing miniskirts, low-cut pants, and high-cut shirts at this time of year. They all allow precious kidney energy to escape and for cold, damp, and wind to get into the body. The main storage points for our deep internal reserves are in the low back (ming men, or gate of vitality) and abdomen (guan yuan, or gate of origin). When these areas are left exposed to cold or somehow compromised, there may be a sense of disconnection from the earth, of not being grounded, spaciness, anxiety, nervousness, or fear.

The heart and kidneys have a close relationship with one another. They provide the main water/fire balance in the body. Water being kidney, fire being heart. In the winter, kidney energy is dominant. If yang is strong and yin is plentiful, there is a water and fire balance that keeps the body and mind healthy. If water and fire are out of balance, it can affect the heart fire adversely. For example, since winter is naturally the high-water season in Chinese medicine, if the yang qi is low and water is high, the excess water can dampen the heart fire. Conversely, if the kidney yang is not held by the yin, it can rise up and harass the heart. In this way, both organ systems and elements need to be considered and kept healthy. In Chinese medicine, the daily use of medicinal wines is recommended in the cold winter months. The wine extracts the active constituents of the herbs which tonify yang, yin, and qi, and is itself medicinal. It acts to warm and circulate the blood, thereby assisting the heart.

Things to do to stay balanced in winter are as follows:

Eat and drink warm, cooked foods and beverages.
Favor hearty soups and stews.
Limit caffeine intake.
Avoid refined sugar.
Practice good hygiene as a preventive for colds and flu.
Exercise.
Get outside each day for fresh air and sunshine.
Keep ears, low back, low belly, and nape of neck covered outside in colder climates.
Wear socks or slippers on cold floors.
Avoid fasting and cleansing.
Establish a meditation practice.

HOME CLEANSING

There are many actions we can take on our own to cleanse and remove toxicity not just from our bodies but from our lives, and sometimes leaving the home and work environment for a time can help us figure out just what needs cleansing. Environment and lifestyle are major contributing factors to physical, mental, and emotional imbalance, and being removed from the daily grind allows one the opportunity to disconnect, however uncomfortable that may be, and reflect upon potential causative factors with regard to familial relationships and lifestyle issues. It is wonderful to take at least a day away for yourself every so often. A road trip to a beautiful place, a weekend away at a retreat center, or time away at a bed and breakfast or even a campground can help you to reflect and gain perspective.

Cleansing, like everything in life, exists in all dimensions of one's being—spiritual, emotional, mental, and physical. Physical cleansing can be dietary, but that is just one aspect of it. Perhaps starting with cleansing the space in which we live would be most helpful. There is an old saying about cleaning the pot before filling it with fresh drinking water. Before a cleanse, during purvakarma, we are encouraged to eliminate difficult-to-digest and addictive substances from our diet. These include meat, sugar, alcohol, and caffeine. But what if before that, we cleanse the structure that houses us.

It is said that our environment, or living space, reflects our inner state. We are all affected by our surroundings, and the age-old practices of feng shui and vastu take into account the best positioning of our home and its objects so that we may live to our full potential in the best mental, emotional, physical, spiritual, and oftentimes financial health. Although there are consultants trained in optimizing the energetic flow in the home or office environment, these practices are entire fields of study, like Chinese medicine, and some people may prefer a simpler way to do this on their own.

There is a wonderful Japanese practice called the "KonMari method," which is a technique used to clear and organize a space.[2] It starts with visualization. People visualize in different ways.

Some can actually close their eyes and see from within, while others get a general sense or a feeling of what something is or could be. Perhaps others can smell, hear, or picture symbols that represent their object of visualization. Whatever works is fine. Just visualize what a preferred space would be for you. Let the clarity of it permeate your mind.

Then, taking your time, physically move from object to object in the space, and hold or touch it. If it brings you joy, keep it. If it does not, ask yourself why you are holding on to it. Perhaps you fear you will need or want it one day, or it holds a special memory. Discern what is healthy for you to keep, what fits with the visualization of your preferred space and the life you wish to live. Inanimate objects are also expressions of qi/prana/life-force energy. Whether you decide to keep or let go of an object, honor it for its place in your life and then find the coolest way possible to rehome what isn't staying. Donations? Gifts? Swap pages? Fireplace on a cold night? Just time to recycle or throw it away? This process can take time. It can take months. Cleansing the body can too.

THREE AYURVEDIC CLEANSES

In the spring, the ideal time for a cleanse, the upward and outward momentum means the emotional energy, mental holding patterns, and the biophysiology resulting from them is less likely to be suppressed. There may be a restlessness, a dissatisfaction with complacency, and an unhappiness with the status quo of one's life. People naturally begin to want to move more on a physical level, to clean out the closets, and to change their diets. This isn't the same as what happens with New Year's resolutions. This is not forced mental striving, making resolutions from obligation or habit, or forcing something to change within; it is the natural flow of spring energy. The timing of the Chinese New Year, also known as the "Spring Festival," makes sense in terms of seasonal flow and what it brings up in us naturally. Go with that. Ask if it's a good time for a dietary or a spatial cleanse and pick the one that is best for you in the moment. Perhaps a little decluttering is right for this time so that the surrounding space becomes an open support that springboards you into a spring or fall cleanse with ease of mind.

It is important to realize that the body is well equipped to cleanse itself without much intervention or willpower on our behalf. The lungs release toxins every time we exhale, the liver and kidneys are also astute at filtering toxins from the blood. The gastrointestinal tract also cleanses itself if given the chance. Oftentimes what we really need when we feel like we need a cleanse or a detox is to hit the reset button by eliminating some bad habits. By just following the basic lifestyle recommendations in the dinacharya (daily routine) section, and integrating a little breathwork and exercise, the body should be able to handle the rest. Tweaking the diet to allow for more time between meals or adding what we need and subtracting what we don't can also do wonders for physical, mental, and emotional well-being. Simple steps in a balanced direction may be all we need to feel cleansed. If you feel drawn to an actual cleansing ritual, however, read on. Ayurveda has just what you may be looking for.

People should not cleanse when they are weak, sick, or overcoming a long illness, have diagnosed medical conditions for which a cleanse is contraindicated, are pregnant, nursing, or trying to conceive, or have recently had surgery. I also recommend that people don't try to do a cleanse when they are freshly grieving, especially the death of a close loved one, or any other time there is physical or emotional upheaval. If you move, wait until you have firmly settled into the new home before cleansing, and if there's a new addition to the family, wait until you've established a set pattern or routine. Too much change can be too much change. It is important to feel anchored before lifting off.

That said, when you know you—or a client—are ready for a cleanse, there are several to choose from that draw from the wisdom of Ayurveda. The first is a simple three-day cleanse. It is a wonderful first-time endeavor or good for someone who isn't sure they can or want to commit to a longer time frame. It is also a good quick cleanse for people needing a boost or who want to do more than one cleanse a year. The second option is for a full week, and the third is for ten days. Beyond that, it is advised to seek professional guidance.

The goal of an Ayurvedic cleanse is to get toxins, including those that are fat soluble, to release and move out of the body. It also helps the individual hit the reset button on their lifestyle and diet. Doing a juice cleanse, as is popular nowadays, will probably just pull water from the tissues, make you feel a little lighter, and cause water-weight loss. Once eating begins again, the weight comes back. In an Ayurvedic cleanse, you eat the whole time, so this doesn't happen. The food, medicinals, and drinks consumed are tridoshic, or constitutionally universally balanced, and easy to digest and help to scrape out the detox channels. The liver and the kidneys will continue to do their work—filtering the blood of toxins and relieving the body of them through urination, respectively.

As in panchakarma, purvakarma, or precleanse actions, are important for getting the body and mind ready to release what is stored within and not healthy. These toxins can be the result of sluggish digestion, by-products of emotional states, stuck metabolic wastes, or pollutants that build up in the system because the liver, kidneys, or lungs are not able to do their jobs properly. They can also be due to environmental toxins that build up from off-gassing upholstery, clothing, rugs, cars, and the pollution we are growing more accustomed to in daily living. Purvakarma (precleansing), which should be done for one to two weeks prior to start of the cleanse, is the same for all of the cleanses outlined below and is as follows:

- Reflect on what you'd like your life to be like, and make an internal commitment to adjust it accordingly.
- Pay attention to your breathing (see the breathwork section in chapter 8)
- Begin a meditation practice of at least a few minutes a day.
- Lighten your regular schedule during the course of the cleanse, making time for contemplation, gentle exercise, breathing, walks in nature, and meditation.
- Give yourself adequate time to rest and go to bed by 10 p.m.
- Begin to eliminate caffeine, sugar, and alcohol from your diet at

least a week before the cleanse begins so that you've finished a detox reaction before the cleanse starts.

- Eliminate meat, poultry, cheese, white/refined flour, fried food, and fish a minimum of four days before the cleanse begins.
- Avoid upsetting situations as much as possible and topics on television or online that may be disturbing like the news, politics, and violence.
- Take ½ teaspoon of psyllium husk in a cup of room-temperature water in the morning.
- Add at least one of the following to your daily routine: yoga, qigong, breathing, tai chi, meditation, yoga nidra.
- Go for daily walks in nature.
- Incorporate dry brushing and tongue scraping into your routine.

In each of the cleanses, you will need the following items:

psyllium husk
white and brown basmati rice
mung dal (yellow mung beans)
ghee (preferably cultured ghee): If you have high cholesterol, you'll also need flax oil.
spices (cumin, coriander, fennel, ginger, cayenne, mustard seed, asafetida [hing])
garshana (dry brushing): Use a brush and/or gloves.
appropriate oil for abhyanga (vata: sesame, pitta: coconut, kapha: almond or sunflower)
brahmi oil
yoga nidra CD
sesame oil if oil pulling
tongue scraper
rejuvenating post-cleanse supplement (chyawanprash)
Triphala

Practice making *kitchari* before the cleanse so you know how to do it and if you like it.

Sample Kitchari Recipe

1 cup mung dal
1 cup white basmati rice
1/4 teaspoon turmeric
1/4 teaspoon cumin
1/4 teaspoon yellow mustard seed
1/2 teaspoon fresh ginger
2 teaspoons ghee
1–3 seasonal, fresh vegetables
Salt and pepper to taste

Combine dal and rice in a pan and rinse and drain it several times.

Add 6–9 cups of water to the pan depending on what you would like the consistency of the rice and dal to be.

Bring the mixture to a boil, then turn it down to a simmer.

Add the turmeric, stir, and let simmer.

In a separate pan combine the ghee, mustard seed, cumin, fresh ginger, and vegetables.

Cook until vegetables are just tender.

Add the vegetable/spice mixture to the rice/dal mix, stir and cook together for another ten minutes.

Serve hot.

You may add a bit more ghee and salt and pepper to taste and some fresh cilantro if you wish.

The ratio of rice to dal can be also be changed, as can the amount of water.

THREE-DAY CLEANSE

For the three-day cleanse, continue to incorporate what you have integrated into your routine from the precleanse. Then for three days you will do three things: eat kitchari for each meal, drink cumin/coriander/ fennel tea between meals, and take Triphala at night. Then follow the post-cleanse section (see page 284).

SEVEN-TO-TEN-DAY CLEANSE

The seven-to-ten-day cleanse protocols are similar, with the exception of the middle part being longer in the ten-day cleanse. I recommend preparing two weeks in advance for these cleanses, maybe even a month, so you can start weaning yourself off of things you don't want freshly in your system or that may be stressful to detox from. For most people, sugar detox can feel like the flu for several days. For this reason, it is best to wean slowly instead of coming off of it cold turkey. Caffeine is the second most difficult thing to clear. This is because it is also addictive and causes withdrawal headaches in some people.

Roasted barley drink is a good antidote for coming off of coffee, as it mimics the taste, body, and feel of coffee. Herbal teas are a good transition from maté, green, white, and black teas. Beginning to integrate the cumin, coriander, and fennel concoction is also a good alternative, as well as adding tulsi to it to help stabilize the mood during the transition. Organic India makes a great tulsi tea, and this can be added in a teabag to the cumin, coriander, and fennel drink.

Do your preparation for the cleanse by following the purvakarma (precleanse) steps above. Integrating all of the dietary changes and the dinacharya (lifestyle/daily routine) changes such as a potentially new meditation practice or dry brushing can be quite a lot to handle all at once. If you know you're going to cleanse in March or April, start shifting your routine slowly in January or February. This will allow you to transition smoothly to the cleanse in the spring. If you plan to do the crash course in cleansing, then if you aren't already meditating, walking in fresh air, exercising, or doing breathing techniques or yoga, you will be completely shifting your entire lifestyle all at once and that may be too much. For beginners, maybe just pick one thing to do—KonMari, perhaps, or meditation or yoga. Or it could be tai chi or breathing. Whatever it is, be consistent with it and ease your way into it slowly.

As with any exercise program or dietary change, always consult with a professional, especially if you know you have preexisting health conditions or don't feel healthy. Again, cleansing is contraindicated during illness, pregnancy, and menstruation. Also, please keep in mind this is a general, safe cleanse regime geared toward a healthy, curious population. A cleanse administered one-to-one with a qualified health care professional would be attuned to an individual's specific needs and constitution.

Purchase all the supplies you will need for the cleanse. Organic India is a great resource for tulsi tea, chyawanprash, and Triphala. Try to get the other ingredients in organic form too. Lisa Deering Temoshok has a wonderful yoga nidra CD; or you can find one you like online. Carve out time in your schedule for a stress-free self-oil massage, extra resting, yoga nidra, cooking kitchari, and drinking teas.

Days 1–3

Begin incorporating internal oleation and kitchari with vegetables into your daily routine. Choose one to three vegetables from your dosha list for your kitchari. Your daily routine should go as follows:

1. Wake by 6 a.m.
2. Go to the bathroom.
3. Scrape your tongue.
4. Brush your teeth.
5. Perform oil pulling.
6. While you're oil pulling you can dry brush.
7. Shower or bathe.
8. Internal oleation: Warm some ghee and sip up to 1 tablespoon (if it gives you the heebie-jeebies or makes you nauseated, skip it). If you have cholesterol issues, use flaxseed oil. Over the course of the first three days, you can increase the intake to 2 tablespoons.
9. Drink a glass of water, either room temperature or warm.
10. Go for a walk, do yoga, meditate, breathe, and so on.
11. Eat kitchari with vegetables.
12. Drink plenty of water throughout your day; half your body weight in ounces is a general rule of thumb.
13. If you encounter cravings or feel hungry, drink some cumin, coriander, fennel, and tulsi (CCFT) tea.
14. Between 11 a.m. and 2 p.m., eat lunch (kitchari with vegetables).

15. Again, drink plenty of water, but not right before or right after a meal. Only sip on hot water, CCF, or CCFT teas during meals.

16. If you encounter cravings or feel hungry, drink some CCF or CCFT tea.

17. Eat dinner (kitchari with vegetables) before 6 p.m. Drink more tea and water.

18. Before bed, take Triphala with warm water as recommended on the label.

19. Massage the feet and scalp with brahmi oil. No need to get a lot of oil in the hair; just put a bit on the fingertips to massage into the scalp. Make sure to thoroughly massage the soles of the feet and around the ankles.

20. Practice yoga nidra.

21. Go to sleep by 10 p.m.

Days 4–6* (or 4–7 if doing the ten-day cleanse)

Changes from days 1–3 are external instead of internal oleation and kitchari without vegetables. Follow the daily routine outlined below:

1. Wake by 6 a.m.

2. Go to the bathroom.

3. Scrape your tongue.

4. Brush your teeth.

5. Perform oil pulling.

6. While you're oil pulling, you can dry brush and add abhyanga (self-oil massage).

7. Shower or bathe.

8. Drink a glass of water, either room temperature or warm.

9. Go for a walk, do yoga, meditate, breathe, and so on.

10. Eat kitchari without vegetables.

11. Drink plenty of water throughout your day; half your body weight in ounces as a general rule of thumb.

---

*On day 6, have hot cereal for breakfast—either rice gruel or black sesame cereal or some other plain, whole-grain cereal—with a bit of ghee in it.

12. If you encounter cravings or feel hungry, drink some CCF or CCFT tea.

13. Between 11 a.m. and 2 p.m., eat lunch (kitchari without vegetables).

14. Again, drink plenty of water, but not right before or right after a meal. You can sip on warm or hot water or the tea during meals.

15. If you encounter cravings or feel hungry, drink some CCF or CCFT tea.

16. Eat dinner (kitchari without vegetables) before 6 p.m.

17. Drink more tea and water.

18. Before bed, take Triphala with warm water.

19. Massage the feet and scalp with brahmi oil. No need to get a lot of oil in the hair; just put a bit on the fingertips to massage into the scalp. Make sure to thoroughly massage the soles of the feet and around the ankles.

20. Practice yoga nidra.

21. Go to sleep by 10 p.m.

Day 7 (or days 8–10* if doing the ten-day cleanse)

On day 7 or days 8–10 you will eat kitchari with vegetables. Choose 1–3 veggies from the dosha list. Your daily routine will go as follows:

1. Wake by 6 a.m.

2. Go to the bathroom.

3. Scrape your tongue.

4. Brush your teeth.

5. Perform oil pulling.

6. While you're oil pulling you can dry brush.

7. Shower or bathe.

8. Drink a glass of water, either room temperature or warm.

9. Go for a walk, do yoga, meditate, breathe, and so on.

10. Eat kitchari with vegetables (choose one to three vegetables from your dosha list).

---

*On day 10 have black sesame or some other whole grain cereal cooked with a little ghee in it and follow the rest of the day's routine from the previous day.

11. Drink plenty of water throughout your day; half your body weight in ounces as a general guideline.

12. If you encounter cravings or feel hungry, drink some CCF or CCFT tea.

13. Between 11 a.m. and 2 p.m., eat lunch (kitchari with vegetables).

14. Again, drink plenty of water, but not right before or right after a meal. Only sip on hot water during meals.

15. If you encounter cravings or feel hungry, drink some CCFT tea.

16. Eat dinner (kitchari with vegetables) before 6 p.m.

17. Drink more tea and water.

18. Before bed, take Triphala with warm water.

19. Massage the feet and scalp with brahmi oil. No need to get a lot of oil in the hair; just put a bit on the fingertips to massage into the scalp. Make sure to thoroughly massage the soles of the feet and around the ankles.

20. Practice yoga nidra.

21. Go to sleep by 10 p.m.

Post-Cleanse

Post-cleanse includes performing rejuvenation practices for at least one to two months. It is advisable to keep abhyanga in the routine at least one day per week. It can be done either in the morning after dry brushing and before showering or at night before bed, if sleeping is an issue. Slowly incorporate more foods into the diet as the days go on. For the first four or five days after the cleanse, lean toward cooked foods only. Whole grain cereals are best for breakfast, and soups are great for lunch or dinner any time of the year.

The body will be very sensitive to excess of any kind. Everything will have more taste, and your tolerance for sweets will have declined. Try to avoid processed foods and leftovers and pay attention to how you feel after you've eaten. Be mindful of portion sizes, your mental state at mealtime, and eating on a regular schedule. Always check in while you're eating to make sure you're paying attention to what you're doing and not just unconsciously cramming food into your body.

The kapha in the stomach possesses intelligence. It knows what will be good for the body and mind as a whole, and what the digestive capacity can comfortably handle. This is what creates the instinctual draw toward certain foods and away from others, which can be observed at a buffet. Even if the food is healthy, there are foods on certain days the body just will not want to eat. Listen to this. If you're really in touch, just reading a menu or visualizing a certain food will cause the body to react. It is oftentimes subtle, but not always. It is the body's innate wisdom communicating with you at almost a subconscious level. Practice listening to this as it is one of the best things a person can do for him or herself, other than healthy breathing.

Your sensitivity to what the body is saying will be heightened after the cleanse. Use the opportunity to hone your perceptive tendencies and follow through with the guidance being received. Gently reincorporate more foods and really listen to yourself. If you do that, you will feel lighter and more energized because what is being ingested will be mostly what your body is telling you it wants. This will be more aligned with what your agni can handle and what you need on any given day and as a result will lead to decreased ama accumulation.

I usually prescribe a post-cleanse rejuvenative supplement or tonic to be taken for at least a month. This is something generally constructed according to a person's constitution. A good alternative for a generalized, tridoshic home cleanse is chyawanprash. Yes, it looks like every herb in the garden mashed together. And it tastes like it too! It is an age-old tonic of herbs made into a fruity amalaki paste with sesame oil, ghee, and honey. It is rejuvenative and supports immunity and digestion. For pitta types with high pitta it may be better to take Shakti Prana "jam," which can be purchased through the Ayurvedic Institute's website. These are best taken first thing in the morning as they are energizing. Take one teaspoonful, then drink a little warm water to wash it down. As with anything, if you have any questions, concerns, or allergies, it is always best to consult with a qualified professional before adding anything new to your diet. Keep in mind that these are guidelines for a home cleanse, so it can be largely self-guided, but always do such things with the insight of a trusted practitioner.

LISTEN TO YOUR BODY

Constipation or a slowing of bowel movements during this cleanse may occur. Please listen to your body and take appropriate action if necessary, like gradually stopping the cleanse if you're uncomfortable in any way. It is always more important to listen to the body and follow its guidance than it is to think you need to finish a cleanse and push through. Your body is always talking to you by way of small aches and pains, gas and bloating, or a general sense that something just isn't right. Achiness and tiredness are also common, especially the first few days if you've just recently cut out sugar. Again, listen to your body. If it's too much then back off on the cleanse and more gently release refined and other sugars before beginning again.

Incorporating meditation and breath awareness into a daily routine should not have any adverse side effects. For some people though, even those two things can be difficult. In those cases, I would not recommend a cleanse at all and would encourage support from a qualified practitioner. Likewise with any of the techniques or suggestions above. For some vikrutis, oil pulling may be contraindicated. If it doesn't feel right, leave it out. Internal oleation may also not be right for you, or taking Triphala. You may have a family to care for and if that's the case this cleanse, especially the 7–10 day version isn't right at all. We are going for balance—if a cleanse would cause more stress, tension, or discomfort I ask that you let it go and simply modify your daily routine.

If you are experiencing blood sugar issues I don't advise a cleanse at all. In fact, if you have any health issues whatsoever please do not do a cleanse without clearing it with your doctor first. As stated earlier, cleansing happens naturally if we allow the body and mind the space and freedom to do as nature intended. This can be a difficult thing to accept after living a life of dieting, fasting, and such. It is the truth, however, and even the most intensely motivated individuals will benefit just from altering their daily routine. What I see the most in the clinic are people who just need to let go of something they are holding on to in order to shift how they feel. I also see people who for one reason or another are not allowing joyful or nurturing practices or experiences into their lives on a regular basis. This is why I recommend self-reflection practices that allow you the space to let your energy and thoughts flow freely so they can be processed, and so you can feel healthier inside and out.

PART III

In the Clinic

11

Integrating Ayurveda and Chinese Medicine

The integration of Chinese medicine and Ayurveda is becoming more popular, particularly in the United States among a small subculture of acupuncturists. It is not uncommon to come across articles in trade publications, websites, or blogs on the similarities of the theories underpinning the two disciplines and ways to practically apply both disciplines clinically. Practitioners are discovering that combining Chinese medicine and Ayurveda can be beneficial to their practice and to their patients/clients. While the previous chapters provided a basic overview and resource for practitioners and their patients, as well as for the lay person wishing to understand these medicines, this chapter is directed more toward the Chinese medicine practitioner or student. This is partly because those practicing Chinese medicine or acupuncture in the Western world will be seeing a higher volume of people than the average Ayurveda practitioner. Also, the concept of detoxification, a field of interest to most Westerners looking to ancient wisdom for healing guidance, isn't as established in Chinese medicine. This chapter is also designed to show Chinese medicine practitioners and students how learning the foundations of Ayurveda may actually help them understand their own medicine more deeply and better serve their community.

The information in this chapter is secondarily provided for

modern, Western-trained Ayurveda practitioners—those who were trained as coaches and bodyworkers, rather than those with BAMS degrees—so that they can better understand the scope of education and emphasis on the clinical science and herbal remedies that Chinese medicine has to offer. It is important for practitioners coming from only a few hundred hours of training in any field to understand that such a training can only offer to scratch the surface of deep and complex medical systems like those of China and India. Even practitioners who have undergone the rigorous training in Chinese medicine or received a BAMS in India continue to learn about and grow into the medicine for the rest of their lives. It is my belief that most Western-trained Ayurvedic practitioners would benefit by referring clients who need herbal medicine to Chinese practitioners for herbs. I also feel that unless well trained in Ayurveda theory, Chinese practitioners, particularly acupuncturists with busy practices, could better serve their clients more completely by referring to Ayurvedic practitioners for ongoing lifestyle maintenance. In order to clearly understand why this is, it is helpful to explore current trends.

GROWING POPULARITY OF ALTERNATIVE MEDICINE

People seem to be leaning toward ancient medicine for three main reasons: the modern accessibility to an abundance of self-help resources and yoga, a rise in chronic illnesses and pain, and dissatisfaction with the modern medical system. I believe that allopathy's limitations in the treatment of the root cause of chronic illnesses and pain conditions, its specialization, long waits to see a doctor, and rushed medical visits are all contributing factors. And I've spoken to doctors who agree. There is no way an average human being can see fifty people a day, fully connect with them, understand the inner and outer environment that may be contributing to their lack of well-being or illness, and use the whole picture to treat accordingly.

In general, acupuncture practitioners are in the room with the client a minimum of a half hour per session. The first session is typically even longer because it includes a detailed health history and Chinese medical assessment of the person and his or her situation. This gives practitioners time for connection, discussion, and understanding. The importance of this cannot be overstated. A number of studies have cited how important clinician-patient communication is to a healing outcome. I hear stories every day that suggest quality of care in allopathy is diminishing and, therefore, quality of life is diminishing as well. There is a propensity to prescribe pharmaceuticals, while an increasing number of people are reluctant to take them or even refuse to take them outright. People are becoming more aware of the fact that they need to research and advocate for themselves with regard to their own medical care. This is unlikely to change anytime in the near future. This is where Chinese medicine and Ayurveda come in.

As more and more insurance companies cover acupuncture, the most recognized bodywork modality in Chinese medicine, more people have access to treatment. Word of mouth about the benefits is increasing, and it is often covered on talk shows and in other media. Doctors are now recommending acupuncture for chronic pain and other conditions, and fertility clinics typically have an acupuncturist on staff, as do many Veterans Affairs (VA) hospitals and substance abuse facilities. Acupuncture and Chinese medicine are no longer just reserved for an elite minority in the West. These ancient modalities are becoming readily available to people of every economic class and belief system.

In addition, many more people are entering into the profession. As acupuncture becomes more popular so does its appeal as a viable career choice. People who don't want to go the allopathic medicine route are choosing acupuncture or Chinese medicine school as an alternative. Chinese medicine training requires a four-year bachelor's degree and several premed prerequisites. Programs are three to five years in length and include thousands of hours of training and clinical experience.

Medical doctors are allowed to practice acupuncture after only a few hundred hours of training, as are physical therapists and veterinarians. While this may not seem fair to those who have invested the time into an acupuncture degree and license, it does show the scope to which acupuncture has reached into mainstream medicine. Many veterinarians are even choosing to focus on acupuncture and Chinese medicine as an alternative to their veterinary practices. Farmers and thoroughbred owners regularly call on acupuncturists or veterinarians with some acupuncture training to treat their animals, and with great success.

Chinese medicine practitioners, including people strictly practicing acupuncture, as well as Ayurvedic practitioners look at the face, nails, belly, tongue, eyes, and hair and take the pulse. Practitioners want to know what their client does for a living, and what their passions and fears are. They want to know what they're eating and how they're sleeping, the state of their digestion, and their level of stress. The living environment is important, as is the mental and emotional environment. These things all contribute to a person's well-being, or lack thereof. There is simply no way to cover this ground in a ten minute consultation.

People choosing to experience acupuncture for themselves, or those who are attending the sessions of loved ones or pets, ask questions during their treatments: Why does that needle need to go there? What is it doing? How does this work? What can I do to help myself between treatments? Because they are asking these questions, the practitioner needs to be able to explain clearly what he or she is doing and why. Having a knowledge of both Chinese medicine and Ayurveda can help a great deal with this challenging task.

As Chinese medicine and its bodywork therapies grow in popularity, so does Ayurveda. Ayurvedic practitioner trainings and its treatment modalities and lifestyle recommendations are becoming more accessible. Traditionally in India, Ayurveda training includes roughly seven years of full-time study. Here in the Western world it's anywhere from 200 hours to a little over 1000 hours of training. There is no regulating body and few prerequisite requirements for admission, so it's appealing to people who are not only naturally drawn to Ayurveda, but have time constraints that don't allow them to pursue studying for several years full time. Many yoga practitioners and massage therapists are drawn to learn Ayurveda as it is an accessible means to help their clients in a different or more complete way. Ayurvedic bodywork is a luxurious and therapeutic complement to any massage therapy practice. Likewise, the theory of Ayurveda is easily interwoven into yoga classes, introducing a growing number of people to its basic concepts.

Yoga is a major gateway to Ayurveda for the average person. Yoga students are being introduced to Ayurvedic language by their yoga teachers en masse. The theory is rather fascinating, makes total sense, and offers insight into who we are. Who wouldn't want to learn more? The naturally inquisitive person then begins to ask questions, read, and do their best to understand and integrate the information they come across. Two of the more fascinating things that initially draw people to Ayurveda are its constitutional theory and its emphasis on dietary therapy. We want to understand ourselves and know what constitutional category we fit into, as well as what to do with that information to make ourselves healthier. The problem is that there are many gray areas in understanding dosha or constitution, and there is so much information it may become overwhelming when doing self-directed study. This is when people seek out Ayurvedic practitioners for help. In fact, Ayurveda has become a subset of yoga trainings today, and many studios are bringing in Ayurveda practitioners to teach workshops for their students.

There is a natural connection between yoga and Ayurveda. Sankhya, one of the six Indian philosophies that Ayurveda is based upon, is the main underlying philosophy of the type of yoga that is most popularly practiced today. Yoga instructors certified by the Yoga Alliance, the United States' yoga industry's self-imposed standardizing body, are required to study Sankhya philosophy. As discussed in chapter 2 (pages 31–32), this philosophy explains the cosmological underpinnings of creation and the nature of existence in both the yogic and Ayurvedic systems of thought. Sankhya philosophy has a great deal of influence on how Ayurvedic medicine is understood, explained to patients, and practiced.

Not only is there a foundational theory of existence link between Ayurveda and Yoga philosophies historically, but we in the West have begun to totally merge them as well. This probably started in the 1960s with the massive influx of Indian philosophy, meditation practice, yoga, and clothing and other goods being imported from India. Ayurveda is becoming increasingly integrated into Western society through the practice of yoga. Most yoga practitioners have some basic Ayurveda theory under their belts and share it with their students. Because of this, the language of Ayurveda is becoming familiar to us. It may not be quite as mainstream as yoga itself, but yoga wasn't always this popular. Ten years ago it was practiced by half as many people as it is today. Like yoga, awareness of Ayurveda is increasing. Well-known author/speaker/physician Deepak Chopra promotes Ayurveda in his books and teachings. He is the cofounder of an integrative clinic that offers Ayurvedic treatment, an informational website, many books, and an app. In addition, the Transcendental Meditation folks have a panchakarma center and a complete secondary education facility right in Iowa. New Ayurvedic teachers and trainings are emerging with greater frequency, especially online. The market for Ayurveda is steadily growing, and our exposure to it is as well—again, largely through yoga.

People—from young children to the elderly—are doing yoga. As of 2012, 20 million people were practicing yoga in the United States alone, and 44 percent of the population either considered themselves beginners or people who wanted to try it. That's nearly half of all Americans either actively practicing or interested in yoga. Nowadays, yoga is coming to be known not only as an exercise program, but as the physical therapy of Ayurveda. By practicing yoga, one is entering a realm of self-discovery, self-awareness, and somatic awareness not present in other forms of exercise. In fact, yoga was originally an esoteric practice designed to help people become more self-aware. Regardless of how denominational or nondenominational a yoga practice is, it has the effect of relaxing the body and mind and creating a greater sense of connection to self and nature. Once people begin to relax, allowing for an expansion of awareness, they begin to notice thoughts, feelings, and beliefs that have been lingering in the background of their consciousness. These things can be mental, emotional, or spiritual in nature.

Once an issue arises, the yogi or yogini tends to want to heal, integrate, release, understand, or work through it. The natural next step is to explore mind/body therapies. There is a natural gravitation toward self-help information, dietary shifts, massage, cleansing, acupuncture, and lifestyle changes. These changes are usually guided by recommendations from others, programs seen on TV, or articles read in magazines or online. This oftentimes leads to an improved sense of well-being but at some point all the information we have accessible to us may become confusing and overwhelming, or we may end up with an imbalance that feels intractable, and this may cause us to seek expert advice.

AYURVEDA CAN ENHANCE CHINESE MEDICINE

Chinese medicine practitioners can greatly benefit from familiarizing themselves with the concepts, language, and lifestyle guidance recommended in Ayurveda. Due in part to the widespread exposure to Indian yoga, it seems that the majority of Westerners have a natural inclination toward the concepts and lifestyle recommendations in Ayurveda. This is particularly the case with cleansing and constitution. There are many reasons for this. For one thing, the Western world has centuries of history with India due to British occupation. Most Indians speak at least some English and we've adopted many things from one another. Also, Western foods are more similar to the cuisine of India than that of China. Most people I see in the clinic are very concerned with diet, healthy lifestyle, losing weight, and their constitution. It's much easier for me to talk potatoes, peas, carrots, cauliflower, garbanzo beans, lentils, and spices with people than it is lotus root, egg yolk, congee, bok choy, cuttlefish, or other medicinal staples cooked into meals that are largely inaccessible to the Western cook unfamiliar with Chinese cooking practices.

Thus, Ayurveda is a very practical approach that can assist the Chinese medicine practitioner in offering lifestyle guidance in the clearest, most comprehensible way possible, which people will be more inclined to follow. That includes offering clients information on how to balance themselves that feels accessible to them and is therefore more likely to become part of their daily routine. This isn't to say that some folks don't have a natural inclination to Chinese culture and theory, but I find clinically that Chinese recommendations feel more foreign to more clients than do Indian ones. In those instances where this is not the case, practitioners can offer lifestyle advice from the Chinese medicine perspective instead.

ACCESSIBILITY OF INFORMATION

As interesting and clinically effective as Chinese medicine is, it is my experience that when my clients see that I also offer educational sessions in Ayurveda, their interest is piqued and they ask lots of questions about what dosha they are or what they should eat. On the table they're interested in what I saw in their tongue, felt in their pulse, and in which meridians need balancing or are affected by what they have going on. Yet when it comes to what they can do for themselves between sessions, they almost always ask specifically in terms of Ayurveda. This may be so for a number of reasons. The popularity of yoga and its role in spreading knowledge of Ayurveda has already been discussed at length, as have the similarities in Western and Indian diets, the modern fascination with cleansing, and the highly developed constitutional theory that Ayurveda offers. These reasons may draw the layperson as well as practitioners of other disciplines into Ayurveda's fold. Another tempting draw toward learning about Ayurveda is the accessibility of the information that Ayurveda offers. Chinese medicine is a treasure trove of wisdom and knowledge on how to treat with acupuncture and herbs, yet there isn't the same degree of access to information available as there is with Ayurveda.

First, Ayurvedic teachings are easier to access for both the layperson and the practitioner. Ayurveda provides a clear, familiar way to understand nature and ourselves that has not been overly watered down, changed, or lost over time. We don't need to do so much work to find out what something means when we're researching a specific topic; it's pretty straightforward in Ayurveda. Second, Ayurvedic theory is easier for the Western mind to follow than Chinese medical theory. Even if they haven't grown up in India, most Westerners can more quickly or easily relate to the logic in Ayurveda than they can to the logic in Chinese medical texts. Chinese texts tend to be riddled with references we simply cannot understand without an insightful teacher. Finally, Ayurveda covers, in detail, dietary recommendations based on constitution, and clearly outlines cleansing and detoxification. These topics are very popular and are not clearly addressed in Chinese medicine. Discussions of them found in the Chinese texts that remain with us today are either incomplete or difficult to interpret.

When studying the Chinese language and learning to transliterate and translate the classics, one gets to see clearly how little straightforward information is actually present. A good friend and former *PARABOLA* publisher, Joe Kulin, pointed out that the foundational Taoist and Chinese medicine texts seemed to be written in a cryptic way, similar to the ancient alchemical texts. It is most likely that these texts were purposely written this way so one would actually need to commit to learning and be diligent with their internal exercises, under the guidance of a master teacher who understood the riddles and vague references contained within the texts. Unfortunately, many of the people who could have passed the information down to us were lost in the Cultural Revolution. There are still people who have an expert experiential understanding of these writings, but they are difficult to find. Many don't have websites and they aren't writing books, at least not in English. In addition, because of cultural influences, many master teachers, particularly those in China, are reluctant to disclose the deepest messages to outsiders or Westerners.

If one wishes to truly understand and interpret the foundational writings of Chinese medicine firsthand, they still need to learn Mandarin, go to China or Taiwan, and actually find a teacher who will share the most precious gems of the medicine with an outsider. There are some Chinese teachers who do teach their Western students, and some Western teachers who do impart wisdom to their Western students.

With Ayurveda, concepts are clearly explained and complete, so there is less struggle and far fewer hours, days, weeks, or maybe even years needed to understand them compared to their Chinese medicine counterparts. There are fewer fundamental discrepancies in Ayurveda than in Chinese medicine as well. For example, most Chinese medicine practitioners are taught that qi is warm. The analogy is that it is like the steam that rises off of cooked rice. I encountered only two people in the years I've been exposed to Chinese medicine who stated that qi is cold. One was an acupuncturist who found a mentor off the beaten path outside a remote Chinese village. The other was a qiqong instructor in Nepal. In Ayurveda, prana is cold, as it is a form of wind or vata. Vata, being made up of space and air, has the intrinsic quality of being cold. It makes perfect sense.

There is always some variation in interpretation of course, based upon what school of thought you come from and your own life experience, regardless of whether you study Chinese medicine or Ayurveda. Some of the Sanskrit writings are up for debate as well. But I would say overall, having skimmed the surface of traditional and simplified Chinese (Mandarin) and Sanskrit, that the Western mind is more inclined to resonate with the flow of Sanskrit in general, and that the writings are less cryptic. The Chinese writings that are not so cryptic are the treatment protocols and diagnostic criteria in the Shang Han Lun, for example. But even in this pivotal text on cold damage, hot debates remain as to whether one should be using cinnamon twig or bark, which is like using two completely different herbs, and both are present in a large portion of the formulas in that text.

The benefit for some and the curse for others is that a seeker drawn more to Taoist thought and ancient Chinese medicine theory, and any student of Chinese medicine, is forced to figure out a lot of the foundational theory for themselves. Chinese medicine training is modeled after Western medicine training and is therefore quite clinically oriented and minimally, if at all, esoteric. This is a shame since the unknown or mysterious is as much a part of medicine as it is of life. How can we say a medicine encompasses all aspects of a person's being if it doesn't take into account all aspects of reality itself? For those wishing to delve into this obscure, almost-lost element of Chinese medicine, there must be a genuine commitment to and love of the theory and a painstaking process of self-discovery and awareness that cannot be shaken. As with anyone who embodies what they do, this can make one a true master at their art. The difficulty with this is that one can get stuck on things for much longer than someone who has many resources that help joggle them more quickly into understanding. Additionally, if we have more access to and a clearer understanding of the details and why they are the way they are, we can more readily offer our understanding, or at least uncorrupted information, to our patients and therefore be of more use to them.

CLEANSING AND DETOXIFICATION

Westerners have a keen interest in cleansing and detoxification. This is evidenced by the abundance of diets, fasts, and fad cleanses on the market. While this concept has its own branch in Ayurveda, it is totally lacking in Chinese medicine. One of my teachers, a fourteen-year resident of Taiwan and a scholar of Chinese medicine and Taoism, who was fluent in translation of simplified and traditional characters, would get so annoyed in class when anyone brought up the concept of detoxification, or toxins, as we tend to refer to them in our culture. It was difficult for us to wrap our heads around the fact that there is, as he emphatically stated, no concept of detoxification or toxicity, as we use the terms today, in Chinese medicine or any of its foundational texts.

Toxins are present in Chinese medicine, but they are the pathogenic factors that create serious fevers, bleeding disorders, and boils. In Chinese medicine there is no system in place for understanding toxins in the way we see them today—as substances that build up in the body that can be cleansed. In fact, one of my Chinese clinic supervisors said we should "eat" the sludge from the tongue each morning as it is viewed as nutrition. One may say that dampness, damp heat, or phlegm are such substances, and that may be so, but the foundational theory on and eradication of these substances from the body-mind in Chinese medicine is nowhere near as comprehensive as in Ayurveda.

As I heard Dr. Daniel Altschuler discuss on numerous occasions throughout my time at the Seattle Institute of Oriental Medicine, the Chinese simply did not have the same concept of cleansing as we do today. This is a huge factor when you're dealing with patients: not because cleansing or detoxification is strictly necessary in the way we view it and are attached to it, but because most clients who are drawn to alternative medicine also feel that they need to cleanse somehow. We can tell them they have heat (inflammation) and/or dampness (ama/toxins/candida overgrowth, etc.), and that we can work to eliminate it through diet, exercise, lifestyle modification, and herbal medicine, but there is no actual theory or preestablished, time-tested, full science with contraindications for treatment or a clearly defined process for how this occurs, how to explain that it works, or how to modify the process based upon the person from a Chinese medicine perspective. In Ayurveda detoxification is its own specialty: panchakarma. That's how elaborate a field it is. Even modern medicine has some sense of detoxification/cleansing; it is being developed in the field of functional medicine, which can also look to Ayurveda for guidance on treating the whole from a constitutional perspective.

CLINICAL VS. EVERYDAY MODALITIES

Overall, Chinese medicine in the West is practiced as a clinically centered modality, and Ayurveda has developed into a practical, everyday, and every-body process. For some people it has even taken on tones of a spiritual path. Both systems recommend self-awareness and meditation, although styles may differ. Both encourage connection and the interconnected nature of reality. Chinese medicine seems to have emerged to focus on being in harmony with nature, while Ayurveda has come to concentrate more on the connection of the individual as he relates to himself and to a greater power. To me, they are ultimately saying the same thing in different ways. The focus on individuality, however, may also be another point that makes Indian medicine feel more natural or accessible to Westerners.

Both medicines focus on seasonal fluctuations and making lifestyle shifts in tune with seasonal change. The problem is that most people see Chinese medicine in the same vein as allopathy: useful for acute symptomatology. This wasn't necessarily intended, but what has emerged as the reality of a Chinese medicine practice is that most people expect to go in for treatment only when things go awry, at least the first few times they try it. This may happen with Ayurveda too, but people tend to view Ayurveda as a long-term process that they engage in daily. They like learning about their constitution and how it interacts with and is influenced by their environment. And why wouldn't they? After all, who doesn't enjoy learning about the most interesting thing in their universe—themselves?

12

The Clinic and Beyond

Chinese medicine and Ayurveda each have specific theories concerning disease causation and progression. But before launching into a discussion of disease etiology, it is important to start with what we bring to the patient as practitioners. Medical training, regardless of genre, usually requires putting the student through very rigorous programming. Education is heavy and entails a lot of work and memorization. Then when clinical rotations happen, the demands placed upon students and interns are tremendous. While this may be the case to a greater extent for someone endeavoring to become a Western medical doctor, it happens more than people may realize to those in Ayurvedic and Chinese medicine programs as well.

Many people enter the field lured by the promise of in-depth alternative medical training. The expectation of a clinical experience may be present, but the reality of the demands of the programs are beyond imagining or preparation. As a student, this doesn't make sense when you're in the heat of it. There is little sleep, a lot of stress, poor eating, bad lifestyle habits, and not much time for family, let alone self. This seems counterintuitive to what the student and eventually, the practitioner, show up to do when they enter the clinic.

All day long we support people in their healing process, and really, in their life process, and then don't practice what we preach. At least while in training. Why shouldn't training involve actually living according to the tenets of the traditional medicine being studied? This question is legitimate. How can a person adequately support someone else along their journey without actually doing it themselves? The answer is that they can't. But as a budding health care professional, the student practitioner must learn how to compartmentalize. They must figure out an internal mechanism by which they can completely suspend their misery and create a whole space for someone else to enter. If this can be done in the midst of their own chaos, then they cannot only do this again when life calls upon them to do so, but once the dust settles, they can do more than hold space. Once the student leaves school and their time and energy demands, at least from that aspect of their lives, decrease, more time can be spent on the self. Then they can not only hold space, they can shine!

True healers aren't just people with a license to practice medicine. They are people who, regardless of their own internal chaos, misery, suffering, stress, angst, anger, frustration, fear, grief, dark nights, and temptation to project show up with centered equanimity for the human being who is waiting for them. This doesn't mean they need to dress in white, stand with their spine completely straight, and behave like an archangel. What it means is that in spite of all their own anguish, they can find the space within themselves, and move, speak, and project from there. They can walk into a room, no matter how rushed they feel, and make the person surrendering to their care and wisdom feel comfortable.

When people are sick, afraid, in pain, desperate, and have exhausted modern medical interventions, which is usually how they are when we see them, they are highly sensitive to what we bring to the table. For many, we are their first alternative medicine experience. All of their hopeful eggs may be in our basket. There is, therefore, a responsibility for us to provide them with the utmost balanced professional and human care possible. If we had not been put through the hell of having to repeatedly put our own stuff aside in order to do this then we might not be able to leave our problems at the door. This would mean doing our patients and our professions a disservice. If medical training were set up to be a utopian experience, it would probably take fifty years to get through it, and the practice of dealing with the harshness of life experienced by everyone who comes through the door would be poor. This is why, I have come to believe, medicine training programs are, quite frankly, sheer hell. We need to practice being a safe space for others and being able to think clearly without internal distraction. It is like developing a muscle. Some people have some level of post-traumatic stress from medical training, I've no doubt. This is not surprising or completely detrimental because by experiencing that stress, they learn how to relate better to people who also suffer from it and guide them through it.

Before bringing theory into the treatment room, we bring ourselves. I believe in the healing power of vibration and resonance and use a tuning fork in my practice. The vibrations of a tuning fork are attuned to specific aspects of being and of material nature. When utilizing these vibrations on acupoints or marma points one is intending to create an equally harmonious resonance in the tissue or aspect of being they are attempting to affect. Likewise, we all emanate vibrations and energetic waves that can be subtly perceived by others. Sometimes the perception is not so subtle. If someone is steaming with anger or rage, we perceive this, and oftentimes it will stimulate a similar spike in our emotional state. When someone emanates great calm, that too resonates with the natural state of internal calm we all possess, and creates more calm.

This is what I mean by creating space to hold another and by being mindful of what we bring into the room with us. If we are able to enter with a vibration that emanates calm and spaciousness, the person we are dealing with can feel this. Then their healing experience in our clinic has already begun. This is more subtle than body language, and it happens well before the first needle is placed or word is spoken. If trust is established and breathing deepened, the path is open to a more healing experience.

The nervous system is very aware, and we are highly sensory creatures and respond automatically to what we feel drawn to or have an aversion to. Science has proven that chronic stimulation of the sympathetic nervous system is taxing to the body and mind. If the parasympathetic nervous system is engaged, i.e., we're in the rest-and-digest mode instead of the fight-or-flight response, we are more likely to heal. This is why it is important for us as medical practitioners to emanate a sense of calm, establish trust, and provide a calm, clean, comfortable atmosphere for our clients or patients. When their minds are at ease and their bodies at greater rest, they will be more open to healing instead of holding patterns in the mind and/or body. Can there be a healing response in the midst of stress or tension? Yes, but in my experience it usually does not come as easily.

A CASE FOR CONNECTION

It was recently all over the news that scientific research supports the theory that a lack of connection to others is at the root of addiction.[1] Actually, this is most likely the primary cause of any disease process, but so far we have technically established that it is the main causative factor involved in the addictive process. The person using the substance to feel better is actually looking for connection. They feel more connected to others or lack the need for connection when they use, which is why they do it. That can be said for any of us. Think about what you do when you feel lonely. Do you go into meditation and contemplate the reality of loneliness and what it means for you in your life? Probably not. Most likely, you call someone or log in to your social media account. We need connection. We have it; we are always connected via atoms and prana, but we need to *feel* it. When we don't feel it, we think we don't have it and then need to numb the sensation of feeling disconnected by gambling, smoking, overeating, watching TV, surfing the internet, gaming, shopping, socializing, partying, or having sex.

Whatever the outlet, lack of connection is a primary causative factor for any mental, emotional, or physical disease. This includes connection to the self. Actually, it is especially true of connection to the self. If we are open and present for whoever we encounter when we walk into the treatment room, there is a greater chance for this primary healing force of connection to occur. Then, if the client feels comfortable and can relax, they are more likely to be made aware of their own inner self-connection. This is primarily why I like to leave people on the table with their needles in instead of chatting the whole time. It gives them space to relax and leaves time for internal connection. This is definitely when the greatest healing occurs.

Subconsciously, if holding patterns are relaxed, then internal communication between cells, tissues, and organs is optimized. This is also a form of connection. Communication can only happen in the midst of connection. I once attended a workshop in which the presenter's primary focus was the role of connection between parts of the body, specifically the organs. He posited that just as we as humans can feel a sense of disconnection, loss, and loneliness, the internal organs can too. He presumed that there is some level of individualized consciousness present in each organ. This is aligned with the idea of wu shen, or the principle of the five spirits, in Chinese medicine. He taught that an internal organ will shrink away, like it is backing into a corner, when it feels disconnected. This causes an actual, physical lessening of the connection with the other organs. The affected organ will then stiffen in its orbit of excursion (the natural rocking rhythm each organ has in the body). This affects fluid and energy flow to and from the organ, which adversely affects the connective tissue and from there all other tissues of the body associated with that organ and anything along the organ's meridian—and there we have the physical basis of disease.

For example, if something happens that causes the gallbladder to retract, it can not only hinder the functioning of the bile, but of the liver, the gallbladder's paired organ. It can impact the sinews, its primary tissue of influence, hamper decision-making, and create stagnation anywhere along the Gall Bladder and Triple Burner channels. This means it can have an adverse effect on anything on the side of the body from the ear to the ribs to the pinky toe. Following from this logic, if you choose to find it to be true, this can happen with people as well. They can feel isolated, and therefore, isolate. From there imbalance continues to manifest. What a gift practitioners bring by being able to provide a space for this process to disengage and unravel!

PATHOGENESIS

Causation is commonly shared between the theories of disease etiology and pathogenesis in both Chinese medicine and Ayurveda. Connection, or disturbance of it, is the main cause of disease. This is called a disturbance or disruption to the flow of qi and/or blood in Chinese medicine. In Ayurveda, it is going against the knowledge of that which makes us connected. This knowledge can be inherent, learned, intuitive, or instinctive and is basically a disruption to the smooth, ordered, correct flow of prana in the body and mind.

External pathogenic factors like wind, cold, damp, heat, or any combination of them (e.g., colds and flus), cannot enter the body if the wei qi, ojas, or immunity is strong. Once in the body, pathogens behave in certain ways based upon the host's strength and internal environment. The primary causative factors for a weakened system usually derive from a mental/emotional imbalance and may manifest externally as wrong diet and lifestyle. When the mind and emotions are not clear, the qi is affected. Other causes of disease include genetic factors, environmental factors, karma, accidents, and possessions or ghosts. Ancient doctors from both fields agree that the majority of illness begins in the mind, and if unchecked, manifests in the body. Disease manifestation and progression, once in the physical body, is called disease pathogenesis.

MODELS OF PATHOGENESIS IN CHINESE MEDICINE

The eight principles of diagnosis discussed in chapter 7 (pages 162–65) are used to assess everyone who walks into the clinic. Practitioners evaluate whether a pathogen or condition is interior or exterior, hot or cold, excess or deficient, and yin or yang. Regardless of the model of pathogenesis and treatment the practitioner decides to use, these parameters are how the client's presentation is assessed. There are two primary schools of thought in Chinese medicine regarding pathogenesis: Shang Han, or cold damage, and Wen Bing, or warm pathogen disease.

Shang Han and the Six Stages

Shang Han means "cold damage." The Shang Han school recognizes that any of the six pernicious influences can cause externally contracted disease. That disease can take the form of cold, heat, wind, damp, dryness, or summer heat. Although this is technically the case, some people still look at Shang Han theory as the pathogenesis of cold-natured pathogens only. Regardless of whether they enter only as cold or cold mixed with another influence or turn to something else once they enter the body, what form an external pathogenic influence (EPI) takes has a lot to do with what season we are in. It also has to do with what internal imbalances existed at the time the ailment was contracted. Shang Han theory is applicable not only to acute externally contracted illness but also to an illness that arises later in life or a chronic illness that may be the result of an initial external invasion. This is sometimes the case in postpartum women, for example, who aren't able to take good enough care of themselves when the body is still open, vulnerable, and deficient, and the psyche is very sensitive.

The eighteen-hundred-year-old Shang Han Lun, or Treatise on Cold Damage, by Zhang Zhong Jing is the pivotal text on cold damage theory and practice. Physician Zhang Zhong Jing had an unfortunate amount of experience in cold disease pathogenic processes. There was an epidemic, not uncommon for premodern China, that affected most of the town he lived in, including his closest family members. He tried his best to save his family, and community and identified the various routes of entry into the body and progression to death or wellness a pathogen may take. His text outlines the myriad manifestations of cold disease, six-channel pattern identification, and treatment protocols including herbal medicine and acupuncture.

According to Zhang Zhong Jing, pathogens enter the body via the channel system and travel in somewhat predictable patterns. Six-channel pattern identification is very useful in the clinic, and many of Zhang Zhong Jing's herbal formulas have come to be known by every Chinese medicine practitioner. His formulations are applicable in a wide variety of circumstances. In fact, many practitioners use only a handful of his formulas, out of the thousands available, for patients.

Many of his formulas are known to even treat specific constitutional types. There is a growing group of practitioners who apply Chinese medicine according to herbal and formula constitutional typing. Each individual is viewed as *chai hui* or a *gui zhi tang* type, for example. They are then given formulas from those families over others when they are prescribed medicinals. As all things evolve and change, so too do the parameters by which theories are thought about and applied, as do their accompanying treatments.

We have already outlined the twelve major channels or meridians. Historically, these twelve were seen as six longer channels. According to the six-stages theory, disease progression occurs through these channels or meridians and their associated organs. In order of cold pathogen disease progression there are three yang channels and three yin channels. The yang channels are as follows: greater yang, or Tai Yang (Small Intestine and Urinary Bladder), yang brightness, or Yang Ming (Stomach and Large Intestine), and lesser yang, or Shao Yang (Triple Burner and Gall Bladder). The yin channels are the great yin, or Tai Yin (Lung and Spleen), lesser yin, or Shao Yin (Heart and Kidney), or terminal yin, Jue Yin (Liver and Pericardium).

The Tai Yang is considered the first in the line of defense against EPIs. If an EPI first enters the Tai Yang channel, the person will usually present with upper back/neck/base-of-the-skull tension. This is due to the contraction of the Tai Yang channel and the stagnation caused by the EPI trying to enter the body. The Yang Ming channel is the next deepest, and this can be affected first as there is the potential for the pathogen to go directly into the mouth. Symptoms may include high fever, thirst, and sweating. Following the Yang Ming stage is the Shao Yang. Symptoms of Shao Yang-type patterns include alternating fever and chills, hypochondriacal pain, irritability, blurry vision, and a bitter taste in the mouth.

The Shao Yang is called the pivot. It is not considered fully exterior like the Tai Yang channel, nor fully interior as are the yin channels. The idea is that if a pathogen enters the yang and leaves, it has never fully entered into the deeper places in the body. The deeper a pathogen goes, the harder it is to treat and the more severe the signs and symptoms.

The Shao Yang is the level that is like a hinge that swings the door between the interior and the exterior of the body. It is a fascinating level. It is where dormant pathogens, or lingering pathogens in Chinese medicine, can hang out.

An example of a dormant pathogen is a retrovirus like herpes, chicken pox, or shingles. It is something that is always there, but not always active. Historically, lingering pathogens were regarded as EPIs that would infiltrate the body in one season and possibly transform within the body and express themselves as an illness in another season. An example would be someone being affected by cold in the winter presenting with a case of severe summer heat in the summer.

Damage to the Tai Yin mostly manifests as spleen deficiency. It can be the result of a mistreated Yang Ming disease, direct impact from a wind cold invasion, or an interior condition that generates cold. Examples of Tai Yin pattern presentation symptoms are abdominal pain and fullness, diarrhea, vomiting, and basic gastrointestinal bug symptoms. Shao Yin patterns usually get hit by something that is coming deeper into the body from the other channels. The Shao Yin can be directly affected by an EPI, but that EPI would have to be very strong, or the person very deficient. They may include fatal illnesses and usually involve a severe heart or kidney deficiency.

Jue Yin patterns are deep, oftentimes sustained, complex, and difficult to treat. There is a lot of wrong-moving energy in Jue Yin patterns, as well as combinations of cold and heat. They may manifest as upper body heat and lower body coldness, cold extremities, diarrhea, vomiting, or hiccups.

Wen Bing

Many believe that Wen Bing theory is an extension of Shang Han theory, or a further development of it. Wen Bing posits that externally contracted pathogenic diseases are warm in nature, and vaguely speaking, there is a yin nourishing and cooling treatment strategy. Generally, from an eight principles perspective, this would mean the disease is hot and yang. This Warm Disease school of thought uses two models for differentiation of patterns: the four levels and the three burners. The four levels model states that a bug will enter the protective level, then the qi level, then the nutritive level, and lastly, the blood. The three burners theory discusses how pathogens enter from the top and work their way down through the body.

Four Levels

When looking at disease pathogenesis and treatment from a Wen Bing perspective, it is important to know two things: what kind of pathogen it is, and what season it was contracted in. The season may actually indicate the type of pathogen. The pathogenic factors and corresponding conditions in Wen Bing theory are: wind heat producing wind warmth, summer heat producing summer heat warmth, damp heat producing the damp warmth, dryness (either warm or cool) producing autumn dryness, and warm toxin producing warm heat. Two of these pathogenic factors can turn into lurking pathogens, as mentioned above in the Shao Yang section. This idea of lurking pathogens is fascinating, and the theory and some of the symptoms closely resemble what is occurring in epidemic proportions with Lyme disease and its related coinfections. These lurkers are EPIs that enter in one season, don't resolve but instead dive deep into the body and hide, then reemerge with voracity when triggered by either another illness, chronically bad lifestyle choices, or severe emotional turmoil. They are spring warmth creating warm heat and lurking summer heat creating damp heat.

In four levels disease progression, one of the above pathogens will enter the body, usually through the nose or mouth. They then progress in somewhat predictable patterns. The order of entry from the most superficial to the deepest and most severe is as follows:

1. Protective level: The wei qi is the body's first line of defense against incoming pathogens. It involves the lungs, throat, nose, and skin. The wei qi circulates between the vessels and the skin, so it is the most superficial level. Primary protective level symptoms are fever, slight chills or cold aversion, and thirst.

2. Qi level: If the pathogen is not expelled from the superficial protective level, it will cause stagnation of qi and this creates a

buildup, almost like friction, that results in heat being generated. This causes a more severe fever, an aversion to heat, and a yellow tongue coating, indicative of the heat.

3. Nutritive level: At this level, called "ying" in Chinese medicine, the pathogen has either passed through the other two levels or entered this one directly. Lurking pathogens can also present with ying-level symptomatology. Profuse sweating can damage the heart spirit and allow for a pathogen to enter the ying level. If you are sick, it's not a good idea to go to hot yoga or sit in a sauna for this reason. Ying-level fevers can feel subjective and seem worse at night. Pathogenic factors in this level can cause insomnia, irritability, and restlessness. Usually the tongue is a deeper red, and there may be thirst with no desire to drink fluids. In ying level, the yin is damaged and the heart spirit is disturbed.

4. Blood level: The blood or *xue* level can be critical. It is the deepest level according to this system of diagnosis. At this level the pathogen can force the blood from the vessels where it congeals, causing blood stasis. This may be a pattern of stroke, heat-induced convulsions, or seizure. There may be vomiting of blood, nosebleed, and bloody stools and urine. Ebola would be an example of a pathogen in the blood level.

Triple Burner Theory

The triple burner was discussed in chapter five, but here's a little review. It is a yang organ that itself lacks form, yet defines boundaries within the body. It has three parts that are stacked one upon another like snowballs in a snowman. Each part has a specific metabolic purpose, and together they help to generate heat and distribute it and fluids through the body. Structures we are aware of today in modern science that may be identified as physical aspects of the triple burner system are the connective tissue, the mesentery, the lymph, the endocrine glands, the interstitial fluid, and the communication pathways in the connective tissue.

The upper burner includes the area of the thorax above the diaphragm, including the lungs and heart. It is responsible for dispersing qi, blood, and nutritive vapor. The middle burner goes from below the diaphragm to the navel and includes the stomach and spleen. It transforms and transports foodstuff. The lower burner is below the navel and includes the kidneys, bladder, and intestines. It is responsible for separating the clear (health-enhancing products of digestion and metabolism) from the turbid (waste products) and eliminating waste from the body. Although the liver is located in the middle burner, it is considered a lower burner organ.

Generally speaking, warm diseases will travel from the upper burner, to the middle, and then to the lower. It is another way that traditional doctors observed pathogens moving through the body and the signs, symptoms, and damage that resulted from this movement. Knowing the tendencies of the pathogen and being able to predict its course combined with an assessment of the individual's strength can help the practitioner to be one step ahead and offer proper treatment. The strategies for upper burner illness are to diffuse the pathogen up and out by using acrid, light, cooling herbals and some sweating. Upper burner patterns usually involve the lungs and present with typical lung symptomatology, like phlegm accumulation or cough which can inhibit functioning in other burners. It may also include the pericardium, which greatly affects the shen.

Middle burner diseases are treated by circulating the qi to improve digestive functioning in order to kill and or move the pathogen out. They include patterns involving the stomach and large intestine, as well as the spleen. These patterns manifest with profound heat, constipation, loose stools, distention, nausea, and shen disturbances. It may seem odd that the large intestine is involved in the pathogenesis of the upper burner sometimes, and the heart shen with that of the middle burner, but in both systems of medicine, it is recognized that one area or pathway is seldom affected in isolation. If it is, it only occurs very early in the onset of most diseases, before a codified disease pattern is even present. Sometimes, though, many systems are affected at once even at the beginning. This is because everything is connected.

With regard to lower burner patterns, the yin and blood are often injured. Although the large intestine is in the lower burner, it is more superficial in terms of how long it takes to be affected by heat and the kind of damage it incurs. When heat enters the large intestine, as in upper and middle burner patterns, we effuse, move qi, and purge. Sometimes we will also drain heat through increasing urination. When blood and yin are involved, a deeper, more tricky problem is created. Lower burner patterns most affect the kidney yin, and this deficiency can easily cause liver wind patterns. These may include palpitations, trembling, spasms, and convulsions. In the case of excess kidney heat, some of it can be drained through the urine, but we mostly need to cool and tonify the yin.

Although there are several patterns of pathogenesis for each of the three burners, it is not important to discuss these in detail at this time. Having a general overview gives one a feel for the theory and methodology. It is important to point out that although the development of these theories may have been in response to an initial pathogenic invasion, practitioners use them for chronic conditions too. The classic texts outline how mistreatment can drive a pathogen deeper and other causes may result in a more chronic issue. Oftentimes damage is done when an invading pathogen lingers in the body, becoming chronic. The initial attack may cause this injury, or a lingering pathogen may be provoked. Trauma such as car accidents, for example, can cause this to happen. The point is that the application exceeds the treatment of acute conditions. Another point is that one model may apply better than the others. Practitioners may see a case that presents textbook as a pattern they've studied or seen before with a mentor. In that scenario they would treat according to that pattern and model.

AYURVEDA AND SAMPRAPTI

Ayurveda, like Chinese medicine, recognizes systematic disease progression. In Ayurveda, it is called "samprapti." I like the simplicity of samprapti, and that it refers to any disease progression, EPI or externally generated. It is a useful tool and another angle from which Chinese medicine practitioners can look when diagnosing. In fact, they can replace the word *dosha* with *pathogenic influence* or *evil* and it will make perfect sense.

In the process of samprapti, a pathogen or causative factor manifests in a specific way, aggravating doshas and adversely affecting dhatus. The physical pathways through which disease manifests are the srotas, the main systems in the body that comprise organs, pathways, openings, body parts, and tissues. Similar to Chinese medicine's meridian networks, each srota has associated organs or structures. One of their primary functions is to transport the material(s) that flows through them. Another is that they contain the agni, or transformative metabolic function, of each tissue they comprise. The srotas are the totality of that which makes them up, what they transport, hold, or carry, and the space in between. The physical body is the srota for the doshas, mind, and spirit.

Disease manifestation begins in the srotas. An ailment may begin in one srota, but others usually become involved. In Ayurveda, an external pathogen will not survive in an inhospitable body. If the doshas and tissues are balanced, it is less likely that bacteria, viruses, fungi, and allergens can settle in, irritate, multiply, spread, or grow. It is not enough to simply eliminate a pathogen by killing it, which is what we do with antibiotics. The doshas and dhatus must be harmonized. Prevention is favored, as is restoring strength and immunity post-illness. Pathogens are seen as disrupting the doshas in Ayurveda, not wreaking havoc on their own.

This manifests as one of the four possible fluctuations that can cause a srota to become imbalanced: (1) there may be too much movement or activity, (2) there may be wrong movement, as in diverticulosis, (3) there could be an acute or chronic obstruction to function, such as external pathogenic invasion, asthma, or the presence of phlegm, and (4) there may be a potential mass or tumor compressing or obstructing the lumina.

Srotas

Although the srotas may be generally equated to the various bodily systems we recognize in today's medicine, they are not complete correlations. They emerge from multiple tissue types, and nourish the dhatus. For a good basic understanding, we can make generalized comparisons.

The *pranavaha* srotas, or air channels, have associations with the trachea, lungs, pulmonary vessels, and the heart. They transport vitality and prana to all regions of the body and most directly correlate on a gross physical level to what we recognize as the respiratory and circulatory systems. They are often disturbed by the suppression of natural urges, excessive intake of dry foods, and excessive physical exertion.

The *annavaha* srotas carry and transform food and mostly correlate to the digestive system. They mainly originate in the stomach. Most digestive problems are the result of some kind of problem in the functioning of the annavaha srotas.

The *udakavaha* srotas are the water metabolism channels, and they are in charge of osmotic pressure balance. They relate to any channel that carries water in the body, so aren't clearly relatable to a single Western counterpart. They originate in the palate and kloma, a region of the throat, and transport water and fluids. Interestingly, they utilize rasavaha and raktavaha srotas (see below) as their vehicles for fluid transport. This is similar to the triple burner of Chinese medicine. Water metabolism issues affect the entire body and may cause swelling, increased heat, and insatiable thirst.

The *rasavaha* srotas originate in the heart and major blood vessels. They participate in plasma and chyle transport and transformation and have a direct link to the lymphatic system and partially to the circulatory system. They supply nutrient material to the entire body including the liver where the blood is made. Imbalance of the rasavaha srotas is often due to the intake of cold, heavy foods and an improper lifestyle and manifests as fatigue.

The *raktavaha* srotas emerge from the liver and spleen, and since they carry blood are most closely related to the circulatory system. They are aggravated by excess oil and heat in the diet and manifest as hot skin disorders and bleeding conditions.

The *mamsavaha* srotas supply nutrition to the muscles, ligaments, and tendons from which they emerge. They supply nutrition to the mamsa dhatu and are most easily injured by a sedentary lifestyle and eating heavy, greasy foods.

The *medavaha* srotas originate in the kidneys and mesentery, specifically the omentum, and supply the adipose tissue. We know excess fatty foods can overwhelm the medavaha srotas and eventually contribute to sugar metabolism issues.

The *asthivaha* srotas govern the skeletal system and originate in the adipose tissue and the hip bones, supplying nutrition to the bones and cartilage. Disturbance to asthivaha srotas can be caused by excessive cold and dry foods and too much movement. If there is an issue with these srotas, the person may have joint and teeth issues and experience excessive fear.

The *majjavaha* srotas supply the nerve tissue, bone marrow, and the brain. They correlate with the nervous system, and originate from the bones and joints. Issues with the majjavaha srotas include deep-seated ailments such as memory issues, fainting, and nervous disorders.

The *shukravaha* srotas are associated with the reproductive system, and they originate from either the testes or the ovaries. Fertility issues are the primary imbalance related to the shukravaha srotas.

In addition to these ten channels there are two others in women that carry the menstrual fluid and the milk during lactation. There are also three elimination channels: one for sweat, one for feces, and one for urine. The sweat channel originates from the skin and fat, the feces channel from the colon and rectum, and the urine channel from the bladder and kidneys. Their symptomatology is pretty straightforward.

Finally there are the *manovaha srotas,* the mind channels. These carry thoughts and originate in the area of the heart.

It is important to know the structural basis for disease manifestation in both Ayurveda and Chinese medicine. In Ayurveda, there is no imbalance without a srota, and the relationship of a srota to what we know in today's medicine helps us to better understand why diseases affect specific organs, organ systems, tissues, and structures.

In Ayurveda, diseases are actually classified according to the srotas, and there are parallels between this srota classification and the external pathogenic theories of the six channels, four stages, and triple burner in Chinese medicine. Although the srotas don't align completely with any one of these Chinese theories, one can see the similarities between them. The triple burner correlations are the easiest to see right off the bat because of the tridosha theory in Ayurveda that recognizes very similar boundaries and functions within those areas. We also see the parallel between the pranavaha srotas (air channels) and the upper burner, the annavaha srotas (food channels) and the middle burner, and the excretory channels and the lower burner. In addition, the function of the udakavaha srotas (water channels), rasavaha srotas, and raktavaha srotas relate to the function of the triple burner as a whole.

Nidan Panchak is what Ayurvedic doctors call disease pattern identification and pathology. It begins with identifying a primary cause. This is called *hetu,* and it is what originally imbalanced the doshas before a disease even manifested. As discussed earlier, it can be due to a number of factors including lifestyle, poor choices, and so on. Then signs and symptoms are examined, including initial and current symptoms, as well as what will aggravate and what will calm them. We look to see if there is too much or too little of something, a wrong flow, or an obstruction of flow. Then the disease pattern can be named, and the pathogenesis can be understood.

Six Stages of Samprapti

We now come back to the discussion of *samprapti,* the term used in Ayurveda for the six-step process in disease manifestation. Any and all diseases, regardless of cause, follow these six stages. Cause in Ayurveda is usually related to one of three factors: making uninformed choices, doing something consciously we know we shouldn't do, and time factors like seasonal changes. Once we know what stage a disease process is in, we can more definitively make a prognosis. The six stages of samprapti are as follows:

1. Accumulation (*sanchaya*): A dosha accumulates. It is the beginning of imbalance. This is when the body will naturally crave what will balance out the accumulating dosha.
2. Provocation (*prakopa*): The dosha that has accumulated did so in its natural location (e.g., vata in the colon). The person experiences some symptoms.
3. Spread (*prasara*): The vitiated dosha flows out from the site of accumulation.

4. Deposition (*sthana samshraya*): The travelling dosha has deposited itself into an area where it shouldn't be. Once disease progresses to this stage it is more difficult to cure. It is a weak spot in the person's physiology, which helps the vitiated dosha gravitate to it. It then gets lodged in the tissue and begins to damage it.

5. Manifestation (*vyakti*): Full-on signs and symptoms may be observed from a subjective and an objective standpoint. There is definite tissue or dhatu involvement, and oftentimes more than one dosha is aggravated. It is also evident at this point which qualities of the imbalance are the most prevalent and need to be addressed.

6. Disease differentiation (*bheda*): A specific disease pattern is now completely evident, and involvement of more than one system or dhatu is present. By this stage, it is more difficult to cure, or is incurable. Symptom maintenance and palliative actions are often utilized.

These stages can be applied to any ailment, in either system. Let's use our knowledge of Chinese medicine, Ayurveda, folk remedies, and modern practices to address some common ailments.

COMMON CONDITIONS

We are plagued by many of the same bodily discomforts, pathogenic processes, and imbalances as the ancients. Below is a modern interpretation of how to deal with these obstacles to feeling healthy when they arise. It is recommended that medical and dental conditions be evaluated by a doctor or dentist, and that the following recommendations be cleared by the appropriate medical practitioner prior to use, including during pregnancy.

Colds and Coughs
Colds, lingering phlegm, and coughs are best prevented to begin with. Utilizing proper hygiene and taking care of yourself are good first steps.

Wash your hands after you touch anything out in public. Wipe your cellphone and computer keys down regularly with an alcohol wipe or something equivalent. If you do need to cough or a sneeze, do it into the corner of your elbow, not your hand. Don't touch anything after you blow your nose before you wash your hands and practice not touching your face before cold and flu season hits. Also, don't lick your fingers when you're out to eat.

There are several Chinese medicine remedies for colds and the resulting lingering coughs that can ensue. I usually employ a combined strategy when dealing with a cold. Yes, it is caused by a pathogen, but it is also an imbalance of the kapha dosha in the upper jiao. We know that zinc helps bind cells preventing the spread of the virus, so take zinc. Zinc drops are available in health food stores. Only use a neti pot when there are symptoms or for maintenance on an irregular basis. Neti pots are sold in health food stores and in some yoga studios. Warm, purified, salinized water is passed from the pot through one nostril and out the other nostril into the sink. A series of yoga-like positions is then done to eliminate all of the water. There is a learning curve for neti pot use. Please follow the instructions on the package and watch a free online tutorial for guidance.

Vitamin C is also good to have during a cold, but not too much. Once the dosage gets into the thousands of milligrams, depending upon your individual makeup, it can get to the point where it causes diarrhea or loose stools. Some people intentionally take high doses of vitamin C in order to do this. They are aware of a connection to what is happening in the sinuses and lungs and the release that can occur through the large intestine. However, this is not usually the proper course of action and may cause the pathogen to be driven deeper into the body. The yang qi, including the spleen yang, can also be depleted, which creates even bigger problems down the road.

Do a steam inhalation with essential oils. The nature of kapha is cold, and the steam helps warm and move it out. A direct steam inhalation can help to open sinuses, clear mucus, and if using a few drops of an aromatic oil like tea tree or eucalyptus, may even help eliminate the pathogen. To do this, bring water to a boil in a saucepan on the stovetop. Place a hot plate on the table and put three or four drops of essential oil in the water. If wearing glasses, take them off, then sit so your face is over the steam and place a towel or shawl over your head. Gently breathe in the steam for a good five minutes. Replace the water and essential oil each time. This can be done twice a day.

At the onset of a cold when the neck and upper back ache, inducing a mild sweat can do wonders. If the pathogen is in the exterior level of the body, the very slight sweat will help open the pores and push it out. To do this, put about five quarter-sized slices of fresh ginger, a clove of chopped garlic, two or three scallions, a pinch of cayenne, two or three red radishes, and salt and pepper to taste in a three quart saucepan of water and bring it to a boil, then reduce the heat and simmer for twenty minutes with the lid at least partially on. There are volatile oils in the ginger you don't want to let escape completely. If you'd like, this decoction can be made with chicken broth, and rice can be added. Once it's done, bundle up in bed or wrap up in a blanket on the couch until you are very warm, and sip on the broth. Once you start to feel a mild sweat coming on, take off the blankets. You can finish the broth; in fact, have a cup three or four times a day if you wish, but don't go through the whole process of inducing a sweat each time. Drink plenty of fluids and keep your feet and the back of your neck warm.

There are two primary formulations in the Chinese medicine cabinet that are also good for the onset of a cold. One is for a wind cold presentation and the other is for wind heat invasion. Wind cold includes mild chills/fever, aversion to cold and wind, and slight upper back, neck, and body ache. We used to be able to prescribe a fabulous formula called Ma Huang Tang, especially when the person did not have a fever with sweat. Unfortunately, the federal government in the United States has withdrawn the access to the main ingredient: ma huang, or ephedra. It used to be misused in some diet pills and to make methamphetamine. Because of illicit drug makers and users, practitioners with the training to use Ma Huang Tang properly, with very positive effects, are prohibited from doing so. Instead, using the broth combined with Gui Zhi Tang, or Cinnamon Twig Decoction, is preferred.

In the case of a wind heat invasion, people will often get a sore throat. Usually it will come on late at night and feel scratchy. At the first sign of this, Yin Qiao San can be taken as directed on the label. This helps effuse the heat and kill the pathogen. If one waits until the pathogen has nestled in the body, this formula will probably not work. It is for a pathogen that is still in the exterior. Drinking plenty of fluids, again, is important. For a cough, one can press acupoint Lung (LU) 5. To find the right location, slide your thumb up the opposite arm along the line that runs from the radial pulse at the wrist (the thumb side of the inner arm) toward the elbow crease, just about a half inch in toward the midline. There will be a band of tight fascia or muscle somewhere in between the wrist and the elbow, but closer to the elbow. Find the "fullest" or tightest, most tender point and press in circular motions with the thumb for a minute or two. It's usually fuller or tighter on one arm than on the other. This can be repeated every few hours. Kidney (KD) 27 is also good for cough. It is just below the collar bone about a half inch lateral to midline and can be lightly tapped.

In order to help clear an external level pathogen, another good point to use is Large Intestine (LI) 4. This is between the thumb and index finger, on the inside of the bone closest to the index finger. Pinch from either side of your hand with your opposite thumb and index finger and press firmly, it will be tender. Keep the pressure on for a minute or so and release. This is useful for sinus issues, jaw tension, and frontal, or around the eye or cheek, headaches. It is also helpful for labor induction so please don't do this if you are pregnant.

In Ayurveda, looking at which dosha is primarily involved is very helpful. Ginger and tulsi teas are great preventatives and also aid immunity after a pathogen has set in. Plenty of fluids and rest are advised. If there is a lot of mucus, cut it by drinking spicy, kapha-clearing teas that contain things like pepper. It's best to eat light, easily digestible foods as the agni may be compromised during illness. A sore throat from postnasal drip can be soothed with a teaspoon of honey. For a more moderate sore throat, gargle with ¼ teaspoon of rock salt, ½ teaspoon of powdered turmeric, and a sprinkle of cayenne in one cup of warm water. Gargle every four to six hours.

Headache

Nine times out of ten when people come into the clinic with a headache it is because they need to drink some water. Any time you have a headache, drink a glass of water. Oftentimes the symptoms will have subsided in ten minutes. If that doesn't work, observe where the headache is. If it is in the front, near the forehead, it is a Yang Ming (Stomach/Large Intestine) channel headache. Doing acupressure on LI 4, as mentioned in the section on colds, can be helpful. If it is around the temples or the sides of the head, it is a Gall Bladder channel headache. In this case, lightly press the temples in a circular motion. You can use a drop of the Chinese remedy "white flower oil" on each temple. Massage it in gently three or four times a day. For Gall Bladder channel headaches you can also do acupressure on point GB 41. This is outside the pinky toe tendon in the depression along the bone (see fig. 12.1).

If the headache is on top of the head this is a Liver channel headache. Use LI 4 with Liver (LV) 3. If you run your finger along the

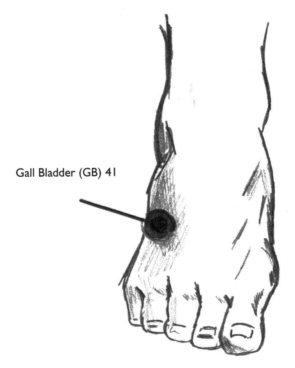

Gall Bladder (GB) 41

Fig. 12.1. Gall Bladder (GB) 41 acupoint

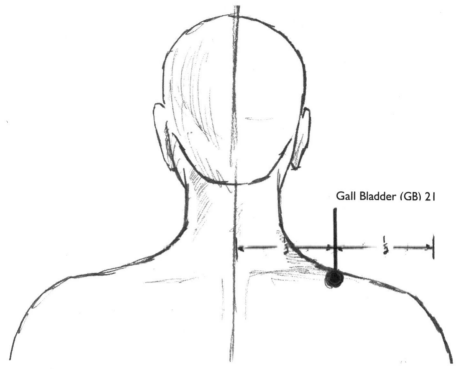

Gall Bladder (GB) 21

Fig. 12.2. Gall Bladder (GB) 21 acupoint

webbing between the big toe and the second toe, LV 3 is in the depression just before the bones come together. (Note that LV 3 is contraindicated during pregnancy.) You can also press KD 1, just opposite it on the sole of the foot at the same time to descend the energy. GB 21 is also good for headaches, especially those that feel worse when you touch them (see fig. 12.2). It is at the top of the muscle, about midway between the outside edge of the shoulder and where the neck meets the body and is also to be avoided if pregnant. Shao Yin headaches are all over the head and include the Heart and Kidney channels. These are due to deficiency, so drink water and rest. Evaluate what is happening in your life and see if you can identify areas where you can improve peace of mind, diet, and sleep.

Occipital headaches, those at the back of the head, are Tai Yang, or Bladder/Small Intestine channel headaches. GB 41 and 21 are both

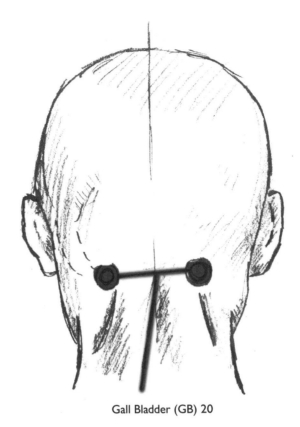

Gall Bladder (GB) 20

Fig. 12.3. Gall Bladder (GB) 20 acupoints

good for this type of headache. Oftentimes these headaches emerge from a tight muscle in the trapezius, somewhere between the shoulder blade and the spine. Rolling on a tennis ball on it to release the pressure or having someone work it out for you can be helpful. In addition, pressing GB 20, on either side of the back of the head just below the bone, may also be helpful (see fig. 12.3). Alternatively, if there is no neck pathology like a disk or vertebral degeneration or a herniation, lying on a still point inducer may help, as may two tennis balls placed in a sock. Knot the sock so the balls can't slip around, place them on the floor, and lie on them for a few minutes to release the muscle tension. They do not go on the spine, but on either side of it at the base of the skull.

Nausea/Heartburn

Nausea can be due to a variety of causes that range from pregnancy hormones and headaches to viral infections. Excess mucus and phlegm from a head cold, sinusitis, or an inflammatory pitta imbalance in the digestive system are also causes, as is stress leading to undigested food being left in the stomach for too long.

An imbalance of stomach acid usually causes heartburn. If there is too little or too much stomach acid, heartburn or acid reflux can result. Follow the guidelines for enkindling agni and for a pitta-pacifying dietary regime. If too much acid, and it really burns or feels like it's coming into your throat, follow a pitta-pacifying or anti-inflammatory diet. Also, eat small meals and do not lie down after eating or gulp fluids. Instead, sip on them consistently throughout the day. For heartburn, some swear by apple cider vinegar, others by sweet apples. I found apples to be extremely helpful in later pregnancy. That, and not overeating, as well as not letting too much time lapse between meals. Spicy, pungent foods can make heartburn worse. Avoid hot chilies and hot sauce.

Shatavari, licorice, and amalaki are a wonderful combination for heartburn. They can be combined in equal parts and made into a tea. It is important to descend the qi so the acid stops splashing. This can be done with acupoints GB 21 (see fig. 12.2 on page 325), Pericardium (PC) 6 (see fig. 12.4 on page 328), Stomach (ST) 44 in the webbing between the second and third toes (see fig. 12.5 on page 328), and GB 41 (see fig. 12.1 on page 324).

For both nausea and heartburn, pressing PC 6 is very helpful. It is on the inner forearm near the wrist crease. With your thumb, glide toward the elbow between the two big tendons. At about an inch away from the wrist, your thumb will fall deeper into the arm. This is PC 6. Press it for a couple of minutes on each side.

For nausea, drinking ginger tea or sucking on a slice of ginger can be helpful. Alternatively, mint tea can help as well. The primary Chinese herbal remedy for temporary nausea (not for pregnancy) is Huo Xiang Zheng Qi Wan. If there is stomach discomfort from overeating, we use Bao He Wan. I usually keep that around during the holidays.

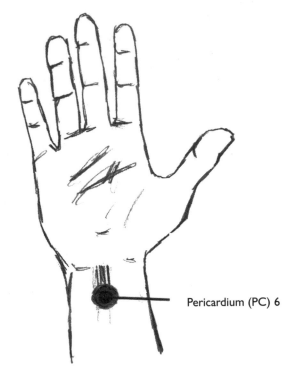

Pericardium (PC) 6

Fig. 12.4. Pericardium (PC) 6 acupoint

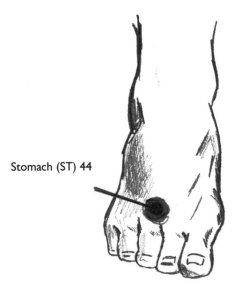

Stomach (ST) 44

Fig. 12.5. Stomach (ST) 44 acupoint

Toothache

Toothaches can be caused by a variety of issues. This recommendation and all the other recommendations in this book are for mild symptoms and for conditions that have been evaluated by a doctor or a dentist. A drop of clove oil mixed in a carrier like olive oil massaged into the tooth and surrounding gum can be very effective in providing relief. Massaging LI 4 (see fig. 12.6), between the index finger and the thumb, is also indicated except during pregnancy. Sometimes people feel tooth pain as a result of sinus pressure. LI 20 (see fig. 12.7) is

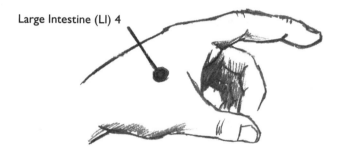

Fig. 12.6. Large Intestine (LI) 4 acupoint

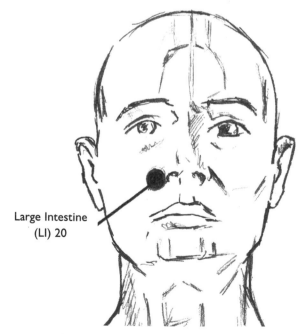

Fig. 12.7. Large Intestine (LI) 20 acupoint

helpful for this. It is located about ¼ inch lateral to each nostril. Just press on it with the fingers. This can help open the nasal passages and is a good point for clearing overall inflammation. Oftentimes gum issues are related to stomach heat, which manifests as hyperacidity of the saliva. Modifying the diet and making oil pulling, where constitutionally appropriate, part of the daily routine can help with many dental issues.

Constipation

Constipation is generally considered a vata disorder, especially if it is chronic. Dryness and apana vayu not moving downward are primary causes. Vata is highly sensitive and stress of any kind can first manifest in holding in the large intestine. Fear would be the root emotional issue triggering this reaction in the body. In Chinese medicine we would say it is qi stagnation, heat, qi and yang deficiency, or dryness. There are a number of formulas in the Chinese pharmacopeia that are helpful for alleviating constipation regardless of the cause. Herbs like rou cong rong help tonify the yang and move the stool in cases of deficiency. There are various seeds such as cannabis seeds for moistening and moving. Chen pi and other citrus peels are helpful for moving the qi in the large intestine. In extreme cases we use senna, da huang, and mang xiao.

In general, if one is prone to constipation there are some everyday things that can be done. One is to eat a few figs or prunes before bedtime. Another is to look at the diet and see where more fiber and prebiotics can be added. Sometimes, taking a probiotic can be helpful as well. Avoid dry food, like processed cereals and dry fruits. Notice if dairy is a trigger. Make sure to get some exercise. A brisk walk with deep breaths twenty minutes a day can do wonders for digestion and managing stress. Triphala can be taken before bed, ¼ teaspoon in hot water. A castor oil pack can be done on the lower abdomen as well.

In addition to good deep diaphragmatic breathing, specific *kriyas,* or cleansing techniques, can be done to keep things moving. Kapalabhati, or skull luster breath, is a wonderful practice for clearing the head, the mind, and moving the qi in the low belly. It is not recommended for those who are pregnant or menstruating or who have high blood pressure or glaucoma. Sit comfortably and with the back straight but relaxed. Take three deep breaths, in and out through the nose. Let the fourth breath come in about half way, then use the low belly to forcefully expel the air through the nose. The tummy will feel like it's pressing in toward your back. Keep pumping the air through like this. As the belly relaxes, the body will naturally inhale about half a breath, then push this air out with the belly. If you feel dizzy or you can't get a breath, please do not continue the practice. Instead, consult with a yoga teacher for guidance. A yoga routine geared toward alleviating chronic constipation is a good idea, and a couple of private lessons with a qualified practitioner can change your life.

Diarrhea/Loose Bowel Movements

Again, looking at diet is very important. Notice if certain foods "go right through you" and avoid them. If there is a burning sensation when passing a stool, or stools are oily, move toward a pitta-pacifying diet. If there is undigested food in the stools and your tongue is pale and shows teeth marks, incorporate more warming, easy-to-digest meals into your diet. In Chinese medicine, the primary reason for loose bowel movements is spleen qi deficiency, which is akin to damaged agni in Ayurveda. Other causes are internal cold or heat. Diarrhea is more extreme than loose bowel movements and is caused by the above issues along with external pathogens like bacteria, viruses, and parasites.

If diarrhea is due to an infection, it is best to let it run its course. This is the body's way of eliminating the pathogen. Once irritated, though, the bowel sometimes remains overactive. Make sure to drink plenty of room temperature fluids and replace electrolytes. Pure huang lian can be administered in pill form for diarrhea. This is a good symptomatic remedy for travelers as it also helps to kill the pathogen. It should be taken with caution, however, as it is very cold and can damage the spleen qi. It should not be used regularly or in cases of deficiency or cold. Nutmeg can bind the stools and can be used for loose bowel movements. Cooked apple seasoned with nutmeg and ghee is nourishing and helps slow down the digestion in cases of deficiency where fats are not an issue. If stools are oily or greasy, eliminate the ghee. Eating white rice with yogurt mixed in, as long as dairy isn't problematic, is a good remedy for diarrhea as well.

Gas/Bloating

It seems that the leading cause of gas and bloating is poor diet and lifestyle, including high stress. Worry injures the agni or spleen qi and weakens the body's capacity to optimally transform and transport food and fluids. Note what foods are causing the gas and bloating and avoid consuming them until the spleen qi or agni are strengthened. Sometimes, a temporary broad-spectrum digestive enzyme is helpful while working to strengthen the digestion. Follow the guidelines in the sections on spleen qi deficiency and agni. Eat at regular times and don't eat when you're upset; calm down first. Avoid overeating or eating before the previous meal is well through the stomach and upper intestine. Don't eat when you're not hungry, unless you're never hungry, in which case take digestive aids twenty minutes before small, easily digestible meals. This may include a thin slice of ginger with a squirt of lime juice and a sprinkle of rock salt or black salt. One may chew on fennel seeds or have CCF tea or fennel tea throughout the day.

If bloating is distracting and uncomfortable, lie on the floor on your back. Pull the knees into the chest and hug in the legs (see fig. 12.8).

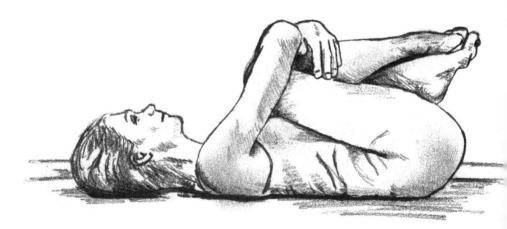

Fig. 12.8. Wind-relieving pose for gas, bloating, and distention

Breathe deep belly breaths while squeezing the legs into the belly. With each exhale, allow the legs to come closer into the body, even if it is just a micro movement. This exercise with help alleviate the bloating by allowing gas to pass. It will happen either in the pose or several minutes after it. Stay in the pose for up to five minutes. Then open the arms to a *T* position on the floor and lower the bent legs to one side. Relax here for ten breaths, then change sides and repeat.

Stress/Anxiety

We all experience stress in one way or another, and there are times in our lives when it's worse than others. There are the major life stressors like ending relationships, moving, incorporating a new family member, changing jobs, dealing with an illness, and mourning the passing of a loved one. In between and in addition to these things are the constant distractions and mental/emotional/physical demands that are unprecedented. Most of us are isolated from nature on a daily basis and forced to sit with poor posture in front of screens. The chronic posture that is naturally adopted in front of the computer screen with hunched back, jutting chin, and shoulders rolling forward is a contributing factor to how we feel stress and the amount of it we endure.

This position promotes the shallow breathing discussed in chapter 8 (page 202), which then turns on the sympathetic nervous system. In addition, nerves may get compressed by stiff muscles in and around the outer clavicle and in the neck. This compression may lead to a rise in blood pressure because of the added pressure of the muscles on the blood vessels, which causes the heart to work harder to pump the blood. Many kinds of back pain and headache are caused by just this posture. Add to it breathing poor quality air, eating on the run, eating non-nutritious foods, and dealing with the demands of family at home, and the stress on the body and mind becomes chronic. Then there are phone texts, social media, politics, and the news—all a recipe for disaster.

The worst thing about it all is that so many people are wrapped up in being stressed that it has become socially unacceptable not to be. This is another stress. Some people can withstand so much stress that they don't even realize how stressed they really are. Oftentimes, the body will take on what the mind has blocked. I find that for many people, shutting off the awareness of just how uncomfortable or miserable they really are is a coping mechanism. These are the people who seem to have the tensest pulse and often suffer from headaches, neck aches, and chronic back pain. When asked about their stress levels, these folks sometimes say that they are managing their stress well. It isn't until they have a few acupuncture treatments or begin yoga or meditation and start to relax that they realize how far from the truth this statement is.

There are several herbal remedies that offer temporary relief from life's pressures. Really, lifestyle needs to be evaluated and changed so that you are operating at a level you can reasonably handle. What is a reasonable level for you may be totally different for others. This can also contribute to stress. If you are more sensitive and adversely affected more quickly than another person, being okay with this and backing off the stressors can be challenging. This is especially true if the other person who may be judging you or you are comparing yourself to is your spouse. If you are judging yourself harshly, the stress will not abate until you stop. If you are judging someone else because you want them to do more than they are, your stress will also not abate until you stop. Adaptogenic herbs can take the edge off the stress and thereby improve stamina and well-being. In Ayurveda we recommend ashwagandha, brahmi, and tulsi. In Chinese medicine, we recommend ginseng and Siberian ginseng. There is also a popular formula for helping one cope with stress in Chinese medicine called "Free and Easy Wanderer." Its name implies the desired effect of taking it.

It is also imperative to take time throughout the day to breathe and focus on the present moment. Being mindful that stress and its associated negative emotional states are present is a way of being present. Know when you feel frustrated, angry, fearful, worried, or anxious. Breathe into it, and its power loosens around the edges. Make a conscious effort to set technology aside. Take off the smart watch, leave the phone in another room, turn off the computer, avoid social media, and don't watch the news. A client and friend who is a successful, mindful financial advisor tells his stressed-out investors to turn off the TV. He believes the news creates a fearful attitude about financial security and causes a lot of unnecessary stress, confusion, and worry.

Do something nurturing for yourself every day. It can be drinking a mindful cup of tea, taking a walk or making a trip to the gym, doing yoga, meditation, or qigong, having a pedicure—it doesn't matter what it is, but do it every day. Even if it's just for five minutes. There is more of you to give if you are actually present, and we can only be present if we are taking care of ourselves. If that doesn't make sense to you right now, that's okay, just do something for yourself every day, however small, and notice how your perspective and reaction to things around you change for the better. Take a moment to sit up straight at your desk and breathe the next breath more deeply than you did the previous one or take a quick walk around the office, taking time to feel your feet on the ground. Gently massage the third eye point between the eyebrows, draw the breath to below the navel, and relax the jaw. These little things all have a tremendous influence on helping one feel less stressed. Any mindful moment you take is a break from pressure.

Back Pain

Back pain is the number one ailment that brings people into the clinic. It may be muscular, arthritic, or disc related. When the back "goes out" so to speak, it is totally incapacitating. Simple movements like standing up, sitting or lying down, or going to the bathroom are major challenges. Life comes to a halt. The author and spiritual teacher Louise Hay believes back pain, specifically low back pain, is related to not feeling supported in life. This is very often true of people who come in for acute low back pain. I find neck pain related to feeling burdened by another. Like any illness or imbalance, the cause of pain may not be simple or rational, but if you can, feel out what emotion or emotions could be triggering the pain. This can be helpful for understanding why your body is doing what it does. You can then begin making changes that can prevent further issues.

In Chinese medicine, any pain is due first to disordered qi. There must be some blockage or lack of flow that results in the pain. Without a blockage in qi, there can be no pain. The two go hand in hand. Bodywork is the number one recommendation for releasing the blockage, restoring proper flow, and alleviating the pain. Acupuncture is wonderful for this. It can relax muscles, reduce inflammation, increase circulation, and even help to put discs back into alignment. Remember, improper flow of qi is what pushed it out of alignment to begin with. Cupping can help to relieve stagnation, as can rubbing aromatic substances into the painful area.

In Ayurveda, we most often use mahanarayan oil. In Chinese practice, we use Zheng Gu Shui, Po Sum On, and Die Da Jiu. There is a specialization in Chinese medicine related to the treatment of musculoskeletal trauma. Various lotions, potions, and patches are useful for the many stages of injury. I have seen the use of Chinese herbs and acupuncture mend a small shattered bone in time to prevent surgery. In addition, several clients have avoided neck surgery by using acupuncture, Chinese liniments, and cupping. One of them is a woman whose neck pain went almost completely away after she broke up with her boyfriend. Weeks prior to the breakup it was recommended that she be operated on by a surgeon.

There is a wonderful back exercise I learned from Frank Bisio and Tom Butler, Chinese medicine practitioners and coauthors of *A Tooth from the Tiger's Mouth: How to Treat Your Injuries with Powerful Healing Secrets of the Great Chinese Warrior*. They call it the "back stretch." Lie on the floor, on a mat or a rug, and bend at the knees so your feet are flat on the floor a few inches forward of your buttocks (see fig. 12.9). Have the legs parallel and hips' width apart. Gently press the small of the back into the floor. Relax any muscles that don't need to be engaged and slightly tuck the chin, not dramatically but enough to mildly lengthen the neck. Straighten the arms toward the ceiling, palms facing each other. Then cross the arms over the chest

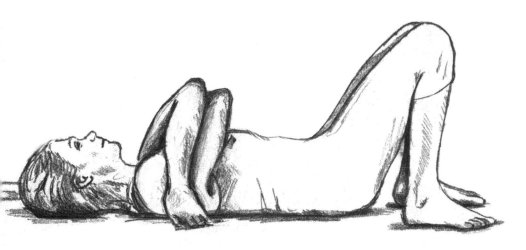

Fig. 12.9. The back stretch

like a gentle hug and relax a bit more. Stay in this posture for a couple of minutes. Then reach the arms up and cross them over the chest in the opposite direction for another few minutes. Work up to twenty minutes total.

This helps strengthen the core, which is often weak in cases of back pain. It does so gently without taxing the back at all. It also helps realign any budding abnormalities in the spinal alignment, including hyper or hypo lordosis or kyphosis. This means the qi or prana is restored to its correct flow. If suffering from an acute back spasm, I don't recommend stretching right away. This can cause the muscle to tighten more in retaliation. If a vertebra is twisted or a disc has gone out of place, don't do any spinal twisting. Depending on the direction of misalignment, it may be worse to do a forward bend, a back bend, or a bend to one side or another. Pay attention to this, seek professional guidance, and take it easy for the time being.

There is plenty of information online and in bookstores for cross-disciplinary practitioners, as well as for the interested lay person. Being mindful and paying attention to how you feel and what your body is saying are the best things you can do for yourself. Breathing well, drinking adequate pure water, and eating and exercising according to your body's recommendations are ideal. Please take change slowly and at a fairly comfortable pace, take time for yourself, and always consult a practitioner if you have any questions or want to learn more. There is nothing more therapeutic than listening to yourself, following your own guidance, and being in the nurturing care of a trusted professional while on the healing journey.

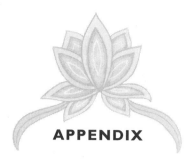

The Hippocratic Oath

I swear by Apollo the physician, and Asclepius, and Hygieia and Panacea and all the gods and goddesses as my witnesses, that, according to my ability and judgment, I will keep this Oath and this contract:

To hold him who taught me this art equally dear to me as my parents, to be a partner in life with him, and to fulfill his needs when required; to look upon his offspring as equals to my own siblings, and to teach them this art, if they shall wish to learn it, without fee or contract; and that by the set rules, lectures, and every other mode of instruction, I will impart a knowledge of the art to my own sons, and those of my teachers, and to students bound by this contract and having sworn this Oath to the law of medicine, but to no others.

I will use those dietary regimens which will benefit my patients according to my greatest ability and judgment, and I will do no harm or injustice to them.

I will not give a lethal drug to anyone if I am asked, nor will I advise such a plan; and similarly I will not give a woman a pessary to cause an abortion.

In purity and according to divine law will I carry out my life and my art.

I will not use the knife, even upon those suffering from stones, but I will leave this to those who are trained in this craft.

Into whatever homes I go, I will enter them for the benefit of the sick, avoiding any voluntary act of impropriety or corruption, including the seduction of women or men, whether they are free men or slaves.

Whatever I see or hear in the lives of my patients, whether in connection with my professional practice or not, which ought not to be spoken of outside, I will keep secret, as considering all such things to be private.

So long as I maintain this Oath faithfully and without corruption, may it be granted to me to partake of life fully and the practice of my art, gaining the respect of all men for all time. However, should I transgress this Oath and violate it, may the opposite be my fate.[1]

TRANSLATED BY MICHAEL NORTH,
NATIONAL LIBRARY OF MEDICINE, 2002

Notes

INTRODUCTION

1. Sharma, *Caraka Samhita,* vol. 1, 19.

CHAPTER 1
THE MAGIC OF ANCIENT MEDICINE

1. Reeves, *Egyptian Medicine,* 51, 53.
2. Reeves, *Egyptian Medicine,* 49.
3. Reeves, *Egyptian Medicine,* 53.
4. Reeves, *Egyptian Medicine,* 26–27.
5. Adams, *On Ancient Medicine,* parts 5, 6, 8–21.
6. Nutton, "Galen of Pergamum," Anatomical and Medical Studies.
7. Nutton, "Galen of Pergamum," Anatomical and Medical Studies.
8. Van Alphen, *Oriental Medicine,* 45.
9. Van Alphen, *Oriental Medicine,* 63.
10. Van Alphen, *Oriental Medicine,* 63.
11. Owen, "Otzi the Iceman."
12. Helmut Kaiser Consultancy, *Traditional Chinese Medicine,* section 1, Initial Situation.
13. Ro, "Enormous Market for Chinese Medicine."
14. Bayer. "Bayer Completes Acquisition of Dihon Pharmaceutical Group."
15. Hatton, "Nobel Prize Winner Tu Youyou."
16. Bloomfield, *Hymns of the Atharva Veda,* sections 1–2.

17. Satake, "India."

18. Association for Traditional Studies, "Evolution of Chinese Medicine," The Nationalist Distrust of Its Own Traditional Medicine.

19. Association for Traditional Studies, "Evolution of Chinese Medicine," The Cultural Revolution and Chinese Medicine.

20. Association for Traditional Studies, "Evolution of Chinese Medicine," The Cultural Revolution and Chinese Medicine.

21. Association for Traditional Studies, "Evolution of Chinese Medicine," Government's Efforts to Document Traditional Medicine.

CHAPTER 2
IN THE BEGINNING:
THE ROOTS OF AYURVEDA
AND CHINESE MEDICINE

1. Violatti, "Confucianism," definition.

2. Chiang, *Historical Epistemology,* 25.

3. Ranade, *Natural Healing,* 29.

4. Das, "Ayurveda-Vedanta," I—Ayurveda as Part of the Vedas.

CHAPTER 3
THE FIVE ELEMENTS

1. Walia, "Vedic Philosophy," Tesla and Ancient Vedic Philosophy and the Properties of Space.

2. Martino, "Water Has Memory," video.

3. Emoto, *Hidden Messages,* xxv.

4. Palep, *Scientific Foundation of Ayurveda,* 65.

5. Joshi, *Ayurveda and Panchakarma,* 38–42.

6. Fountain, "Earth's Hidden Ocean."

CHAPTER 4
CONSTITUTION

1. *TrueAyurveda* (blog), Ritucharya: The 6 seasons and lifestyle, diet, and your Yoga practice.

2. Maciocia, *Diagnosis,* 15.

3. Maciocia, *Diagnosis,* 16.

4. Maciocia, *Diagnosis,* 19.

5. Maciocia, *Diagnosis,* 19.

6. Maciocia, *Diagnosis,* 19–20.

CHAPTER 5
ANATOMY:
NUTS AND (LIGHTNING) BOLTS

1. Milbradt, "Bonghan Channels."

2. Sharma, *Caraka Samhita,* vol. 2, 387–91.

3. Murthy, *Vagbhata's Astanga Hridayam,* 422.

4. Robertson, *Applied Channel Theory,* 422.

5. Robertson, *Applied Channel Theory,* 423.

6. Robertson, *Applied Channel Theory,* 423.

7. Robertson, *Applied Channel Theory,* 423.

CHAPTER 6
CONSCIOUSNESS

1. Blackmore, *Consciousness,* 5.

2. Massar, "Q&A," What are the possible implications for us/for humankind?

3. Chalmers, *Conscious Mind,* xii–xiv.

4. Lad, *Marma Points,* 32.

CHAPTER 8
PREVENTION AND MAINTENANCE

1. Sharma, *Caraka Samhita,* vol. 1, 123.

2. Elkaim, "Truth," The Uber Simple Hydration Equation.

3. National Association for Holistic Aromatherapy (website).

CHAPTER 9
TASTE AND NUTRITION

1. Bradley Yantzer, email messages to author, February 5 and 12, 2017.

CHAPTER 10
CLEANSING AND THE SEASONS

1. Murthy, *Vagbhata's Astanga Hridayam,* vol. 1, 33.

2. Kondo, *Life-Changing Magic,* 1.

CHAPTER 12
THE CLINIC AND BEYOND

1. Weiss, "Opposite of Addiction," What Causes Addiction?

APPENDIX
THE HIPPOCRATIC OATH

1. North, "Greek Medicine."

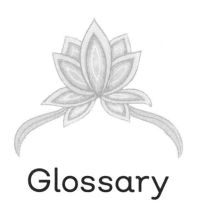

Glossary

abhyanga: Ayurvedic therapeutic oil massage. Term commonly used to describe self-oil massage or that done by one or more practitioners as a stand-alone treatment or as a therapy in panchakarma.

acupoint: Intersection point along an acupuncture meridian that allows for multitissue communication. Acupoints are needled in acupuncture and manipulated in acupressure therapy to establish a smooth flow of qi and blood through the body and to balance the mind.

agni: Metabolic fire in Ayurvedic medicine that transforms raw materials into nourishment and nutrition. It includes, but is not limited to, enzymatic activity, bile, and stomach acid.

ahamkara: Individual self-awareness that arises from mahat, or universal intelligence. Also known as ego.

Akasha: Space; in Ayurvedic theory, the original element from which all others are derived.

ama: The term in Ayurveda used to describe toxins. Usually these are accumulated metabolic wastes and the residual effect of emotional states and traumas in the tissue.

apana vayu: One of the five subforms of the vata dosha in Ayurveda. It is responsible for the downward and outward movement of prana vata, and for elimination, menstruation, and birth.

asana: Literally, "seat" in Sanskrit, asanas are the poses most yoga classes consist of.

astanga: Meaning "eight-limbed" in Sanskrit, it is the name for the Yoga philosophy of the scholar/philosopher Patanjali, documented in his Yoga Sutras. Today this term has also come to mean several series of sequential yoga poses that originated in Mysore, India.

aura: The sometimes visible energy field that surrounds the form of anything that is alive.

bagua: A circular arrangement of eight trigrams used in Taoist cosmology to represent the eight fundamental principles of reality.

brahmi: An herb in the Ayurvedic pharmacopoeia that is used to calm the nervous system.

burner: A region of the body whose contents work together to serve a general physiological function. In Chinese medicine there are three burners which function as an organ called the triple burner, triple warmer, or san jiao.

chakra(s): Vortices of energy and information that emanate from a central axis in the core of the body and both energize the body and mind as well as project from them. Each chakra is said to have a seed syllable sound that activates or balances it, a color, a deity, and physiological and mental/emotional functions and characteristics associated with it.

channel: Also called a meridian, a channel is a passageway for qi, or vital life-force energy to circulate throughout the body.

Charaka: An Ayurveda Vidya who authored one of the two major foundational texts of Ayurvedic medicine, the Charaka Samhita.

chyawanprash: A nutritious jam made from a mixture of honey, ghee, sesame oil, herbs, spices, and other ingredients including amalaki.

cuneiform: The written language of the Sumerians. Cuneiform is believed by most to be the first written language.

dharana: One of the eight limbs of Patanjali's astanga yoga. It is the stage before dhyana, meditation, and after pratyahara, sense withdrawl. Dharana is a mental state of complete concentration on a single object.

dhatu: A dhatu is a tissue type in Ayurveda. An example would be mamsa, which is muscle tissue.

dhyana: The second-to-last limb in Patanjali's astanga yoga. It is the state that arises spontaneously as a result of dharana, or complete concentration upon a single object. Dhyana is meditation. It is a misnomer to call our modern-day meditation practices meditation. Meditation, as it is referred to today, is actually dharana. Dhyana is the last step before Samadhi.

dinacharya: Dinacharya is the daily regimen one is recommended to follow in Ayurveda.

eight principles: The eight principles are the basic assessment criteria a Chinese medicine practitioner uses to formulate a clearer picture of a client's imbalance(s). They are yin/yang, interior/exterior, cold/hot, and deficiency/excess.

emesis: Vomiting therapy used in Ayurvedic medicine to rid the body of ama and accumulated kapha dosha.

five phase theory: Also called five element theory in Chinese medicine as the elements (wood, fire, metal, earth, and water) are the controlling forces at work in the activity of the five phases. The five phases can be viewed throughout nature and are at the root of some Chinese systems of constitutional analysis. Whether used for constitutional purposes or not, the five phases are useful for diagnosis and treatment.

four levels: The four levels are a Chinese diagnostic parameter by which a practitioner can assess the depth and severity of an external pathogen, particularly wind-heat. From there, the practitioner can correctly treat the person.

garshana: In Ayurveda, it's the practice of dry brushing. It involves rubbing or "brushing" the skin in a specific pattern with a silk glove or some type of loofah. This is done to increase circulation and assist in the body's natural detoxification processes.

gu qi: This is the qi generated from the digestive process. It is a result of the activity of the spleen qi.

gua sha: Gua sha is a method of treatment in Chinese medicine in which the practitioner firmly rubs or "scrapes" the skin with a blunt instrument such as a Chinese soup spoon or, traditionally, with a piece of water buffalo horn. It is used to alleviate stagnation and release the exterior.

guna: A guna can be one of two things, either a quality of material nature or a particular mental quality. In terms of the twenty qualities of matter, there is a spectrum upon which every quality of nature can be measured. The presence or absence of a particular quality and its quantity is indicative of the nature of an object and its functioning. The three gunas that are part of the mental qualities are a separate thing. These three gunas are sattva, rajas, and tamas. These are states of the mental/emotional nature and translate roughly to calmness, activity, and inertia.

hun: The hun is one of the spirits in Chinese medicine that is associated with the liver organ. It is the spirit that leaves the body at death and goes on, like the soul or consciousness in other traditions.

ida: Ida is one of the principal nadis or channels in Yoga anatomy. Ida nadi traverses the left side of the body, and is roughly akin to the feminine, lunar principle in nature. It is often correlated to passive activities and creativity.

jiao: See "burner."

kapha: Kapha is one of the three doshas in Ayurveda. It is associated with the principle of stability in nature and the earth and water elements.

kitchari: Kitchari is a staple of Ayurvedic cuisine. It is an easily digestible, nutritive gruel or congee usually made with mung dal and rice.

kosha: Kosha means, "sheath." There are five koshas that make up the individual. They are said to be stacked within one another like a Russian doll. The five koshas are the food sheath (physical body), pranic sheath (vital or energetic body), mental sheath (mental/emotional body), intellect sheath (wisdom body), and bliss sheath (transcendent consciousness).

kundalini: Kundalini is a powerful creative and vital force that is stored in the human body at the base of the spine. It is usually activated through rigorous spiritual practice, and sometimes by hallucinogenic substances or instantaneous life-altering experiences. Its release brings a profound shift in spiritual awareness and awareness of the self.

marma: A marma in Ayurveda is like an acupoint in Chinese medicine. It is an intersection where communication between tissues is heightened, as well as access to deeper structures within the body. These points are interaction points between the interior and exterior world.

marma therapy: Marma therapy is a bodywork modality in Ayurveda. Similar to acupressure, it involves the manipulation of marmani to effect healing in the body and mind. In addition to touch, poultices, herbs, and oils may be applied to marma points.

marmani: Plural for marma, marma points.

meridian: See "channel."

moxa: Moxa is dried mugwort used in moxibustion.

moxibustion: The Chinese therapy by which moxa is burned either directly on the skin or over acupoints to effect healing in the body. It is particularly useful for tonifying yang.

mudra: *Mudra* means "seal." It is a subtle lock in the body that's held to redirect or control the flow of prana throughout the body and mind. It is also the hand positions used to direct subtle prana flow in the mind.

nadi(s): Sanskrit for "flow," "channel," or "vibration." Similar to acupuncture channels or meridians, they are pathways for the flow of prana.

niyamas: The second limb of Patanjali's astanga yoga. Niyamas are recommended states to be internally cultivated for healthy living. The five niyamas are: purity, contentment, self-discipline, self-study, and surrender to a greater power.

pakua: See "bagua."

panchakarma: The therapeutic modality of Ayurvedic medicine dealing with detoxification of the tissues. It is often a precursor to rasayana, or rejuvenation therapies. It means "five actions."

pestilential qi: In Chinese medicine it is the qi responsible for certain illnesses, like a pathogen.

pingala: Pingala is one of the principle nadis or channels in Yoga anatomy. Pingala nadi traverses the right side of the body, and is roughly akin to the masculine, solar principle in nature. It is often correlated to heat and activity.

pitta: One of the three doshas in Ayurveda. Associated with the transformative principle in nature and the fire and water elements.

pneuma: In Greek, it means "breath" and has been used to indicate the soul, spirit, and vital force.

po: One of the five shen or spirits in Chinese medicine, called the corporeal soul. It is associated with the lungs and is responsible for the formation and growth of the physical body.

pragya parad: Sanskrit for "the mistake of the intellect," and refers to the underlying cause of disease.

prakriti: In Indian philosophy, the foundational material energy from which all matter manifests.

prakruti: The true nature of a person's constitution. This usually does not change throughout the lifetime.

prana: Vital life force, vitality, and one of the five subforms of the vata dosha.

pranayama: Yogic breathing practices designed to control the flow of prana. The fourth limb of Patanjali's astanga yoga.

pratyahara: The fifth limb of Patanjali's astanga yoga. It means sense withdrawal, drawing attention internally, or not feeding the senses so that one may focus in preparation for meditation.

purusha: The primordial consciousness that arises with prakriti at the beginning of existence.

purvakarma: Preparatory practices to be implemented prior to the Ayurvedic cleansing modalities of panchakarma.

rajas: One of the three gunas of the mind. It is a more active, turbulent, passionate mind state.

rasa: The word *rasa* means many things in Sanskrit. In Ayurveda it means "taste" and it is also a fluid tissue type (dhatu) that equates roughly to the plasma in the blood.

ritucharya: Seasonal cycles and the lifestyle guidance that goes along with them.

samadhi: A state of consciousness in which one is considered to be fully self-aware, and in later stages, cosmically aware. Synonymous terms from other traditions might be *nirvana, satori, enlightenment,* or *rapture.*

samana vayu: The inward movement of prana that is associated with vitality. Samana vayu is located in the navel area, and governs agni.

samprapti: Pathogenesis in Ayurveda. The process of disease manifestation.

Sankhya: One of the foundational philosophies of Ayurvedic medicine.

sattva: One of the three gunas of the mind, refers to a calm, peaceful state of equanimity.

shakti: Power, vital force. Sometimes used as a synonym for the term *prana.*

shen: Spirit, or mind in Chinese medicine.

sheng cycle: The generating cycle in five phase theory.

sitali pranayama: A cooling form of breathwork in yoga.

six pernicious influences: The qualities of pathogenic qi that cause imbalance. The six pernicious influences are: wind, cold, damp, heat, summer heat, and dryness.

srota(s): A channel system in Ayurveda that has major physiological function in the body or in the mind. Examples are the arteries in the circulatory system or the intestines in the gastrointestinal tract.

Sushruta: A famous doctor in Ayurveda who wrote one of the two seminal treatises on the medicine that contains information on surgical techniques, the Sushruta Samhita.

sushumna: The central nadi or channel in the body that runs through the spine. It is the nadi kundalini shakti rises through, and is therefore associated with higher states of awareness and enlightenment.

sutra: *Sutra* means "thread" in Sanskrit. A sutra is a collection of wisdom teachings in which each thought is strung upon the thread of the entire composition like a pearl on a necklace.

tamas: One of the three gunas of the mind, it is the state of inertia, often associated with ignorance.

tan tien(s): In qigong practice, the three primary energy centers in the body representing the earth, humanity, and the heavens. They are sites of vitality and transformation. The lower tan tien (below the navel) stores jing/essence, the middle (at the heart center) stores and transforms shen/spirit, and the upper (at the third eye) is responsible for higher awareness.

ten thousand things: A common phrase used in the Chinese tradition to refer to all that is.

three burners theory: Three burners theory is a diagnostic model that recognizes the movement of pathogens as going from the top down in the body.

Three Treasures: The Three Treasures in the Chinese system are the jing/essence, qi/vital life force, and shen/spirit.

tridoshic: When a person's prakruti or original constitution is equally balanced in quantity between vata, pitta, and kapha.

Triphala: An Ayurvedic remedy containing three fruits that is useful for bowel regulation and detoxification.

triple burners: The three regions of the body in Chinese medicine, also called san jiao or triple warmers, that are responsible for circulation of fluids, yang qi, and transformation.

udana vayu: In the Indian tradition, one of the five forms of vata. Udana is situated in the throat and governs upward movement of prana. It governs communication, expression, and metabolism.

Unani: Islamic or Arabian traditional medicine that, like Ayurveda and Chinese medicine, is still in use today.

vaidya: A senior or master Ayurveda doctor.

vata: The dosha in Ayurveda that is comprised of ether and air and governs movement.

vayu: A subset of vata. There are five, and each is responsible for a specific movement of qi in the body and helps govern physiological processes.

Vedanta: A philosophy from India that emphasizes self-reflection. It recognizes an ultimate reality that manifests itself as illusion and that our minds are reflections of the illusion.

vikruti: Acquired constitution. The constitutional traits one presents at the moment that are indicative of a straying from balance, or one's original constitution, prakruti.

vipaka: The post-digestive effect of a substance.

virya: The thermal quality of a substance.

vyana vayu: One of the five forms of vata responsible for the spreading and diffusing movement of prana. It is present throughout the body and is responsible for overall bodily communication and regulation of the other four vayus.

wei qi: The defensive qi affiliated with immunity. It circulates close to the surface in order to protect us from incoming external pathogens.

Wen Bing theory: Warm disease school of thought in Chinese medicine that teaches that communicable diseases are primarily warm in nature or turn warm upon entering the body.

Wu Xing theory: See "five phases."

yamas: Ethical practices and the first limb in Patanjali's astanga yoga. They include not harming, not stealing, truthfulness, not coveting, and celibacy, or control of the senses.

yi: One of the five shen/spirits of Chinese thought. Yi is intellect and is associated with the spleen and the earth element.

Yin Qiao San: A Chinese herbal formula that, when taken at the onset of wind heat invasion, can help the body push the pathogen back out of the body.

yoga nidra: The yoga of sleep. Largely done lying down, it encourages the mind to settle into the state between sleep and wakefulness so that subconscious and unconsciousness blockages can clear.

Yoga vs. yoga: *Yoga* with a capital "Y" is used in this text to denote the philosophy and practice of India employed by those wishing to achieve self-realization, cosmic consciousness, samadhi, kundalini awakening, or enlightenment. When *yoga* is spelled with a lower case "y," it indicates the common usage of the term, as in "yoga class." This type of yoga is focused on the physical and mental and, although it is recommended to be done under the guidance of a teacher, does not require the guidance of a guru.

yogi: A yogi is someone who practices Yoga. In the west we use *yogi* to describe a yoga practitioner, and some people further differentiate with a female form of the word *yogi, yogini*.

yuan qi: Source qi or original qi.

zhi: One of the five shen/spirits in the Chinese tradition. It is the will, and is associated with the kidneys and the water element.

Bibliography

Association for Traditional Studies. "The Evolution of Chinese Medicine." Accessed January 15, 2015. www.traditionalstudies.org/evolution-of -chinese-medicine.

Bayer. "Bayer Completes Acquisition of Dihon Pharmaceutical Group Co., Ltd. in China: Transaction Strengthens Consumer Care Business and Moves Bayer HealthCare to a Leading OTC Position in Key Growth Country." Published November 3, 2014. www.investor.bayer.com/en/nc /news/archive/investor-news-2014/investor-news-2013/?tx_news_pi1%5 Bnews%5D=1757&cHash=9b9057878c8eb98706120f25fe607a62.

Bhattacharya, Bhaswati. *Everyday Ayurveda: Daily Habits That Can Change Your Life in a Day.* Gurgaon, India: Random House, 2014.

Blackmore, Susan. *Consciousness: An Introduction.* London: Oxford University Press, 2003.

Bloomfield, Maurice, trans. *Hymns of the Atharva Veda: Together with Extracts from the Ritual Books and the Commentaries.* Accessed February 2, 2016. http://www.sacred-texts.com/hin/av.htm.

Chalmers, David. *The Conscious Mind: In Search of a Fundamental Theory.* Oxford, U.K.: Oxford University Press, 1997.

Chiang, Howard. *Historical Epistemology and the Making of Modern Chinese Medicine.* London: Oxford University Press, 2015. Accessed July 7, 2016. https://books.google.com/books?id=atfJCgAAQBAJ&pg=PA25& lpg=PA25&dq=new+culture+movement+and+chinese+medicine

&source=bl&ots=3u80PzNlb&sig=aEkfZ1EC8VaQ14i0A84zcD7fb2
o&hl=en&sa=X&ved=0ahUKEwj3tYelobXTAhVl2oMKHfb6CRQQ
6AEISjAG#v=onepage&q=new%20culture%20movement%20and%20
chinese%20medicine&f=false.

Das, Atmatattva. "Ayurveda-Vedanta: The Vedanta of Life Science." Accessed September 10, 2015. http://www.sanskritimagazine.com/ayurveda /ayurveda-vedanta-the-vedanta-of-life-science.

Elkaim, Yuri. "The Truth about How Much Water You Should Really Drink." Accessed September 8, 2016. http://health.usnews.com/health-news /blogs/eat-run/2013/09/13/the-truth-about-how-much-water-you-should -really-drink.

Emoto, Masaru. *The Hidden Messages in Water.* New York: Atria Books, 2005.

Fountain, Henry. "The Earth's Hidden Ocean." Accessed September 9, 2015. https://www.nytimes.com/2014/06/17/science/the-earths-hidden-ocean .html?_r=0.

Hatton, Celia. "Nobel Prize Winner Tu Youyou Helped by Ancient Chinese Remedy." Published October 6, 2015. http://www.bbc.com/news /blogs-china-blog-34451386.

Helmut Kaiser Consultancy. "Traditional Chinese Medicine (TCM): In China and Worldwide 2015–2016–2017–2018–2019–2020–2025 with History 2012–2014." Updated March 2017. http://www.hkc22.com /ChineseMedicine.html.

Hippocrates. *On Ancient Medicine.* Translated by Francis Adams. Accessed July 20, 2015. http://classics.mit.edu/Hippocrates/ancimed.html.

Joshi, Sunil. *Ayurveda and Panchakarma: The Science of Healing and Rejuvenation.* Twin Lakes, Wis.: Lotus Press, 1997.

Kondo, Marie. *The Life-Changing Magic of Tidying Up: The Japanese Art of Decluttering and Organizing.* New York: Random House, 2014.

Lad, Vasant, and Anisha Durve. *Marma Points of Ayurveda: The Energy Pathways for Healing Body, Mind, and Consciousness with a Comparison to Traditional Chinese Medicine.* Albuquerque: The Ayurvedic Press, 2008.

Liu, Guohui. *Warm Pathogen Diseases: A Clinical Guide.* Seattle, Wash.: Eastland Press, 2005.

Maciocia, Giovanni. *Diagnosis in Chinese Medicine: A Comprehensive Guide.* London: Churchill Livingstone, 2004. Accessed August 12, 2015. www.redwingbooks.com/assets/skins/redwing_skin/content /DiaChiMedMac_E.pdf.

Martino, Joe. "Study Shows Water Has Memory: German Scientists Expand on Dr. Emoto's Work." Published December 20, 2015. www.collective -evolution.com/2015/12/20/study-shows-water-has-memory-german -scientists-expand-on-dr-emotos-work.

Massar, Patricia, and Mareike Gutschner. "Q&A," What are the possible implications for us/for humankind? Accessed April 15, 2016. www.elsevier .com/connect/q-and-a-2-renowned-physicists-on-the-controversial -theory-of-consciousness.

Milbradt, David. "Bonghan Channels in Acupuncture." Accessed August 31, 2015. http://acupuncturetoday.com/mpacms/at/article.php?id=31918.

Mitchell, Craig, Feng Ye, and Nigel Wiseman. *Shang Han Lun: On Cold Damage; Translation and Commentaries.* Brookline, Mass.: Paradigm Publications, 1999.

Murthy, K. R. Srikantha. *Vagbhata's Astanga Hrdayam: Text, English Translation, Notes, Appendix and Indices.* Varanasi: Chowkhamba Krishnadas Academy, 2007.

National Association for Holistic Aromatherapy. Accessed October 3, 2016. http://naha.org/membership/find-an-aromatherapist.

North, Michael. "Greek Medicine: 'I Swear by Apollo Physician . . .': Greek Medicine from the Gods to Galen." Accessed August 30, 2015. www.nlm .nih.gov/hmd/greek/greek_oath.html.

Nutton, Vivian. "Galen of Pergamum: Greek Physician." Accessed July 15, 2015. www.britannica.com/biography/Galen-of-Pergamum.

Owen, James. "5 Surprising Facts about Otzi the Iceman: Scholars Continue to be Amazed by the Ancient Man Found Frozen in the Alps." Published October 18, 2013. http://news.nationalgeographic.com /news/2013/10/131016-otzi-ice-man-mummy-five-facts.

Parcak, Sarah. "Help Discover Ancient Ruins—before It's Too Late." (TED) Accessed February 2, 2017. www.ted.com/talks/sarah_parcak _help_discover_ancient_ruins_before_it_s_too_late/transcript ?language=en.

Palep, H. S. *Scientific Foundation of Ayurveda*. Delhi: Chaukhamba Sanskrit Pratishthan, 2004.

Ranade, Subash. *Natural Healing through Ayurveda*. Sandy, N.Mex.: Morson, 1992. Accessed October 12, 2015. https://books.google.com/books?id =PFyBHvc0C5EC&pg=PA29&dq=mimamsa+role+in+ayurveda&hl =en&sa=X&ved=0ahUKEwiO3ZXcionLAhUJHD4KHZ99COgQ 6AEIKjAC#v=onepage&q=mimamsa%20role%20in%20ayurveda&f =false.

Reeves, Carole. *Egyptian Medicine*. Buckinghamshire, U.K.: Shire Publications, 2001.

Ro, Sam. "The Enormous Market for Chinese Medicine Is Booming." Published November 29, 2012. www.businessinsider.com/chinese -medicine-booming-2012-11.

Robertson, Jason, and Wang Ju-Yi. *Applied Channel Theory in Chinese Medicine: Wang Ju-Yi's Lectures on Channel Therapeutics*. Eastland Press, Seattle, 2008.

Satake, Alison, and Andi McDaniel. "India: A Second Opinion; Ayurveda 101 and Related Links." Accessed February 2, 2016. www.pbs.org /frontlineworld/stories/india701/interviews/ayurveda101.html.

Sharma, R. K., and Bhagwan Dash. *Caraka Samhita: Text with English Translation and Critical Exposition Based on Cakrapani Datta's Ayurveda Dipika*. Varanasi: Chowkhamba Sanskrit Series Office, 2003.

Shoba, Kumudini. *Ayurveda: Ancient Wisdom, Modern Life*. Prague: Service Plants, 2012.

Svoboda, Robert, and Arnie Lade. *Tao and Dharma: Chinese Medicine and Ayurveda*. Twin Lakes, Wis.: Lotus Press, 1996.

TrueAyurveda (blog). https://trueayurveda.wordpress.com/?s=ritucharya.

Van Alphen, Jan, and Anthony Aris. *Oriental Medicine: An Illustrated Guide to the Asian Arts of Healing*. Boston: Shambhala, 1996.

Violatti, Cristian. "Confucianism: Definition." Published August 31, 2013. www.ancient.eu/Confucianism/.

Walia, Arjun. "The Influence Vedic Philosophy Had on Nikola Tesla's Idea of Free Energy." Published July 23, 2014. www.collective-evolution

.com/2014/07/23/the-influence-vedic-philosophy-had-on-nikola-teslas
-idea-of-free-energy/.

Weiss, Robert. "The Opposite of Addiction Is Connection: New Addiction
Research Brings Surprising Discoveries." Posted September 30, 2015. www
.psychologytoday.com/blog/love-and-sex-in-the-digital-age/201509
/the-opposite-addiction-is-connection.

Index